Racism and African American Mental Health is an absolute must read for all clinicians who aim to effectively employ CBT strategies with African American clients—clients who endure harsh and overwhelming societal challenges but who also possess considerable untapped strengths. Dr. Steele superbly integrates the unique reality of African American clients into the CBT paradigm. She does so in a nuanced manner that is needed but rarely if ever taught in graduate coursework or in 'multicultural' training. Clinicians at every level of professional development, from early career to advanced, will benefit from the theoretically informed and practical insights and tools in this comprehensive book.

> **Rheeda Walker**, PhD, author of *The Unapologetic Guide to Black Mental Health* and *No Racial Elephants in the Therapy Room*

Racism and African American Mental Health is a tour de force that reimagines psychotherapy from an African-centered cultural perspective in order to help Black Americans create narratives of strength and resilience to counter experiences of systemic oppression. This is one of those rare and wise books that deserves to be read by every mental health professional in North America. Whatever your familiarity with African American culture, racism, and psychological empowerment, every chapter enriches your understanding. Therapists who wonder about the benefits of discussing race in therapy or how and when to do it have steady guidance here. Questions to ask about racial experiences and processes for responding with cultural sensitivity are clearly illustrated. Detailed case examples and therapist-client dialogues show the depth of impact offered by culturally informed treatment strategies. Guided activities throughout the book allow readers to measure their own gaps and growth. I highly recommend this engaging book as one every therapist will want to read and reread, no matter what racial and cultural identities you and your clients hold.

> **Christine A. Padesky**, PhD, co-editor of *Dialogues for Discovery: Improving Psychotherapy's Effectiveness* and author of *The Clinician's Guide to CBT Using Mind Over Mood*

Wow, I loved this book! Packed with thought-provoking exercises, rich case examples, authentic therapist-client dialogues, and practice-oriented interventions, this book is a treasure and much-needed resource for all therapists. Definitely a must read that therapists will be using for many years to come!

> **Pamela A. Hays**, PhD, author of *Addressing Cultural Complexities in Counseling and Clinical Practice: An Intersectional Approach*

HI0234905

Racism and African American Mental Health is a groundbreaking book that delves into the intersection of racism and mental health in the African American community. Dr. Steele combines culturally relevant insights and expertise with research in this field to provide a powerful analysis of the negative impacts of racism on the mental health of African Americans and the ways in which CBT can be appropriately incorporated into treatment plans. At my nonprofit, The AAKOMA Project, and in my professional work with the Dr. Alfiee Org, I constantly highlight the need for nuanced approaches to mental health research and care in support of Black people, and other people of color (with all of our beautiful, intersectional identities). This book is a must read for anyone seeking to understand and better center the unique needs of African Americans, the impact of racism on mental health, and the ways in which CBT can be used to mitigate exposure to racism in culturally relevant ways.

Alfiee M. Breland-Noble, PhD pioneering psychologist, mental health thought leader, and founder of The AAKOMA Project

Racism and African American Mental Health

Racism and African American Mental Health examines the psychological impacts of racism within the African American community and offers a culturally adapted model of cognitive behavior therapy for more culturally relevant case conceptualization and treatment planning with this population.

Readers of this text will gain a greater understanding of how manifestations of racism contribute to the development of psychological distress among African Americans and learn specific strategies to address the negative automatic thoughts and maladaptive beliefs that develop in response to racism.

Reflection questions and guided practice are incorporated throughout the text to assist readers with application of the strategies discussed in their own clinical settings.

Janeé M. Steele, PhD, is a licensed professional counselor, counselor educator, and diplomate of the Academy of Cognitive and Behavioral Therapies. Dr. Steele is also the owner of Kalamazoo Cognitive and Behavioral Therapy, PLLC, where she provides therapy, supervision, and training in CBT, and co-author of *Black Lives Are Beautiful: 50 Tools to Heal from Trauma and Promote Positive Racial Identity*.

Clinical Topics in Psychology and Psychiatry

Much of the available information relevant to mental health clinicians is buried in large and disjointed academic textbooks and expensive and obscure scientific journals. Consequently, it can be challenging for the clinician and student to access the most useful information related to practice. **Clinical Topics in Psychology and Psychiatry** includes authored and edited books that identify and distill the most relevant information for practitioners and presents the material in an easily accessible format that appeals to the psychology and psychiatry student, intern or resident, early career psychologist or psychiatrist, and the busy clinician.

Series Editor: Bret A. Moore, PsyD, Boulder Crest Retreat, Virginia, USA

For more information about this series, please visit: www.routledge.com/Clinical-Topics-in-Psychology-and-Psychiatry/book-series/TFSE00310

Racism and African American Mental Health

Using Cognitive Behavior Therapy to Empower Healing

Janeé M. Steele

Foreword by Judith S. Beck

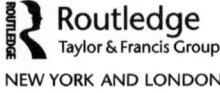

Routledge
Taylor & Francis Group

Designed cover image: dmfoss © Getty Images

First published 2025
by Routledge
605 Third Avenue, New York, NY 10158

and by Routledge
4 Park Square, Milton Park, Abingdon, Oxon, OX14 4RN

Routledge is an imprint of the Taylor & Francis Group, an informa business

British Library Cataloguing-in-Publication Data
A catalogue record for this book is available from the British Library

ISBN: 978-1-032-05050-8 (hbk)
ISBN: 978-1-032-05049-2 (pbk)
ISBN: 978-1-003-19630-3 (ebk)

DOI: 10.4324/9781003196303

Typeset in Times New Roman
by SPi Technologies India Pvt Ltd (Straive)

To my husband, De Vanne Burch, Sr., whose support has been instrumental in more ways than can be counted.

To my father, Matt Jenkins, who along with my husband, De Vanne, was willing to listen and provide feedback on various aspects of this text.

To my colleagues and mentors in CBT, Scott Waltman, Mudita Badahur, Lizbeth Gaona, Jamie Schumpf, Hollie Granato, Carmella Tress, and Lisa Bolden. Thank you for all of the many ways you've supported and encouraged me.

To my mother, Joslyn Jenkins, my sister, Stephanie Jenkins, and my aunts and uncles, Dwanna Ogles, Diane Ogles, Ken Ogles, Ellis Ogles, and Russell Hardaway who always love and support me.

Contents

Series Editor's Foreword

Racism and African American Mental Health: Using Cognitive Behavior Therapy to Empower Healing is the latest volume in one of Routledge's most popular series, Clinical Topics in Psychology and Psychiatry (CTPP). The overarching goal of CTPP is to provide mental health practitioners with practical information on psychology and psychopharmacological topics. Each volume is comprehensive but easy to digest and integrate into day-to-day clinical practice. It is multidisciplinary, covering topics relevant to the fields of psychology, social work, counseling, and psychiatry, and appeals to the student, novice, and senior clinician. Books chosen for the series are authored or edited by national and international experts in their respective areas, and contributors are also highly respected clinicians. The current volume exemplifies the intent, scope, and aims of the CCTP series.

In *Racism and African American Mental Health*, Janeé M. Steele, Ph.D. provides a unique look and perspective on how racism impacts the psychological health of African Americans. Drawing upon the modest research on the topic, Dr. Steele highlights the myriad harmful effects of racism within this community and how so many clinicians are unaware of these effects and how to address them in treatment. Utilizing the core principles of cognitive behavior therapy, Dr. Steele introduces the reader to a culturally appropriate framework for understanding symptom presentations of African American individuals as well as culturally sensitive and effective means with regard to evaluation and treatment. Upon completing this book, the reader will be well-versed in the research supporting the effective use of CBT with African American clients as well as the inherent limitations of the CBT approach with diverse groups (an area that is often neglected in texts on CBT). As a clinician herself, Dr. Steele understands the critical importance of establishing a strong working therapeutic alliance, which can only be accomplished by understanding the many cultural influences that affect both the client and therapist. Of particular importance and uniqueness, Dr. Steele helps the clinician better understand how their own racial worldview impacts clinical outcomes with African American clients by engaging in reflection exercises.

I am convinced that *Racism and African American Mental Health* will become one of the lead textbooks in training students and clinicians in how to effectively apply CBT theory and techniques through a culturally and racially sensitive and well-defined framework. In other words, it will make therapists who work with African American clients more effective. I anticipate that *Racism and African American Mental Health* will become a required reading in graduate psychotherapy training programs of all sizes, shapes, and theoretical orientations. More importantly, it will improve the quality of life for countless African Americans who seek treatment for the psychological distress that stems from the interpersonal, institutional, and structural racism they face on a daily basis.

Bret A. Moore, Psy.D., ABPP
Series Editor
Clinical Topics in Psychology and Psychiatry

Foreword

Racism and African American Mental Health: Using Cognitive Behavior Therapy to Empower Healing is a very important book in the evolution of CBT. Janeé Steele has meticulously researched how CBT needs to be adapted for African American clients who have been exposed to racism, often from a very early age. Research shows that repeated encounters with racism are associated with trauma, low self-esteem, clinical depression, and anxiety, and, at its most dangerous, suicidality. African Americans continually experience significant stress and distress related to bias and discrimination in personal, school, or work encounters, either endured or witnessed. Additionally, structural racism has led to many negative social determinants and systemic inequities. African Americans often encounter significant barriers to mental health treatment and receive inadequate care. Fortunately, CBT, appropriately adapted as described so clearly in this thoughtful, pragmatic book, has been shown to be effective in empowering African American clients to overcome these challenges, even when they have internalized anti-Black attitudes and beliefs. Later I will describe some of the conceptual additions and treatment techniques that are essential when working with this population.

But first, to go back in history, my father, Aaron T. Beck, MD, and colleagues conducted the first randomized CBT research study and co-authored the first CBT treatment book (*Cognitive Therapy of Depression*) in the late 1970s. My father did not know at that time whether CBT would prove to be effective for populations other than the ones he, his colleagues, and his trainees at the University of Pennsylvania were treating. But time has shown that CBT has evolved and its efficacy has been demonstrated for a wide range of psychiatric disorders (even schizophrenia and bipolar disorder), psychological problems, and medical conditions with psychological components. It has been adapted for a wide range of populations: individuals of various ages, cultures, gender identities, and socioeconomic levels. And it is used in a wide variety of settings: schools, residential and vocational programs, medical facilities, correctional settings, community centers, private practice, and others. It is the most highly researched and widely practiced psychotherapy in the world.

It is important to note that from the beginning, Dr. Beck emphasized two foundational principles of CBT. One was that therapists need to conceptualize clients according to a cognitive framework, which posits that the meanings clients put to their experiences are related to their emotional, behavioral, and physiological responses and that the themes in these meanings (that is, their automatic thoughts about situations) are related to their underlying beliefs about themselves, their worlds and other people, and the future. The second foundational principle was that it is essential for therapists to build a strong therapeutic alliance with clients so they will be willing to collaborate with their therapist and engage in the hard work of therapy, both in and out of sessions. Dr. Steele has done an admirable job in describing how to maintain these two core principles and vary their implementation for the African American population by intentionally including social influences and exploration of race (and racism) in case conceptualization and ongoing conversations with clients.

Dr. Steele details how continual exposure to racism and aversive racist experiences, especially the depiction of African Americans as inferior, can cause psychological distress and lead some African American clients to internalize racism. They may see themselves in a negative light; for example, they may believe that they don't measure up and/or that they are powerless in the face of discrimination. Research indicates that clients may not bring up their concerns about racism in therapy, though. When they don't, CBT therapists need to initiate these kinds of discussions by directly asking African American clients about their experiences with racism and discrimination and then explore how these kinds of experiences might be related to their specific current difficulties or to obstacles to achieving their aspirations. Failure to do so can decrease the impact of treatment. Failure to do so sensitively can lead to ruptures in the therapeutic relationship and premature termination.

This book is faithful to core conceptual and treatment components of CBT. But crucially, it adds a sociocultural lens when conceptualizing clients who have experienced racism, enhancing our understanding of why our African American clients often have a strong negative reaction to certain situations, why they may have developed certain coping strategies, why they may be vigilant for harm from others (especially the culturally and politically dominant group), and why they often feel unempowered. It focuses on the importance of adapted psychoeducation, problem-solving, cognitive restructuring, and skills training when clients have experiences of blatant or indirect racism. Equally important is an emphasis on creating opportunities for racial empowerment, including consciousness raising and building racial pride. Transcripts that contrast a traditional CBT approach with a culturally-sensitive CBT approach are wonderful illustrations of how therapists can significantly improve outcomes with African American clients.

Judith S. Beck, PhD
President, Beck Institute for Cognitive Behavior Therapy
Clinical Professor of Psychology in Psychiatry,
University of Pennsylvania

Introduction to Cognitive Behavior Therapy and Its Use with African American Clients

On November 6, 2021, ten-year-old Isabella Tichenor died by suicide. "Izzy," as she was affectionately known to her family members, was reportedly subject to racial harassment because of her race and disability. Each day as she went to school, she was taunted by peers who called her racist names and stated that she smelled and needed to wash her hair, all because of the color of her skin. Eventually, the bullying became too much, and the young girl took her own life (Alessandrini, 2023).

The death of ten-year-old Izzy highlights the impact of racism on the psychological wellbeing of African Americans and the communities to which they belong. While this impact is illustrated anecdotally through stories like Izzy's, empirical evidence to support the assertion that African Americans experience daily psychological distress due to racism continues to grow. In fact, several decades of research show a relationship between racism and trauma, depression, anxiety, low self-esteem, and even suicidality (Carter et al., 2017). In their study of 1,200 African American men ages 18 to 93, for example, Goodwill et al. (2021) found that Black men who reported more frequent encounters with racial discrimination were more likely to experience symptoms of depression and thoughts of suicide at some point during their lifetime. Similarly, Brooks et al. (2020) found that while discrimination resulted in emotional distress for both the Black and White participants of their study, for Black adults, perceived discrimination is a statistically significant predictor of suicidality, even more so than feelings of depression and other non-discriminatory stressors.

In spite of the longstanding and clearly documented relationship between racism and mental health among African Americans, many therapists remain challenged in their ability to address racism during therapy (Knox et al., 2003). One significant barrier has been the paucity of theoretically based approaches within the counseling and psychology literature to assist therapists with countering the psychological effects of racism (Hanna & Cardona, 2013). Over the past decade, however, scholars have increasingly recognized the utility of cognitive behavior therapy (CBT) in addressing

DOI: 10.4324/9781003196303-1

racism and its psychological correlates among African Americans (M. T. Williams et al., 2022). In particular, CBT's emphasis on personal empowerment, attention to client strengths and support systems, and affirmation of one's own sense of identity have been found to make this form of therapy especially well-suited for addressing the psychological distress, sense of powerlessness, and internalized anti-Black attitudes that may occur as a result of racism (Hays & Iwamasa, 2006). Moreover, the active, problem-focused, and time sensitive nature of CBT (Wenzel, 2019) may also be attractive to African American clients who generally experience more barriers to treatment such as lack of childcare or the inability to take time off from work (NeMoyer et al., 2019).

My primary goal in writing this book is to help therapists increase their ability to explore racial oppression and empower healing in African American clients suffering the psychological effects of racism. Accordingly, this book builds on previous descriptions of culturally responsive CBT with African Americans by (a) describing psychological phenomena occurring in the African American community as a result of racism and how understanding of these phenomena may aid in case conceptualization, (b) exploring recently proposed cognitive models of racism, and (c) providing specific examples of cognitive, body-centric, and empowerment intervention techniques therapists can immediately implement with their clients. In this chapter, I provide an introduction to CBT and its use with African American clients, highlighting key terms and theoretical constructs. For readers who may be new to CBT, I also discuss some of the basic tenets of the approach and provide an overview of session structure, assessment practices, and key intervention strategies in CBT.

Reflection 1.1: Initiating discussions on race and racism can be difficult regardless of one's status or experience as a clinician. Even as an African American therapist, I struggle at times with how to discuss these topics during therapy, fearing that I might offend clients or say the wrong thing. What are some of the fears you have around discussing race and racism with your African American clients? How might these fears affect your work with this population?

Components of Culturally Sensitive CBT

CBT is an effective treatment for a variety of psychological disorders. For example, meta-analytic reviews show empirical support for CBT in the treatment of mental health concerns such as depression (López-López et al., 2019), anxiety (Zhang et al., 2019), obsessive-compulsive disorder (Brauer et al., 2011), post-traumatic stress disorder (Mavranezouli et al., 2020), substance use disorder (Polak et al., 2021), psychosis (Turner et al., 2020), anger management (Fernandez et al., 2018), insomnia (Parsons et al., 2021), and recently, hoarding disorder (Tolin et al., 2015). While it is beyond the scope of this text to review the breadth of this research, in sum, these studies suggest CBT offers long-term effectiveness and relapse prevention, is superior to many alternative forms of treatment, and in some instances, produces outcomes better than or similar to those achieved through psychopharmacological intervention (Butler et al., 2006).

Given its efficacy, CBT is often described as the gold standard of psychological care (D. David et al., 2018). Yet, with increased recognition of the ways in which culture influences the therapeutic process, scholars have identified a need for greater cultural sensitivity in CBT (Hays & Iwamasa, 2006; Rathod et al., 2015). For example, while CBT focuses primarily on the restructuring of negative thoughts, it also emphasizes the importance of the therapeutic alliance, which is facilitated through basic counseling skills such as warmth and empathy (Matu, 2018). Perceptions of therapist empathy and the strength of the therapeutic alliance, however, are both influenced by the therapist's ability to broach race during therapy with clients from diverse racial/ethnic backgrounds (Day-Vines et al., 2018; Fuertes et al., 2006). *Broaching* is defined as "a consistent and ongoing attitude of openness with a genuine commitment by the counselor to continually invite the client to explore issues of diversity" (Day-Vines et al., 2007, p. 402). This entails raising the subject of race and racism when exploring client concerns, as well as broaching racial dynamics within the therapeutic relationship itself. While many therapists believe clients will initiate these conversations if they are relevant, most clients rely on the therapist to do so.

Other race-related factors such as racial microaggressions from the therapist and missed opportunities to respond empathetically to racial content also have a significant effect on the therapeutic alliance (Comas-Díaz, 2006; Owen et al., 2014; Tao et al., 2015). *Microaggressions* are subtle, often unintentional, statements that reflect prejudiced or discriminatory messages about various minority groups (Sue et al., 2007). Owen et al. (2014) found that clients' perceptions of these statements during therapy were negatively related to the working alliance, even after controlling for clients' current psychological well-being, number of sessions, and therapist racial and ethnic status; yet, these researchers also found that therapists who took opportunities to discuss the occurrence of microaggressions had higher quality alliances when compared to client/therapist dyads wherein the microaggressions were not discussed. Essentially, therapists who make prejudiced or discriminatory statements during sessions cause ruptures to the therapeutic alliance even when these statements are subtle or unintentional. These ruptures can be repaired, however, when therapists openly discuss any inadvertent microaggressions.

The findings discussed above reinforce the idea that in order to build strong therapeutic alliances with clients from racially diverse backgrounds, therapists must approach therapy in a way that openly acknowledges race and reflects a core understanding of clients' lives as racial beings (Calloway & Creed, 2021). Researchers have also recognized a need for greater cultural sensitivity in CBT in terms of case conceptualization and treatment planning (Graham et al., 2013; J. M. Steele, 2020). Recently, Graham et al. (2013) identified enhanced psychoeducation, adapted cognitive restructuring, and modified exposure situations as specific techniques therapists can implement to meet this need. *Enhanced psychoeducation* involves connecting concepts discussed during psychoeducation directly to clients' lived experiences as members of marginalized groups. Consider Michelle, a 37-year-old African American woman suffering from performance anxiety. Michelle, who was the only person of color at her job, reported excessive worry and worsened performance while being observed by her supervisor and co-workers. Typical psychoeducation in Michelle's case would consist of information about social anxiety, its cognitive model, symptoms, and treatment. Enhanced psychoeducation, however, might also include information on culture-specific factors of anxiety such as stereotype threat (i.e., the fear of conforming to negative stereotypes about one's social group), as some of Michelle's difficulties may have reflected self-inflicted pressure to disconfirm negative stereotypes about African Americans being lazy and unintelligent (E. J. R. David, 2009; C. M. Steele & Aronson, 1995).

Enhanced psychoeducation situates clients' concerns within their broader social context, normalizing clients' experiences and providing insight needed for more effective problem solving (Graham et al., 2013). *Adapted cognitive restructuring* can also help clients explore their concerns in a way that is sensitive to their cultural values, life experiences, and context. Traditionally, cognitive restructuring focuses on teaching clients to examine the rationality of their thinking through Socratic questioning (Matu, 2018). Questioning clients' experiences of discrimination and other race-related concerns, however, can be invalidating and may exacerbate their symptoms. In contrast, adapted cognitive restructuring focuses on: (a) validating the painful emotions that arise in the face of these experiences, (b) acknowledging that we live in a society where these painful experiences occur, and (c) challenging negative thoughts about self that occur in response to these experiences rather than the experiences themselves (Graham et al., 2013, p. 104). Use of adaptive cognitive restructuring with our case illustration, Michelle, for example, would first focus on validating the vulnerability and anxiety she experiences in her predominantly White work setting. Subsequently, her therapist could then use Socratic questioning to help Michelle identify and challenge negative thoughts or self-appraisals she may be experiencing in the situation, being careful to avoid questioning that would imply Michelle's concerns about being the only person of color at work are irrational or distorted.

The last strategy identified by Graham et al. (2013), *modified exposure situations*, refers to exposure activities that are designed in consideration of the client's cultural worldview. In CBT, exposure activities are implemented based on the understanding that avoidance of anxiety provoking situations limits a client's ability to disconfirm their worry and fears, which ultimately makes the fear stronger (American Psychological Association, 2017). Accordingly, exposure activities typically consist of exercises that help clients take small, incremental steps toward engaging in feared situations. A benefit of these exercises is that they increase clients' confidence in their ability to cope with threatening outcomes and reduce their sense of uncertainty. In the case of Michelle, traditional exposure activities might focus on helping her to become more comfortable being the center of attention while being observed. Modified exposure exercises in this situation, however, would focus on achieving this objective while also considering the reality that African Americans are, in fact, judged more harshly than their White counterparts as it relates to work ethic (DeSante, 2013). This would include designing fear hierarchies with activities that gradually increase the level of attention focused on Michelle as she simultaneously gives herself messages that affirm her racial identity and attribute her anxiety to stereotype threat rather than to the risk of failure.

Finally, in CBT, treatment considerations such as the use of psychoeducation, cognitive restructuring, and exposure therapy are heavily dependent upon the therapist's conceptualization of the client's concerns (J. S. Beck, 2020). CBT theorizes that our life experiences, particularly our childhood experiences, lead to core beliefs that influence our automatic thoughts in daily situations. In my own clinical work, I have observed that in addition to early life experiences, societal influences also have an effect on clients' automatic thoughts and their underlying cognitions (J. M. Steele, 2020; J. M. Steele & Newton, 2022). Influences of particular relevance to the African American community are those that perpetuate messages of White superiority and Black inferiority, for example, the underrepresentation of African Americans in the higher echelons of society or media portrayals that offer a distorted representation of African Americans and reinforce racial negative stereotypes (Bailey et al., 2014; Prilleltensky & Gonick, 1996). These influences, along with individual childhood experiences, are significant because they affect the beliefs African Americans develop about themselves, other people, and their world, as well as the assumptions and rules they use to guide their subsequent behavior in response to these beliefs. Accordingly, culturally responsive CBT not only requires sensitivity in the therapeutic relationship and adaptations to the interventions utilized with culturally diverse clients—it also necessitates an understanding of the societal influences and psychological phenomena unique to the cultural experiences of these clients.

To summarize, culturally sensitive CBT with African Americans requires therapists to be intentional in their exploration of how race and racism influence client concerns. This involves being mindful of the impact of race on the therapeutic alliance and contextualizing interventions used during therapy to include relevant aspects of the client's racial worldview. Accordingly, therapists should be comfortable responding to racial content during sessions and take opportunities to initiate conversations about race when they present themselves. Likewise, interventions used during therapy should also attend to the experience of race and racism in the lives of these clients. This can be accomplished with strategies such as enhanced psychoeducation, adapted cognitive restructuring, and modified exposure situations, as well as the integration of sociocultural considerations into the cognitive conceptualization process (Graham et al., 2013; J. M. Steele, 2020).

Key Terms

This section defines key terms used throughout this text. One difficulty some therapists have in developing the competence necessary to address racism with African American clients is that many multicultural concepts have differing or idiosyncratic definitions, which creates challenges for therapists when it comes to translating the ideas associated with these terms into clinical practice (Ridley et al., 2021). When working with African American clients, terms of particular relevance include *culture, race, ethnicity, racism,* and *racial trauma.* Brief definitions of these constructs are provided below; however, most are discussed in greater depth in Chapter 2. Before reading each definition, write down your own meanings for these terms and compare how you define each term to how it is defined below. How accurate are your definitions? How might the way you define these terms influence your understanding of your clients' worldview and your conceptualization of their problems?

Culture

Culture refers to the norms, values, attitudes, and behaviors of groups of people who share "demographic variables (e.g., age, sex, place of residence), status variables (e.g., social, educational, economic), affiliations (formal and informal), [or] ethnographic variables such as nationality, ethnicity, language, and religion" (Pedersen, 1991, p. 7). Given this broad definition, it is generally understood that individuals may belong to more than one cultural group and some cultural identities may be more salient than others (Sue et al., 2019). Moreover, some cultural identities may be influenced by one or more other intersecting identities. African American women, for example, share unique cultural experiences based on their intersecting ethnic and gender identities (Crenshaw, 1989). The salience of each intersecting identity may shift depending on the situation or may result in "double jeopardy," wherein individuals are placed at additional disadvantages due to their multiple marginalized identities (Sue et al., 2019).

Race

Race refers to groups of people who share physical characteristics such as skin color, facial features, and other hereditary traits (Cokley, 2007). In the United States, these groups are labeled White, Black or African American, Asian American, American Indian/Alaska Native, and Native Hawaiian/Pacific Islander (U.S. Census Bureau, 2021). Because members of various racial groups are distinguished by their physical characteristics, some individuals mistakenly believe that race is a biological construct. Advances in the study of genetics, however, indicate that there is no biological basis for race, as 94 percent of human genetic variation is found within members of the same race, while only 6 percent of this variation exists between races (Burns & Vaughn, 2021). Accordingly, most contemporary conceptualizations of race describe it as a social construct that was initially developed during the late 17th century to justify slavery, colonialism, and the conquest of people defined as inferior at the time (Smedley & Smedley, 2005). Yet, while the idea of race as a biological construct has long been debunked, race remains a salient factor in the lives of individuals today given its psychological, educational, and political consequences (Cokley, 2007).

Ethnicity

Ethnicity refers to groups of people who share various cultural traits that distinguish them from other groups of people (Smedley & Smedley, 2005). Some of these traits include shared language, place of origin, religion, history, traditions, and beliefs. Psychologically, ethnicity derives its significance as a source of culture, identity, and status (Phinney, 1996). In fact, for people of color, ethnicity is often the primary source of the cultural norms transmitted across generations, so much so, that the terms ethnicity and culture are frequently used interchangeably. Positive feelings about one's ethnic group membership (i.e., one's ethnic identity) offers strong protection against the psychological impacts of racial prejudice and discrimination by contributing to one's self-esteem and sense of belonging. Unfortunately, ethnicity also has significance because of its association with status, which, for people of color, equates to less power and the experience of racial prejudice and discrimination (Phinney, 1996). While ethnicity has some relationship to race, members of the same racial group may belong to different ethnicities. The most common Black ethnicities in the United States include

African American, Jamaican, Haitian, Nigerian, and Dominican (U.S. Census Bureau, 2021). Individuals who are Black share common experiences based on their racial experiences and shared African descent; however, these individuals also have unique histories, languages, customs, norms, and traditions based on their ethnicities.

Racism

Racism refers to the transformation of racial prejudice into systems of oppression through the use of power directed against members of racially marginalized racial groups (Carter, 2007). Broadly, racism may be expressed covertly or overtly, and may occur at interpersonal, institutional, or internalized levels. *Interpersonal racism* refers to conscious or subconscious discrimination against a person or group because of race, while *institutional racism* refers to racist policies and practices within various institutions (Evans et al., 2021). *Internalized racism,* on the other hand, refers to a negative view of oneself based on the perceived inferiority of one's own race or ethnicity (Graham et al., 2016). Regardless of its form, racism is a significant source of psychological distress for people of color and often impacts the overall nature their presenting concerns (D. R. Williams, 2018).

Racial Trauma

Racial trauma refers to mental and emotional injury caused by repeated encounters with racial bias, hostility, discrimination, or harassment (Carter, 2007). These encounters, known as *race-based events*, result in racialized trauma when they are experienced as sudden, out of one's control, and highly negative or emotionally painful. Individuals with racialized trauma fear for their safety and often become hypervigilant, or "on guard" for new or repeated threats to their safety. These individuals may also withdraw from their friends and family, have difficulty trusting others, and experience distressing symptoms such as nightmares, flashbacks, and intrusive thoughts. Essentially, racialized trauma is stressor-related disorder that carries with it the same cognitive, emotional, behavioral, and physiological symptoms as other trauma disorders. Therefore, in order to effectively address racialized trauma, therapists must have a good understanding of the overall nature of trauma and its treatment.

Activity 1.1: Developing a List of Terms

This section reviewed just a few of the key terms relevant to racism and African American mental health. Other terms related to identity, privilege, and bias also have relevance during therapy with African American clients.

Examples of these terms include *intersectionality*, *White privilege*, and *implicit* or *unconscious bias*. Lists of these terms are available widely on the Internet. You can easily find them by entering the phrase "diversity terms" into a Google search. Try conducting your own search to find a list of terms you can bookmark for future reference. Which of these terms are most unfamiliar? What additional knowledge or training can you pursue to increase your understanding of these terms and their impact on the lived experiences of African American clients?

Culturally Sensitive CBT With African American Clients

Now that culturally sensitive CBT and relevant key terms have been reviewed, let's discuss the integration of these concepts into CBT with African American clients more specifically and with attention to the effects of racism. Other researchers (e.g., Bryant & Harder, 2008; E. C. Ward & Brown, 2015; Zigarelli et al., 2016) have explored the use of CBT with African Americans; however, these approaches do not always address the impacts of racism. Racism has unique psychological correlates that require specific considerations during therapy with African American clients (Carter & Sbrocco, 2018; Greer et al., 2018; Kelly, 2019; Neblett et al., 2018). Based on a review of the literature, these considerations can be summarized into the following points:

1. Psychological phenomena experienced by African Americans follow cognitive models similar to other clinical issues.
2. Cognitive conceptualization requires consideration of individual and societal influences.
3. Treatment planning to address racialized trauma should include empowerment goals.

Psychological Phenomena Experienced by African Americans Follow Cognitive Models Similar to Other Clinical Issues

In CBT, explanations of the development and maintenance of symptoms associated with various psychological disorders are known as *cognitive models*. The cognitive model of depression, for example, states that early life experiences lead to the development of negative thoughts about oneself, the world, and the future, which when triggered by critical incidents in an individual's life, lead to negative automatic thoughts and their corresponding affective, behavioral, cognitive, motivational, and physiological responses (A. T. Beck et al., 1979). A benefit of cognitive models is that they provide therapists with frameworks they can use to conceptualize the connections between a client's thoughts, feelings, behaviors, and physical symptoms. This allows therapists to pinpoint what needs to be addressed during treatment planning. This benefit also provides clients with additional insight, which can be cathartic in itself.

Similar to other clinical issues, psychological phenomena experienced by African Americans also follow specific cognitive models (J. M. Steele, 2020). Watts-Jones's (2002) seminal discussion of internalized racism, for example, revealed a cognitive model wherein maladaptive thinking (i.e., the shame associated with being of African descent) leads to negative psychological (i.e., self-degradation and self-alienation) and behavioral (i.e., secrecy) responses that have a negative impact on overall wellbeing and health. Bailey et al. (2014) also delineated cognitive, as well as behavioral aspects of internalized racism that included: "(1) belief in a biased representation of history; (2) alteration of one's physical appearance; (3) internalization of negative stereotypes about African Americans; and (4) changing one's hair texture and style to fit a more European aesthetic" (p. 145). In this description, belief in a biased representation of history and internalization of negative stereotypes represent cognitive processes within an individual, while changing one's appearance and hair are corresponding behavioral reactions.

Other examples of psychological phenomena specific to the African American experience include stereotype threat (C. M. Steele & Aronson, 1995), which was mentioned earlier in this chapter, cultural mistrust (Terrell et al., 2009), working twice as hard (DeSante, 2013), and colorism (Belgrave & Allison, 2019). The cultural relevancy achieved through integration of these psychological considerations into case conceptualization has several advantages. First, understanding the ways in which racism and discrimination affect clients' perceptions of events and the meanings they attribute to them can help minimize the occurrence of inadvertent racial microaggressions on the part of the therapist. For example, therapists who understand that African Americans are often afforded less credibility and as a result have to "work twice as hard," especially in professional settings, can be more careful to avoid examining situations in ways that invalidate the experiences of these clients. Second, additional insight on the impact of racism on one's psychological distress can help clients who may have been attributing their difficulties to personal flaws or weaknesses develop alternative explanatory models for their problems. Lastly, as many of the psychological concerns unique to African Americans are situated in the sociopolitical context of this population, recognition of these factors during therapy can provide indications for meso- or macro-level environmental interventions, which may further enhance treatment outcomes among this community (Vera, 2020).

Cognitive Conceptualization Requires Consideration of Individual and Societal Influences

As mentioned earlier in this chapter, treatment planning in CBT is largely based on the therapist's conceptualization of the client's concerns. Experiences that inform the underlying cognitions in the conceptualization have origins in both individual and societal influences. Individual factors that influence the development of core beliefs, for example, include discord among family members, difficult peer relationships, and adverse life conditions such as the death of a loved one, illness, or abuse (J. S. Beck, 2020). As an ethnic group, however, African Americans share a societal context that also influences how they see themselves and the world (Kelly, 2019). The legacy of slavery has a particularly profound impact on the psychological well-being of African Americans, as the racial ideologies that were initially created during the 1700s to justify slavery continue to have a deleterious effect on African Americans through the ongoing proliferation of messages that depict African Americans as inferior to other racial groups. Although studies on this topic are limited, research conducted by Adams-Bass et al. (2014) found that African American youth internalize negative stereotypes received through the media even when these youth generally have a positive private regard for their racial group. In a similar study, L. M. Ward (2004) found that stronger identification with White television characters, which are generally featured more prominently throughout the media, results in lower total self-esteem among African American adolescents. Likewise, Gordon (2016) found that media use contributes to lower academic performance, lower self-perceptions, and less interest in college-oriented careers among African American college students. Based on the findings of these studies, it is clear that negative media portrayals not only have an effect on African Americans' perceptions of self, but also have an effect on factors that ultimately influence overall quality of life such as academic performance and career aspirations.

Other societal influences that serve as antecedents to the development of negative core beliefs include colorblind racial ideologies, poverty, segregated schools and neighborhoods, and exposure to crime and violence. Intentional exploration of these influences during cognitive conceptualization reinforces the idea that clients' negative perceptions of themselves may reflect racist messages received from society rather than actual deficits in their character or ability. Exploration of societal influences also elicits important data that may be used during the implementation of interventions designed to modify core beliefs. Consider historical reviews of core beliefs (J. S. Beck, 2020), for example. Instead of focusing solely on personal experiences that may have influenced how core beliefs originated and have been maintained over the years, guiding clients in exploration of how the messages they've received from society may have also contributed to the development and maintenance of core beliefs over time can provide additional evidence clients can use to challenge their beliefs. Restructuring beliefs in this way gives clients permission to relinquish old beliefs and the freedom to develop new, more positive core beliefs.

Treatment Planning to Address Racialized Trauma Should Include Empowerment Goals

One of the psychological consequences of racism is a feeling of disempowerment, which ultimately contributes to clinically significant outcomes such as depression and anxiety. Among the many clients with racial trauma I have seen in my own clinical practice, the sense of hopelessness and worry they experience as a result of perceived powerlessness is often the most psychologically and emotionally distressing aspect of their race-based stress. Helping clients regain their sense of empowerment can have substantial therapeutic effects by reducing depression, anxiety, and other symptoms associated with racialized trauma. Accordingly, treatment planning when addressing racial trauma should consist of traditional CBT goals and interventions surrounding cognitive restructuring, as well as broader empowerment goals, which focus on consciousness-raising and claiming one's voice and power in a system of oppression.

Empowerment is "the process of increasing personal, interpersonal, or political power so that individuals, families, and communities can take action to improve their situations" (Gutiérrez, 1995, p. 229). While empowerment occurs across various levels and within several domains, therapists can focus on psychological empowerment as an expression of self-worth and a means to further facilitate healing from racialized trauma. *Psychological empowerment* is broadly defined as awareness of factors that impinge upon one's ability to structure their life and committed action to initiate change in these factors (Curtis-Tweed, 2003; Zimmerman, 1995). Findings suggest that for racial and ethnic minorities such as African Americans, psychological empowerment is not only a significant contributor to overall psychological wellbeing, but to health, educational, economic, and other social outcomes as well (Cooper & Conklin, 2015). From a CBT perspective, empowerment goals can also produce effects similar to traditional behavioral activation by prescribing changes in behavior that result in increased feelings of accomplishment and self-determination.

In conclusion, therapists must have a broad understanding of the societal context in which African Americans experience racism in order to effectively conceptualize and treat its psychological impact on these clients. This treatment should include traditional cognitive restructuring and behavioral modification goals, as well as broader empowerment goals. However, while racism and resulting symptoms of racialized trauma are concerns for many African American clients, these concerns are not always explicitly stated or readily apparent during therapy. The following dialogue, which is divided into two parts, illustrates this point. Consider the differences between the two approaches taken in each part of the dialogue and be sure to respond to the prompts and reflection questions interjected throughout the dialogue in order to begin application of the ideas presented so far in this chapter.

Meet Bilal: Part 1

Bilal is a 22-year-old African American man who was referred to therapy by his primary care physician due to an ongoing history of depression. Primary symptoms endorsed by Bilal at intake included sadness, angry outbursts, irritability, feelings of worthlessness, anxiety, frequent headaches and stomach complaints, and thoughts of suicide. Bilal, who is a senior in college, attributes his current difficulties with depression to hopelessness about finding a job after graduation and fear of letting his family down. The excerpt below is taken from Bilal's first session with his therapist as she attempts to gather information needed to conceptualize his case and devise an initial treatment plan. As you read the excerpt, think about the ideas presented so far in this chapter and reflect on any evidence or omission of cultural sensitivity in the therapist's dialogue with Bilal.

Therapist: Bilal, I understand that you've been experiencing problems with depression and anxiety for some time now. I'd like to spend some time today learning more about your concerns and how I can help.

Bilal: Okay.

Therapist: Great. When did your current feelings of depression begin?

Bilal: I guess I'd say they started at the beginning of this school year. I'm a senior majoring in geosciences. I get good grades, but I am having a hard time connecting with other people. Most students are completing internships or working with faculty on projects. I'm just by myself.

Therapist: Okay, I hear that you're feeling pretty isolated at school right now.

Bilal: Yes, but it's been that way my whole life. I've always been kind of a nerd and never really fit in with the kids who were doing things I was interested in like cosplay and sci-fi.

Therapist: So, fitting in has been something you've struggled with for a long time.

Bilal:	Yeah, and no matter what I do to fit in, it never works. I get good grades, but people still treat me like I don't know anything. It's like I have to be twice as good as everybody else for people to take me seriously. My father tells me he had to deal with the same thing during the '60s but that doesn't make me feel any better.
Therapist:	I imagine a lot of frustration and hopelessness in that situation.
Bilal:	Right. I could deal with it when it was only affecting classwork but now that graduation is almost here, I am getting worried I don't have the hands-on experience I need to show I can be a good scientist. I probably won't get a good job.

Debriefing the Case of Bilal

During the session with Bilal, several of the challenges in culturally sensitivity in CBT described above are present, particularly as it relates to the therapeutic alliance and conceptualization of client issues. Recall research discussed previously describing the importance of the therapeutic alliance during therapy with racially diverse clients. Generally, the therapeutic alliance is facilitated through skills such as empathy and active listening; however, during therapy with racially diverse clients the therapeutic alliance is also dependent upon the therapist's ability to broach race and culture (Day-Vines et al., 2018; Fuertes et al., 2006). In the excerpt of the session with Bilal, the therapist demonstrates her ability to be empathetic and use active listening through the implementation of basic counseling techniques such as reflection of content and reflection of feeling; however, at least two opportunities to broach race or respond to racial content were missed during the session. Early in the session, Bilal mentioned his geosciences major and noted that he has difficulty connecting with others in his field. In her response, the therapist failed to acknowledge the underrepresentation of African Americans in science majors and to validate the isolation he might be experiencing due to his identity as an African American man. A little later in the session, Bilal mentioned working twice as hard as others in his program and that his father experienced similar challenges. Here, the therapist missed yet another opportunity to acknowledge a racial experience commonly shared among African Americans (i.e., working twice as hard) and the long history of this in the African American community. While these types of missed opportunities do not always harm the relationship between the client and the therapist, they do increase the chances of a loss of credibility or other ruptures to the therapeutic alliance occurring (Comas-Díaz, 2006; Owen et al., 2014; Tao et al., 2015). They also prevent the therapist from obtaining data that may be useful in understanding precipitants to Bilal's concerns or factors leading to the development of his core beliefs.

At this point, Bilal's therapist has two primary options for the continued direction of the session. The first option is to probe the thoughts contributing to Bilal's chief complaints, looking for cognitive distortions and other patterns of maladaptive thinking. For example, in response to the thought "I probably won't get a good job," the therapist could make a statement such as "It sounds like you feel pretty negative about the future" and use this as a segue to psychoeducation on negative automatic thoughts and their impact on one's mood and behavior. From there, the therapist could then set the expectation that she and Bilal would begin to explore ways to challenge and reframe these and other negative thoughts at the next session, implementing techniques such as Socratic questioning and thought records.

While the approach described above is typical of a first session in CBT, focusing exclusively on Bilal's cognitions while ignoring entry points to broach the racial and cultural content of the session would represent a violation of the components of culturally sensitive CBT discussed at the beginning of this chapter. A second option focused on initiating a conversation around the potential impact of racism and Bilal's African American identity on his presenting concerns, however, would reflect greater cultural responsiveness in the session and ideally lead to some of the benefits of cultural sensitivity in therapy including a greater sense of validation and overall satisfaction with services (Meyer & Zane, 2013). The excerpt below continues the earlier dialogue between Bilal and his therapist, demonstrating how a therapist might validate and explore Bilal's experience with racism while also engaging in guided discovery of the cognitions contributing to his current psychological distress.

Meet Bilal: Part 2

Therapist: Bilal, I understand that students who are underrepresented in certain fields often experience isolation or outright discrimination in their programs. How might discrimination and racism be related to the difficulties you're having with your classmates and professors?

Bilal: I think they're definitely related. For example, I think the fact that I can't even get an interview for an internship in spite of my qualifications is because of racism. Everyone has heard of the studies showing that applicants with African American sounding names have a harder time finding a job. If my name was Kyle instead of Bilal, I would have received at least some interest in my resume by now.

Therapist: Bilal, thank you for sharing that. I know racism can be a difficult subject to talk about.

Bilal: Yeah.

Therapist: I also recognize it can be even more difficult to talk about this subject with a White person. I want you to know that while I may never be able to fully appreciate what it's like to experience racism, I recognize that racism is deeply painful. I am committed to acknowledging the impact racism has on your life and exploring that pain with you.

Bilal: Thank you. That makes me feel a little better.

Therapist: Good. So, what I am hearing so far is that as one of the few African American men in your program, you've experienced isolation and discrimination from your classmates and professors. It's your senior year and you haven't gotten much field experience because of this discrimination. You're worried that you will continue to have difficulties finding an internship and that this might affect your ability to get a job long-term. I think I even heard you say, "I probably won't get a good job," is that correct?

Bilal: Yes.

Therapist: And how do you feel when you have that thought?

Bilal: I feel really sad. And afraid.

Therapist: Thank you, Bilal. The thoughts and feelings that you're having are actually a good example of something we call the cognitive model...

Debriefing the Case of Bilal: Part 2

Two of the more important tasks of a first session in CBT include (1) building trust and rapport (i.e., the therapeutic alliance) with clients and (2) educating them about the cognitive model (J. S. Beck, 2020). The therapist demonstrated culturally sensitive approaches to each of these tasks as she continued the session with Bilal. In part 1 of the session, the therapist used basic skills such as reflection of feeling and empathy to build rapport with Bilal but missed several opportunities to broach the racial themes present in the discussion of his presenting concerns. In part 2, however, the therapist capitalized on opportunities to broach race, exploring the impact of racism on Bilal's presenting concerns and acknowledging differences between the racial worldviews of Bilal and the therapist. It is likely that broaching race early in the therapeutic relationship in this way would not only strengthen the therapeutic alliance by validating Bilal's experience as a racial being but would also remove taboos around open discussion of race and racism. According to King and Borders (2019), this approach provides an alternative to "race-neutral counseling as usual" and encourages continued discussion of race throughout the remainder of the relationship (p. 349).

While the therapist was intentional in broaching the topics of race and racism in her work with Bilal, she was also careful to focus on the primary goal of an initial session in CBT, which is to help the client gain a basic understanding of the cognitive model. According to J. S. Beck (2020), this goal is achieved best when therapists use the client's own examples to illustrate the connection between their thoughts and reactions. At the conclusion of the excerpt, we see the therapist begin this process as she draws attention to the thought "I probably won't get a good job." Continued exploration of this thought for the purpose of educating the client on the cognitive model would likely consist of use of a diagram or some other instructional aid to illustrate the relationship between Bilal's thoughts and his feelings. A key point here is that although culturally sensitive CBT emphasizes direct exploration of race and racism during therapy with African American clients, adherence to the basic tenets and principles of the theory must also be maintained.

Activity 1.2: Continuing the Case of Bilal

Imagine you were the therapist in the session with Bilal. Review the excerpts in parts 1 and 2 of the session and identify ways you would have broached race and racism in response to Bilal's statements. After developing your responses, reflect on the following questions:

- What challenges did you have in identifying broaching statements for the session with Bilal? What additional knowledge might you need to obtain?
- As you imagined yourself making your broaching statements, what emotions were elicited? What sensations did you feel in your body?
- What fears may have given rise to the emotions and physical sensations you experienced when imagining broaching race and racism with Bilal?
- What steps can you take to address any challenges or fears you have concerning exploration of race and racism during therapy with African American clients?

A CBT Refresher

Given that some readers may lack familiarity with the basic principles and techniques of CBT, this section provides a brief overview of the primary constructs associated with the theory and discusses session structure, assessment practices, and key intervention strategies in CBT. CBT is a broad term used to describe theories of counseling that focus on the connection between thoughts and feelings (DiGiuseppe et al., 2018). The earliest forms of the CBT were originated by Albert Ellis and Aaron Beck in the early 1960s. Since that time, several iterations of the theory have been developed, including trauma-focused CBT (Cohen, 2006), acceptance and commitment therapy (Hayes et al., 2011), dialectical behavior therapy (Linehan, 1993), and mindfulness-based therapy (Kabat-Zinn, 2013). While these and other forms of CBT emphasize differing theoretical constructs and interventions, each approach is based on the assumption that cognition affects mood and behavior, and changes in mood and behavior can be achieved through changes in cognition (DiGiuseppe et al., 2018).

The approach to CBT taken in this text is based largely on the work of Aaron Beck. Beck, who recently celebrated his 100th birthday, began his career during the 1950s as a psychiatrist and fully trained psychoanalyst (J. S. Beck, 2020). His initial theory of cognitive therapy was formulated after a series of experiments he developed to test the psychoanalytic view of depression failed to produce the empirical results he expected. Depression from the psychoanalytic perspective is hypothesized to be an expression of unconscious anger toward the self (Matu, 2018). The results of Beck's experiments, however, suggested that depression is more so the result of negative patterns of thinking about oneself, the world, and the future (A. T. Beck et al., 1979). The form of treatment Beck went on to develop based on this understanding has become the most widely researched and empirically validated form of therapy available today (Butler et al., 2006). The paragraphs below highlight the primary elements of CBT from a Beckian perspective.

Cognitive Model

CBT is based on the idea that our reactions—that is, our feelings, behaviors, and physiological responses—are not caused by what happens to us, but by how we think about what happens to us (J. S. Beck, 2020). This idea is called the *cognitive model*. Imagine a situation in which a woman suddenly cancels dinner plans with two friends at the last minute. One friend thinks, "She always does this, she doesn't care about me at all," causing that friend to feel sad and depressed. That friend even cries about the situation and feels sick to her stomach. Conversely, the other friend thinks, "It would be nice to have some extra time to myself" and feels happy about the canceled plans. This friend orders dinner and decides to engage in her favorite self-care activity over the course of the evening. Although the situation was the same, the thoughts of the first friend led to emotional and physiological distress, while the thoughts of the second friend led to a response that was functional and adaptive. Clients can begin to experience a reduction in the symptoms leading them to seek therapy when they learn to adopt thinking styles similar to those of the second friend. For this reason, clients are introduced to the cognitive model and made aware of its importance early in CBT. This introduction typically occurs through psychoeducation and interventions that teach clients how to recognize and replace negative thinking in their lives.

Automatic Thoughts

Automatic thoughts are what we call the negative, unintentional thoughts that occur during various situations in life (Matu, 2018). While these thoughts typically take the form of words and phrases, they may also consist of mental pictures or memories (Greenberger & Padesky, 2015). Whether these thoughts occur as words, images, or memories, a primary feature of automatic thoughts is their fleeting nature. Automatic thoughts often occur so quickly, we don't realize we've even had them. Yet, according to the basic premise of the cognitive model, these thoughts are the primary source of the distressing emotions that lead clients to seek therapy. Accordingly, early sessions in CBT focus on (a) helping clients increase their awareness of these thoughts and (b) teaching clients how to develop alternative ways of thinking. In considering this task, it is important to keep in mind that some automatic thoughts are reasonable given the situations clients face. For example, in the face of repeated discrimination and racism in the workplace, it would make sense to have thoughts focused on the injustice of the situation. In these cases, therapists should be careful to avoid examining thoughts in ways that invalidate the client's experience. Instead, therapists should help clients identify and challenge any additional automatic thoughts that reflect negative self-appraisals or surplus powerlessness as a result of the situation (Prilleltensky & Gonick, 1996). When automatic thoughts are true, it can also be helpful to focus on problem-solving or empowerment (J. S. Beck, 2020; J. M. Steele, 2020).

Cognitive Distortions

Cognitive distortions are patterns of negative, non-adaptive ways of thinking (Matu, 2018). Examples of cognitive distortions include *catastrophizing*, which refers to beliefs that what has happened or will happen will be absolutely terrible and result in the worst outcome possible; *mind reading*, or assuming that you know what other people are thinking; *mental filtering*, which refers to focusing on the negatives while ignoring the positives; and *should statements*, which refer to statements about what you or others "should," "ought," or "must" do (Dozois & A. T. Beck, 2008; Freeman et al., 2004). Helping clients identify and label cognitive distortions gives them an additional tool for assessing their thoughts. Accordingly, many CBT interventions encourage clients to label their cognitive distortions when identifying the negative automatic thoughts that contribute to their distress. Examples of these interventions include thought records and Socratic questioning.

Core Beliefs

Core beliefs refer to the central ideas about oneself that underlie automatic thoughts and lead to errors in thinking (J. S. Beck, 2020). They may be negative or positive, and typically develop in response to early childhood experiences and societal messages about one's racial group (J. M. Steele, 2020). According to J. S. Beck (2020), negative core beliefs generally fall into three categories: (1) helplessness, (2) unlovability, and (3) worthlessness. Helplessness core beliefs reflect ideas about personal incompetence, vulnerability, and inferiority (Schaffner, 2021). Examples of these core beliefs include "I am incompetent" and "I am a victim." Clients with unlovability core beliefs, on the other hand, perceive themselves as unlikable and incapable of intimacy. Examples of beliefs in this category include "I am unattractive" and "I am bound to be rejected." Lastly, clients with worthlessness core beliefs perceive themselves as inherently bad and/or a burden to others. Examples of these beliefs include "I am worthless" and "I don't deserve to live."

Elsewhere, Dozois and A. T. Beck (2008) more broadly categorized core beliefs into just two themes reflecting competency and desirability. In Chapter 6, I discuss five categories of core beliefs commonly developed specifically in response to racism. These categories include inferiority, inadequacy, personal blame, powerlessness, and belief in a just world (J. M. Steele & Newton, 2022). Given that an internalized sense of inferiority is a primary psychological outcome of racism, core beliefs reflecting inferiority and inadequacy are especially prominent among clients who experience racial prejudice and discrimination. For example, African Americans who spend most of their lives in predominantly White school and work settings often experience a sense of rejection from their White counterparts (Tatum, 1997). This sense of rejection might be expressed as the core belief "I don't fit in" and reflect the larger personal inadequacy and inferiority themes characteristic of internalized racism. For some individuals, negative core beliefs are only active during discrete episodes of psychological distress. However, because of the pervasive and insidious nature of racism in our society, clients who experience negative core beliefs in response to racial stressors may find their beliefs are activated on a more frequent and ongoing basis.

Intermediate Beliefs

Intermediate beliefs are the attitudes, rules, and assumptions clients develop in response to their negative core beliefs (J. S. Beck, 2020). Essentially, intermediate beliefs describe mindsets, guidelines, and "if-then" conditions clients develop to prevent their core beliefs from being true. Let's continue with the example above to illustrate intermediate beliefs. In the example, the client developed the core belief "I don't fit in" in response to the sense of rejection she has experienced in predominantly White school and work environments. Her attitude in this situation has been "It's terrible when others don't accept me," while her rule has been "I have to 'play the game' or be stereotyped." This attitude and rule are further delineated by the conditional assumption "If I look and act similar to my peers, I'll fit in and be okay; but if I don't look and act similar to my peers, I'll be ostracized and rejected." While fitting in with peers is a normal developmental task to some extent, the desire to be like others can result in a sense of self-alienation or even self-hatred when it requires rejection of the cultural norms and aesthetics of the racial group to which one belongs. Therefore, when explored within the context of racism, helping clients articulate and modify intermediate beliefs can be a powerful intervention, as doing so targets both thoughts and behaviors that contribute to any internalized racism or racialized trauma occurring as a result of their experiences.

Compensatory Strategies

Compensatory strategies refer to the methods clients use to cope with what they perceive as personal weaknesses. According to J. S. Beck (2020), most compensatory strategies are actually normal behaviors that are overused at the expense of more functional strategies. Examples of compensatory strategies include perfectionism, people pleasing, being overly controlling, seeking recognition, avoiding confrontation, and their opposites (i.e., purposely appearing incompetent, distancing oneself from others, and abdicating control to others). In Chapter 6, I also discuss specific compensatory strategies commonly developed in response to racism. These strategies include avoidance, conformity, overperformance, and learned helplessness (J. M. Steele & Newton, 2022). For example, the client with internalized racism and the core belief "I don't fit in" might use a compensatory strategy of conforming to White social norms and standards of beauty to cope with their perception of personal inadequacy. Generally, addressing compensatory strategies involves helping clients (a) increase awareness of their maladaptive compensatory strategies and (b) develop more positive and adaptive ways of coping. When dealing with racism, an additional goal for therapy involves helping clients learn to cope in ways that are self-affirming and empowering.

Cognitive Conceptualization

Cognitive conceptualization can be likened to a map that depicts the relationship between the client's core beliefs, conditional assumptions, and automatic thoughts (J. S. Beck, 2020). This map consists of data describing (a) the client's relevant childhood experiences, (b) their central beliefs about themselves, (c) attitudes and rules they use to navigate the world in light of their beliefs, (d) cognitive, affective, and behavioral strategies they use to adhere to their rules, and (e) examples of how such data are translated into negative automatic thoughts and reactions in daily situations. In CBT, cognitive conceptualization is considered a critical aspect of therapy as it not only provides the framework for understanding the client's problems but also directs the interventions used during treatment (Matu, 2018). While cognitive conceptualization begins during the first session, it continues throughout therapy as more is discovered about the client's automatic thoughts and the deeper-level cognitions underlying these thoughts (J. S. Beck, 2020). Given the ongoing nature of cognitive conceptualization, any interpretations or hypotheses formed during the conceptualization process should be viewed as tentative and therapists should regularly check-in with clients to determine the accuracy of the conceptualization, modifying it as necessary.

Activity 1.3: Test Your Knowledge

The sections above provided an overview of primary constructs in CBT. Test your comprehension of each construct by completing the statements in the right column with the most appropriate response from the column on the left.

1. Overperforming in occupational, academic, or social settings to meet real or perceived expectations greater than those held for members of the dominant racial group and adjusting one's speech, appearance, and behavior to be more similar to the dominant culture are examples of

   _____

2. Perceptions such as "I am not good enough" or "I am inferior" that develop in response to negative childhood experiences and societal messages are examples of

   _____

3. Thoughts such as "They're going to think I don't know what I am talking about" and "No one ever listens to me" that occur while leading the morning staff meeting are examples of negative _____

4. The therapist's understanding of the relationship between the client's core beliefs, intermediate beliefs, compensatory strategies, and automatic thoughts is known as

   _____

5. The assumption "If I work twice as hard, then I'll be accepted" is an example of one's

   _____

6. "I shouldn't let these people get to me" is an example of a _____

7. The idea that our emotional, behavioral, and physiological reactions are caused by our perceptions of events is known as

   _____

a. Automatic thoughts
b. The cognitive model
c. Intermediate beliefs
d. Core beliefs
e. Cognitive distortion
f. Cognitive conceptualization
g. Compensatory strategies

Session Structure

Because CBT from the Beckian perspective relies heavily on the cognitive conceptualization of each individual client, manualized approaches are typically not utilized in treatment. Nevertheless, therapy from this approach generally adheres to specific objectives for the beginning, middle, and end of sessions (J. S. Beck, 2020). At the beginning of sessions, therapists pay close attention to facilitation of the therapeutic alliance, emphasizing skills that build rapport with the client such as active listening, warmth, and authenticity. Therapists also work to strengthen the alliance at this point in the session by conducting a mood check. *Mood checks* are quick assessments of symptoms the client has experienced in the time since the last session. They can be taken by client report or through use of a standardized assessment such as the Beck Anxiety Inventory (BAI; A. T. Beck, 1990) or the Generalized Anxiety Disorder-7 (GAD-7; Spitzer et al., 2006). Following the mood check, the therapist collaborates with the client to establish an agenda for the session. According to J. S. Beck (2020), this can be accomplished by asking questions such as, "What happened in between this session and last session that I should know?" "What would you like to talk about today?" and "What problem would you like my help in solving today?" Then, before moving on to discussion of the issues listed on the agenda, the therapist makes a bridge between the current and previous sessions to check for application of previously discussed concepts by asking questions such as "What did you get done?" "What did you learn from that?" and "Is there anything you have done this week that would be helpful to keep doing?" These questions not only reinforce the importance of completing homework in between sessions, but they also alert the therapist to any obstacles that might be interfering with treatment, as well as any additional items that should be included on the agenda (Wenzel, 2019).

Once the agenda for the current session is established, the middle of the session in CBT is spent gathering information about the problems identified on the agenda, using the cognitive model as an organizing framework (Dobson & Dobson, 2013). During this time, therapists may implement specific strategies such as Socratic questioning or collaborate with clients to develop behavioral experiments to test their thinking in real world situations outside of therapy. As strategies and interventions are implemented, therapists should be sure to teach clients what they are doing so that clients are eventually able to be their own therapists. This includes providing psychoeducation on the techniques used during therapy, helping clients to summarize their insights, and collaborating with clients to create action plans as they become aware of ways to solve their problems. *Action plans* are homework assignments clients complete outside of therapy to help them apply and practice the new learning and skills they acquire during sessions

(Wenzel, 2019). To further facilitate application and practice of new learning and skills, clients should also be encouraged to take their own therapy notes for review outside of session.

As sessions draw to a close in CBT, therapists should focus on (a) helping clients further summarize and explain insights gained as a result of the session and (b) finalizing the action plan to be completed before the next session. According to J. S. Beck (2020), this can be done by asking questions such as "What do you want to remember?" "What would be important for you to remind yourself of this week?" and "What else should be added to your action plan for this week." As clients share their insights, therapists should make sure clients have an accurate summary of what happened in the session and correct any misunderstanding of the concepts presented in the session or feedback given by the therapist. Additionally, as they confirm their action plans, therapists should remind clients to give themselves credit every time they complete something on the plan. This affirms the progress clients are making toward their goals and increases their motivation to complete assignments outside of session. Therapists can also implement a strategy called *covert rehearsal* at this point in the session, which includes asking questions such as "What thoughts or feelings might interfere with you completing the activities on your action plan?" and "What could you tell yourself or do in those moments?" This further increases the likelihood clients will complete the action plan outside of session.

Finally, experts believe that since many of the impacts of racism and racialized trauma live in the subconscious parts of the brain that activate the body in the face of danger, thinking or talking about trauma alone is not enough to promote healing (Menakem, 2017). Therefore, it may be helpful to integrate various mindfulness approaches that address the body's response to traumatic stress into the regular session structure of CBT when addressing racism and racialized trauma with African American clients. At the beginning and end of the sessions, this may include guiding clients in a breathing or relaxation exercise to help them calm down and discharge negative energy that may have surfaced as a result of processing their experiences with racism. For clients with more severe symptoms of racialized trauma, this may also include use of grounding techniques such as the 5-4-3-2-1 method to manage any dissociative symptoms that may occur during therapy while discussing race-based events.

Assessment

While the structure described above broadly applies to all sessions in CBT, additional considerations are made during the assessment phase of therapy. Novice counselors often think of assessment as a process that occurs during the first one or two sessions of treatment. However, in CBT, assessment is not limited to the first few initial contacts with clients (J. S. Beck, 2020). Instead, assessment is a critical part of therapy that begins in the first session and is weaved throughout the remainder of the therapeutic process as the therapist continues to gather data needed to refine their conceptualization of the client's presenting concerns (Matu, 2018). With that said, it is important to spend time collecting as much assessment data as possible at the start of the counseling relationship in order to make a diagnosis, begin formulation of the client's cognitive conceptualization, and develop an initial treatment plan. This data includes information about the nature of the client's present-ing concerns and symptoms, as well as their duration, severity, and impact on client functioning. Relevant histories and information necessary for a biopsychosocial evaluation should also be taken at this time. This includes (a) the client's psychiatric, medical, developmental, educational, vocational, family, and substance use histories, (b) their expectations for therapy, and (c) any strengths, adaptive coping strategies, and protective factors that may assist with the treatment process (J. S. Beck, 2020).

There are many quantitative and qualitative tools available to help thera-pists collect information during the assessment phase of therapy. Common quantitative measures specific to CBT include the Beck Depression Inventory-II (BDI-II; A. T. Beck et al., 1996) and the Beck Anxiety Inventory (BAI; A. T. Beck, 1990). Other atheoretical quantitative measures commonly used for assessment include the Patient Health Questionnaire-9 (PHQ-9; Kroenke et al., 2001), the Generalized Anxiety Disorder-7 (GAD-7; Spitzer et al., 2006), and the Outcome Questionnaire-45.2 (OQ-45.2; Beckstead et al., 2003). While these and other empirically validated tests have been found to be psychometrically reliable and valid assessments of the constructs they purport to measure, it is important to keep in mind that the results of these assessments may be influenced by social desirability, fatigue, or the test-taker's general attitude toward the assessment. Therefore, good assessment practice necessitates a balance between the use of quantitative instruments and an in-depth clinical interview. The Cultural Formulation Interview (CFI; American Psychiatric Association, 2013) is a popular and comprehensive tool many therapists use to obtain qualitative information about the client's mental health and the impact of culture on their presenting concerns. This tool, located in the Emerging Measures and Models section of the *Diagnostic and Statistical Manual of Mental Disorders-5* (DSM-5; American Psychiatric Association, 2013), emphasizes four areas of assessment: (1) Cultural Definition of the Problem; (2) Cultural Perceptions of Cause, Context, and Support; (3) Cultural Factors Affecting Self-Coping and Past Help Seeking; and (4) Cultural Factors Affecting Current Help Seeking. Details concerning each of the four areas of the CFI are provided later, in Chapter 6.

The CFI offers therapists insight into the cultural lens through which clients view, explain, and cope with their problems (American Psychiatric

Association, 2013). When considering the impacts of racism, however, therapists must also be intentional in their exploration of symptoms associated with race-based traumatic stress within their clients. One of the most well-researched and empirically validated assessments of race-based traumatic stress is a measure titled the Race-Based Traumatic Stress Symptom Scale (RBTSSS, Carter et al., 2013). According to the scale's authors, race-based traumatic stress can be conceptualized and assessed along seven clusters of symptoms that occur after a race-based event. These factors include Depression, Intrusion, Anger, Hypervigilance, Physical Reactions, Low Self-Esteem, and Avoidance. Levels of symptomatology within the seven clusters are assessed using Likert-type scale items that yield quantitative scores for each cluster; however, the assessment also includes an initial qualitative component in which clients are asked to describe three of the most memorable events of racism they have experienced in their lives. This combination of quantitative and qualitative approaches accomplishes several aims. First, the quantifiable measure of the seven clusters aids therapists' understanding of the nature and severity of symptoms clients experience as a result of race-based traumatic stress, which increases the therapist's ability to attend to these issues in treatment planning more directly. Second, the inclusion of a qualitative component that allows clients to share stories about their experiences with racism sends the message that it is safe to explore race within the context of the therapy dyad and may improve the overall cultural sensitivity in the therapeutic relationship as the therapist listens to and validates the client's experiences (M. T. Williams et al., 2018). Finally, use of a standardized measure such as the RBTSSS may be beneficial for therapists who experience some discomfort broaching topics related to race and racism as the assessment is easily administered and creates space to initiate these conversations.

Reflection 1.2: Think about your current assessment practices with African American clients. To what extent do you seek to obtain information about the impact of race and racism on the client's social context and presenting concerns? What are some immediate steps you can take to increase your intentionality in assessing for the presence of racial stressors in your clients' concerns?

Key Interventions

This final section of the chapter reviews key CBT interventions, as well as other relevant strategies found to be effective in the treatment of racialized trauma. As previously mentioned, individuals with racialized trauma experience many of the same emotional, cognitive, behavioral, and physiological symptoms as people dealing with other forms of trauma. Of particular importance are the core reactions to race-based traumatic stress, which include intrusion, arousal, and avoidance or psychic numbing (Carter, 2007). According to research, these reactions occur primarily as the result of dys-regulated activity in the amygdala, hippocampus, and sympathetic nervous system as the brain responds to stimuli that is perceived to be physically or emotionally threatening and the body and the brain become locked in a natural feedback loop (Wolkin, 2016). Because of this mind/body connection in trauma, effective therapy requires interventions focused not only on cognitive and emotional healing, but on reprograming of the body/mind connection as well. In therapy, this involves two types of approaches—bottom-up approaches and top-down approaches (van der Kolk, 2014). *Bottom-up approaches* are designed to help clients cope with their raw emotions and defense reactions using body-centric mindfulness strategies such as breathing and relaxation exercises. *Top-down approaches*, on the other hand, are designed to help clients think differently about their problems using therapies such as CBT. Socratic questioning, thought records, the downward arrow technique, behavioral experiments, behavioral activation, and graduated exposure activities are the top-down strategies applied to the case illustrations in this text. Mindfulness and relaxation strategies are the bottom-up approaches discussed as a way address the core reactions of racialized trauma.

Socratic Questioning

Socratic questioning, also referred to as *Socratic dialogue* or *guided discovery*, is a structured format of questioning that helps clients monitor their thoughts and emotions, evaluate their thinking, and respond to situations that occur in life in an adaptive way (Matu, 2018). In CBT, Socratic questioning is typically utilized as one of the primary tools of cognitive restructuring (i.e., the process of noticing and changing one's thinking). Accordingly, this intervention should be introduced only after clients have a firm understanding of the cognitive model and that their thinking in specific situations affects their mood and behavior. Use of Socratic questioning involves asking clients a series of open-ended questions that help them look for evidence to challenge unhelpful thinking patterns and identify solutions to their problems. Examples of these questions include "What is the evidence for this thought?" "What is the evidence against this thought?" and "What could I do if this thought were true?" Socratic questioning can also be applied more broadly to help clients deconstruct the role of race in their thinking. Examples of questions that can be used in this process include:

- When did you first realize yourself as a racial being?
- What did being Black mean for you at that time?
- What are the advantages and disadvantages of being Black?
- What are the stereotypes associated with being Black?

- How did you learn these stereotypes?
- Where did these stereotypes come from?
- How do these stereotypes affect the way you see yourself and people in your racial group?
- What are some alternative explanations for these stereotypes?
- What would you like to believe about yourself outside of these stereotypes?
- What evidence is there to support these beliefs?

Thought Records

A *thought record* is a specific type of journaling activity that helps clients utilize the cognitive model on a daily basis (J. S. Beck, 2020). Typically, thought records are in chart format, with sections for clients to record situations, feelings, negative automatic thoughts, and new, more functional thoughts. This process helps clients increase insight into the automatic thoughts contributing to their mood, and to be more active in challenging and replacing these thoughts. Like Socratic questioning, thought records should not be introduced into therapy until clients have gained an adequate understanding of the cognitive model (Matu, 2018). Use of a complete thought record also requires clients to have developed an adequate ability to reframe their negative automatic thoughts. Therefore, therapists may consider starting clients with a partial thought record that only includes sections to record situations, emotions, and negative automatic thoughts. Clients can use these partial thought records for homework assignments and then work with the therapist to identify alternative thoughts during sessions. This assists clients who initially have trouble developing alternative thoughts and helps mitigate incorrect use of the tool.

Downward Arrow Technique

While Socratic questioning and thought records focus on helping clients identify, challenge, and replace negative automatic thoughts, the *downward arrow technique* is designed to help uncover the core beliefs that lead to negative automatic thoughts in daily situations (J. S. Beck, 2020). To implement the downward arrow technique, the therapist first listens for automatic thoughts that seem to reflect negative core beliefs. The therapist then asks the client what meaning the automatic thought would have to the client's life if it were true, continuing this process until one or more core beliefs are revealed. For example, Kaila was a 24-year-old African American woman I saw in clinical practice for approximately one year. Kaila was active in the Black Lives Matter movement and, within the year that I saw her, became increasingly anxious and depressed in response to the murders of Ahmaud Arbery, Breonna Taylor, and George Floyd. While discussing news coverage of these events, Kaila reported having the automatic thought "No one cares about Black people." Suspecting that this thought reflected an underlying core belief of helplessness, I implemented the downward arrow technique, saying to Kaila, "If this is true, that no one cares about Black people, what meaning does this have for you?" Kaila responded saying, "It means more of the same. That people can do whatever they want to Black people and get away with it." Continuing with the downward arrow technique, I then asked, "And what does that mean, that people can do whatever they want to Black people and get away with it?" to which Kaila replied, "It means I'm not safe." In this instance, only two questions were needed before I was able to uncover the negative core beliefs leading to Kaila's automatic thought. In some cases, however, more questions may be required, or clients may provide feeling responses rather than an indication of the meaning associated with the thought. In these situations, J. S. Beck (2020) recommends therapists vary their inquiry using questions such as "If that's true, so what?" "What's so bad about..." "What's the worst part about..." and "What does that mean about you?"

Behavioral Experiments

Behavioral experiments refer to activities that are designed to: (a) help clients test the validity of their cognitions, (b) help clients construct and test new, more adaptive cognitions, and (c) provide therapists with data that can be used to elaborate on their formulation of the client's cognitive conceptualization (Rouf et al., 2004). The most common behavioral experiments are known as active experiments (Rouf et al., 2004). Active experiments are those in which the client identifies an unhelpful cognition and then identifies how they might deliberately think or act differently in the problem situation. For example, a client who thinks "I will be mocked if I share my feelings with others" may devise an experiment where they practice sharing feelings with a few individuals whom they believe might be capable of responding to their story in a respectful manner. If at least one of the individuals offers an appropriate response, the client can then move on, developing additional experiments to test a new, more adaptive thought such as "Not everyone should be trusted with my feelings, but there are some individuals I can trust." If clients experience such intense distress that they are not able to perform their own direct tests, therapists can begin by using other approaches to behavioral experiments such as role-play or observation.

Behavioral Activation

Behavioral activation is an intervention that is designed to have a positive impact on mood by increasing client engagement in activities that offer a sense of pleasure and accomplishment (J. S. Beck, 2020). Most often, behavioral activation is used in the treatment of disorders such as depression and anxiety. Clients who are depressed or anxious tend to withdraw socially and avoid activities that would typically elicit positive emotions. Over time, this results in a worsening of mood due to the ongoing isolation and absence of pleasurable activities in the client's life. Behavioral activation can help reverse this pattern by increasing the amount of time clients spend engaged in pleasure and mastery. To use behavioral activation as an intervention, therapists should first ask clients to monitor how they currently spend their time. This includes recording the activities they engage in on a daily basis and rating the amount of pleasure and accomplishment they feel as a result of completing each activity on a scale of 1 to 10. After gaining a baseline of their current activity levels, therapists should then ask clients to draw conclusions from what they have recorded and identify activities that would introduce more pleasure and accomplishment in their lives. Next, the client and therapist should work together to strategically schedule activities throughout each day in order to increase the number of opportunities clients have to feel good. For clients who have difficulty recalling the types of activities from which they previously derived pleasure and satisfaction, it may be helpful to first spend time creating a list of activities to choose from. Additionally, some clients may have difficulty experiencing pleasure or accomplishment due to critical or otherwise negative automatic thoughts (J. S. Beck, 2020). In these instances, identifying and challenging negative thoughts that may be interfering with the intervention can also be beneficial.

Graduated Exposure Activities

Graduated exposure activities are used primarily in the treatment of anxiety disorders. One of the core elements of anxiety disorders, such as generalized anxiety disorder and social anxiety disorder, is avoidance of situations that produce worry or fear (American Psychiatric Association, 2013). However, limited exposure to anxiety-provoking situations reduces one's ability to disconfirm their worry and fears and ultimately makes the fears even stronger. Graduated exposure activities are designed to help clients identify small, incremental steps they can take to engage in anxiety-inducing social situations. Over time, these activities help clients reduce the amount of worry they have and increase their tolerance of the distress they experience in anxiety-provoking situations. One specific example of a graduated exposure activity is the fear hierarchy, wherein the client creates an anxiety situation list and identifies goals for addressing each situation, starting with the least challenging (Leahy et al., 2012). Another similar example is the fear ladder, wherein the client takes a specific goal they have developed to reduce their anxiety and then identifies small, incremental steps they can take toward accomplishing that goal (Clark & A. T. Beck, 2012). As discussed at the beginning of this chapter, any exposure activities used while addressing racialized trauma should be modified in consideration of the client's cultural worldview (Graham et al., 2013).

Mindfulness and Relaxation Strategies

Because emotional and psychological distress can have physiological manifestations, the physical sensations clients experience in their bodies can be important alert signals. For example, when experiencing race-based stress, clients may not be aware of the negative thinking contributing to their distress but may be alert to bodily sensations such as stomachaches, chest pains, or muscle tension (Carter, 2007). *Mindfulness strategies* refer to techniques that are designed to help clients become more aware of and observe these internal experiences without evaluating or judging them as signs of weakness. This allows clients to have greater self-compassion and to be more intentional in implementing tools from their box of coping strategies when necessary. In a similar way, *relaxation strategies* also serve as coping mechanisms by providing a way for clients to safely discharge negative energy associated with racialized trauma (Menakem, 2017). Examples of mindfulness and relaxation strategies include meditation, mindfulness of breath, mindfulness of emotion, progressive muscle relaxation, body scan, grounding, and guided imagery. While mindfulness and relaxation strategies are widely recognized trauma interventions, therapists should note that there has been some stigma associated with these practices in the African American community generally, and with meditation practices in particular (Watson-Singleton et al., 2019). For example, some within the African American community believe meditation involves subscribing to certain religious philosophies or communicating with spirits. Others believe mindfulness and meditation practices are incompatible with prayer or reliance on God. Therefore, when integrating mindfulness and relaxation strategies into treatment planning with African American clients, therapists should be careful in their use of language and frame mindfulness in a culturally sensitive way, for example, describing meditation as awareness or relaxation focused on nonjudgmental attention to one's thoughts, emotions, and physiological sensations (Watson-Singleton et al., 2019).

Outline of the Remainder of this Book

In this chapter, I discussed the use of CBT as an approach to address the impact of racism among African Americans and reviewed primary constructs associated with CBT more broadly. The next two chapters offer a more in-depth look at racism and mental health in the African American community, focusing on definitions, psychological consequences, and cultural strengths African Americans may call upon as resources to cope with the stress of racism. Chapters 4 and 5 present an overview of the dispositions and skills necessary to build culturally sensitive therapeutic relationships and maximize the effectiveness of CBT when working with clients from diverse racial, ethnic, and cultural backgrounds. Chapters 6, 7, and 8 continue exploration of the use of CBT to address the impact of racism on African American clients, highlighting specific strategies to challenge the negative automatic thoughts and maladaptive beliefs that develop in response to racial oppression. The final chapters illustrate how the concepts discussed throughout the book might be used with African American clients experiencing depressive, anxiety, and post-traumatic stress disorders. Throughout the book, reflection questions, guided practice, and case vignettes are incorporated into each chapter to assist readers with application of the ideas presented in the text into the users' own clinical setting.

References

Adams-Bass, V. N., Stevenson, H. C., & Kotzin, D. S. (2014). Measuring the meaning of Black media stereotypes and their relationship to the racial identity, Black history knowledge, and racial socialization of African American youth. *Journal of Black Studies, 45*(5), 367–395. https://doi.org/10.1177/0021934714530396

Alessandrini, K. (2023, August 9). Utah school district to pay $2M settlement to family of 10-year-old Black girl who died by suicide. *Blavity.* https://blavity.com/utah-school-district-pay-2m-settlement-black-girl-died-suicide

American Psychiatric Association. (2013). *Diagnostic and statistical manual of mental disorders* (5th ed.). American Psychiatric Association. https://doi.org/10.1176/appi.books.9780890425596

American Psychological Association. (2017). *What is exposure therapy?* https://www.apa.org/ptsd-guideline/patients-and-families/exposure-therapy

Bailey, T.-K. M., Williams, W. S., & Favors, B. (2014). Internalized racial oppression in the African American community. In E. J. R. David (Ed.), *Internalized oppression: The psychology of marginalized groups* (pp. 137–162). Springer Publishing Company, Inc.

Beck, A. T. (1990). *Manual for the Beck Anxiety Inventory.* Pearson.

Beck, A. T., Rush, A. J., Shaw, B. F., & Emery, G. (1979). *Cognitive therapy of depression.* Guilford Press.

Beck, A. T., Steer, R. A., & Brown, G. K. (1996). *Manual for the Beck Depression Inventory-II.* Pearson.

Beck, J. S. (2020). *Cognitive behavior therapy: Basics and beyond* (3rd ed.). Guilford Press.

Beckstead, D. J., Hatch, A. L., Lambert, M. J., Eggett, D. L., Goates, M. K., & Vermeersch, D. A. (2003). Clinical significance of the Outcome Questionnaire (OQ-45.2). *The Behavior Analyst Today, 4*(1), 86–97. https://doi.org/10.1037/h0100015

Belgrave, F. Z., & Allison, K. W. (2019). *African American psychology: From Africa to America* (4th ed.). Sage Publications, Inc.

Brauer, L., Lewin, A., & Storch, E. (2011). A review of psychotherapy for obsessive-compulsive disorder. *Mind & Brain: The Journal of Psychiatry, 2*(1), 38–44.

Brooks, J. R., Hong, J. H., Cheref, S., & Walker, R. L. (2020). Capability for suicide: Discrimination as a painful and provocative event. *Suicide & Life-Threatening Behavior, 50*(6), 1173–1180. https://doi.org/10.1111/sltb.12671

Bryant, C. E., & Harder, J. (2008). Treating suicidality in African American adolescents with cognitive-behavioral therapy. *Child & Adolescent Social Work Journal, 25*(1), 1–9. https://doi.org/10.1007/s10560-007-0100-2

Burns, M. A., & Vaughn, K. R. (2021). Race metatheory: Toward a dissolution of a calamitous concept. *Professional Psychology: Research and Practice, 52*(5), 487–493. https://doi.org/10.1037/pro0000416

Butler, A. C., Chapman, J. E., Forman, E. M., & Beck, A. T. (2006). The empirical status of cognitive-behavioral therapy: A review of meta-analyses. *Clinical Psychology Review, 26*(1), 17–31. https://doi.org/10.1016/j.cpr.2005.07.003

Calloway, A., & Creed, T. A. (2021, July). Enhancing CBT consultation with multicultural counseling principles. *Cognitive and Behavioral Practice.* Advance online publication. https://doi.org/10.1016/j.cbpra.2021.05.007

Carter, M. M., & Sbrocco, T. (2018). Cognitive behavioral models, measures, and treatments for anxiety disorders in African Americans. In E. C. Change, C. A. Downey, J. K. Hirsch, & E. A. Yu (Eds.), *Treating depression, anxiety, and stress in ethnic and racial groups: Cognitive behavioral approaches* (pp. 179–202). American Psychological Association.

Carter, R. T. (2007). Racism and psychological and emotional injury: Recognizing and assessing race-based traumatic stress. *The Counseling Psychologist, 35*(1), 13–105. https://doi.org/10.1177/0011000006292033

Carter, R. T., Johnson, V. E., Roberson, K., Mazzula, S. L., Kirkinis, K., & Sant-Barket, S. (2017). Race-based traumatic stress, racial identity statuses, and psychological functioning: An exploratory investigation. *Professional Psychology: Research and Practice, 48*(1), 30–37. https://doi.org/10.1037/pro0000116

Carter, R. T., Mazzula, S., Victoria, R., Vazquez, R., Hall, S., Smith, S., Sant-Barket, S., Forsyth, J., Bazelais, K., & Williams, B. (2013). Initial development of the Race-Based Traumatic Stress Symptom Scale: Assessing the emotional impact of racism. *Psychological Trauma: Theory, Research, Practice, and Policy, 5*(1), 1–9. https://doi.org/10.1037/a0025911

Clark, D. A., & Beck, A. T. (2012). *The anxiety & worry workbook: The cognitive behavioral solution.* Guilford Press.

Cohen, J. A. (2006). *Treating trauma and traumatic grief in children and adolescents.* Guilford Press.

Cokley, K. (2007). Critical issues in the measurement of ethnic and racial identity: A referendum on the state of the field. *Journal of Counseling Psychology, 54*(3), 224–234. https://doi.org/10.1037/0022-0167.54.3.224

Comas-Díaz, L. (2006). Cultural variation in the therapeutic relationship. In C. D. Goodheart, D. Carol, A. E. Kazdin, E. Alan, & R. J. Sternberg (Eds.), *Evidence-based psychotherapy: Where practice and research meet* (pp. 81–105). American Psychological Association.

Cooper, A. A., & Conklin, L. R. (2015). Dropout from individual psychotherapy for major depression: A meta-analysis of randomized clinical trials. *Clinical Psychology Review, 40*, 57–65. https://doi.org/10.1016/j.cpr.2015.05.001

Crenshaw, K. (1989). Demarginalizing the intersection of race and sex: A Black feminist critique of antidiscrimination doctrine, feminist theory, and antiracist politics. *University of Chicago Legal Forum, 1.* https://chicagounbound.uchicago.edu/cgi/viewcontent.cgi?article=1052&context=uclf

Curtis-Tweed, P. (2003). Experiences of African American empowerment: A Jamesian perspective on agency. *Journal of Moral Education, 32*(4), 397–409. https://doi.org/10.1080/0305724032000161295

David, D., Cristea, I., & Hoffmann, S. G. (2018). Why cognitive behavioral therapy is the current gold standard of psychotherapy. *Frontiers in Psychiatry, 9*(4). https://doi.org/10.3389/fpsyt.2018.00004

David, E. J. R. (2009). Internalized oppression, psychopathology, and cognitive-behavioral therapy among historically oppressed groups. *Journal of Psychological Practice, 15*(1), 71–103.

Day-Vines, N. L., Ammah, B. B., Steen, S., & Arnold, K. M. (2018). Getting comfortable with discomfort: Preparing counselor trainees to broach racial, ethnic, and cultural factors with clients during counseling. *International Journal for the Advancement of Counselling, 40*(2), 89–104. https://doi.org/10.1002/jcad.12304

Day-Vines, N.L., Wood, S. M., Grothaus, T., Craigen, L., Holman, A., Dotson-Blake, K., & Douglass, M. J. (2007). Broaching the subjects of race, ethnicity, and culture during the counseling process. *Journal of Counseling & Development, 85*(4), 401–409. https://doi.org/10.1002/jcad.12069

DeSante, C. D. (2013). Working twice as hard to get half as far: Race, work ethic, and America's deserving poor. *American Journal of Political Science, 57*(2), 342–356. https://doi.org/10.1111/ajps.12006

DiGiuseppe, R., Venezia, R., & Gotterbarn, R. (2018). What is cognitive behavioral therapy? In A. Vernon & K. A. Doyle (Eds.), *Cognitive behavior therapies: A guidebook for practitioners* (pp. 1–35). American Counseling Association.

Dobson, D. J. G., & Dobson, K. S. (2013). In-session structure and collaborative empiricism. *Cognitive and Behavioral Practice, 20*(4), 410–418. https://doi.org/10.1016/j.cbpra.2012.11.002

Dozois, D. J., & Beck, A. T. (2008). Cognitive schema, beliefs, and assumptions. In K. S. Dobson & D. J. Dozois (Eds.), *Risk factors in depression* (pp. 121–143). Academic Press.

Evans, A. M., Hemmings, C., Ramsay-Seaner, K., & Barnett, J. (2021). Perceived racism and discrimination among people of color: An ethnographic content analysis. *Journal of Multicultural Counseling and Development, 49*(3), 152–164. https://doi.org/10.1002/jmcd.12221

Fernandez, E., Malvaso, C., Day, A., & Guharajan, D. (2018). 21st century cognitive behavioural therapy for anger: A systematic review of research design, methodology and outcome. *Behavioural and Cognitive Psychotherapy, 46*(4), 385–404. https://doi.org/10.1017/S1352465818000048

Freeman, A., Pretzer, J., Fleming, B., & Simon, K. M. (2004). *Clinical applications of cognitive therapy* (2nd ed.). Springer.

Fuertes, J. N., Stracuzzi, T. I., Bennett, J., Scheinholtz, J., Mislowack, A., Hersh, M., & Cheng, D. (2006). Therapist multicultural competency: A study of therapy dyads. *Psychotherapy: Theory, Research, Practice, Training*, *43*(4), 480–490. https://doi.org/10.1037/0033-3204.43.4.480

Goodwill, J. R., Taylor, R. J., & Watkins, D. C. (2021). Everyday discrimination, depressive symptoms, and suicide ideation among African American men. *Archives of Suicide Research*, *25*(1), 74–93. https://doi.org/10.1080/13811118.2019.1660287

Gordon, M. K. (2016). Achievement scripts: Media influences on Black students' academic performance, self-perceptions, and career interests. *Journal of Black Psychology*, *42*(3), 195–220. https://doi.org/10.1177/0095798414566510

Graham, J. R., Sorenson, S., & Hayes-Skelton, S. A. (2013). Enhancing the cultural sensitivity of cognitive behavioral interventions for anxiety in diverse populations. *The Behavior Therapist*, *36*(5), 101–108.

Graham, J. R., West, L. M., Martinez, J., & Roemer, L. (2016). The mediating role of internalized racism in the relationship between racist experiences and anxiety symptoms in a Black American sample. *Cultural Diversity and Ethnic Minority Psychology*, *22*(3), 369–376. https://doi.org/10.1037/cdp0000073

Greer, T. M., Brondolo, E., Amuzu, E., & Kaur, A. (2018). Cognitive behavioral models, measures, and treatments for stress disorders in African Americans. In E. C. Change, C. A. Downey, J. K. Hirsch, & E. A. Yu (Eds.), *Treating depression, anxiety, and stress in ethnic and racial groups: Cognitive behavioral approaches* (pp. 287–311). American Psychological Association.

Greenberger, D., & Padesky, C. A. (2015). *Mind over mood: Change how you feel by changing the way you think* (2nd ed.). Guilford Press.

Gutiérrez, L. M. (1995). Understanding the empowerment process: Does consciousness make a difference? *Social Work Research*, *19*(4), 229–237.

Hanna, F. J., & Cardona, B. (2013). Multicultural counseling beyond the relationship: Expanding the repertoire with techniques. *Journal of Counseling and Development*, *91*(3), 349–357. https://doi.org/10.1002/j.1556-6676.2013.00104.x

Hayes, S. C., Villatte, M., Levin, M., & Hildebrandt, M. (2011). Open, aware, and active: Contextual approaches as an emerging trend in the behavioral and cognitive therapies. *Annual Review of Clinical Psychology*, *7*(1), 141–168. https://doi.org/10.1146/annurev-clinpsy-032210-104449

Hays, P. A., & Iwamasa, G. Y. (2006). *Culturally responsive cognitive-behavioral therapy: Assessment, practice, and supervision*. American Psychological Association.

Kabat-Zinn, J. (2013). *Full catastrophe living: How to cope with stress, pain and illness with mindfulness meditation*. Piatkus Books.

Kelly, S. (2019). Cognitive behavior therapy with African Americans. In G. Y. Iwamasa & P. A. Hays (Eds.), *Culturally responsive cognitive behavior therapy: Practice and supervision* (pp. 105–128). American Psychological Association. https://doi.org/10.1037/0000119-005

King, K. M., & Borders, L. D. (2019). An experimental investigation of White counselors broaching race and racism. *Journal of Counseling & Development*, *97*(4), 341–351. https://doi.org/10.1002/jcad.12283

Knox, S., Burkard, A. W., Johnson, A. J., Suzuki, L. A., & Ponterotto, J. G. (2003). African American and European American therapists' experiences of addressing race in cross-racial psychotherapy dyads. *Journal of Counseling Psychology*, *50*(4), 466–481. https://doi.org/10.1037/0022-0167.50.4.466

Kroenke, K., Spitzer, R. L., & Williams, J. B. (2001). The PHQ-9: Validity of a brief depression severity measure. *Journal of General Internal Medicine*, *16*(9), 606–613. https://doi.org/10.1046/j.1525-1497.2001.016009606.x

Leahy, R., Holland, S. J. F., & McGinn, L. K. (2012). *Treatment plans and interventions for depression and anxiety disorders*. Guilford Press.

Linehan, M. (1993). *Skills training manual for treating borderline personality disorder*. Guilford Press.

López-López, J. A., Davies, S. R., Caldwell, D. M., Churchill, R., Peters, T. J. et al. (2019). The process and delivery of CBT for depression in adults: A systematic review and network meta-analysis. *Psychological Medicine*, *49*(12), 1937–1947. https://doi.org/10.1017/S003329171900120X

Matu, S. A. (2018). Cognitive therapy. In A. Vernon & K. A. Doyle (Eds.), *Cognitive behavior therapies: A guidebook for practitioners* (pp. 75–108). American Counseling Association.

Mavranezouli, I., Megnin-Viggars, O., Daly, C., Dias, S., Welton, N. J., et al. (2020). Psychological treatments for post-traumatic stress disorder in adults: A network meta-analysis. *Psychological Medicine*, *50*(4), 542–555. https://doi.org/10.1017/S0033291720000070

Menakem, R. (2017). *My grandmother's hands: Racialized trauma and the pathway to mending our hearts and bodies*. Central Recovery Press.

Meyer, O. L., & Zane, N. (2013). The influence of race and ethnicity on clients' experiences of mental health treatment. *Journal of Community Psychology*, *41*(7), 884–901. https://doi.org/10.1002/jcop.21580

Neblett, E. W. Jr., Sosoo, E. E., Willis, H. A., Bernard, D. L., & Bae, J. (2018). Cognitive behavioral models, measures, and treatments for depressive disorders in African Americans. In E. C. Change, C. A. Downey, J. K. Hirsch, & E. A. Yu (Eds.), *Treating depression, anxiety, and stress in ethnic and racial groups: Cognitive behavioral approaches* (pp. 73–97). American Psychological Association.

NeMoyer, A., Alvarez, K., & Alegría, M. (2019). Understanding mental health disparities. In M. T. Williams, D. C. Rosen, & J. W. Kanter (Eds.), *Eliminating race-based mental health disparities: Promoting equity and culturally responsive care across settings* (pp. 9–25). Context Press/New Harbinger Publications.

Owen, J., Tao, K. W., Imel, Z. E., Wampold, B. E., & Rodolfa, E. (2014). Addressing racial and ethnic microaggressions in therapy. *Professional Psychology: Research and Practice*, *45*(4), 283–290. https://doi.org/10.1037/a0037420

Parsons, C. E., Zachariae, R., Landberger, C., & Young, K. S. (2021). How does cognitive behavioural therapy for insomnia work? A systematic review and meta-analysis of mediators of change. *Clinical Psychology Review*, *86*, 1–14. https://doi.org/10.1016/j.cpr.2021.102027

Pedersen, P. B. (1991). Multiculturalism as a generic approach to counseling. *Journal of Counseling & Development*, *70*(1), 6–12. https://doi.org/10.1002/j.1556-6676.1991.tb01555.x

Phinney, J. S. (1996). When we talk about American ethnic groups, what do we mean? *American Psychologist*, *51*(9), 918–927. https://doi.org/10.1037/0003-066X.51.9.918

Polak, K., Reisweber, J., & Meyer, B. L. (2021, November). Transcending self therapy: Four-session individual integrative cognitive-behavioral treatment: A case report. *Psychological Services*. Advance online publication. https://doi.org/10.1037/ser0000539

Prilleltensky, I., & Gonick, L. (1996). Polities change, oppression remains: On the psychology and politics of oppression. *Political Psychology*, *17*(1), 127–148. https://doi.org/10.2307/3791946

Rathod, S., Kingdon, D., Pinninti, N., Turkington, D., & Phiri, P. (2015). *Cultural adaptation of CBT for serious mental illness: A guide for training and practice*. Wiley Blackwell. https://doi.org/10.1002/9781118976159

Ridley, C. R., Mollen, D., Console, K., & Yin, C. (2021). Multicultural counseling competence: A construct in search of operationalization. *The Counseling Psychologist*, *49*(4), 504–533. https://doi.org/10.1177/0011000020988110

Rouf, K., Fennell, M., Westbrook, D., Cooper, M., & Bennett-Levy, J. (2004). Devising effective behavioural experiments. In J. Bennett-Levy, G. Butler, M. Fennell, A. Hackmann, M. Mueller, & D. Westbrook (Eds.), *Oxford guide to behavioral experiments in cognitive therapy* (pp. 21–58). Oxford University Press.

Schaffner, A. K., (2021, June 6). Identifying and challenging core beliefs: 12 helpful worksheets. *Positive Psychology*. https://positivepsychology.com/core-beliefs-worksheets/

Smedley, A., & Smedley, B. D. (2005). Race as biology is fiction, racism as a social problem is real: Anthropological and historical perspectives on the social construction of race. *American Psychologist*, *60*(1), 16–26. https://doi.org/10.1037/0003-066X.60.1.16

Spitzer, R. L., Kroenke, K., Williams, J. B., & Lowe, B. (2006). A brief measure for assessing generalized anxiety disorder: The GAD-7. *Archives Internal Medicine*, *166*(10), 1092–1097. https://doi.org/10.1001/archinte.166.10.1092

Steele, C. M., & Aronson, J. (1995). Stereotype threat and the intellectual test performance of African-Americans. *Journal of Personality and Social Psychology*, *69*(5), 797–811. https://doi.org/10.1037/0022-3514.69.5.797

Steele, J. M. (2020). A CBT approach to internalized racism among African Americans. *International Journal for the Advancement of Counselling*, *42*(3), 217–233. https://doi.org/10.1007/s10447-020-09402-0

Steele, J. M., & Newton, C. S. (2022). Culturally adapted cognitive behavior therapy as a model to address internalized racism among African American clients. *Journal of Mental Health Counseling*, *44*(2), 98–116. https://doi.org/10.17744/mehc.44.2.01

Sue, D. W., Capodilupo, C. M., Torino, G. C., Bucceri, J. M., Holder, A. M. B., Nadal, K. L., & Esquilin, M. (2007). Racial microaggressions in everyday life: Implications for clinical practice. *American Psychologist*, *62*(4), 271–286. https://doi.org/10.1037/0003-066X.62.4.271

Sue, D. W., Sue, D., Neville, H. A., & Smith, L. (2019). *Counseling the culturally diverse: Theory and practice* (8th ed.). John Wiley & Sons, Inc.

Tao, K. W., Owen, J., Pace, B. T., & Imel, Z. E. (2015). A meta-analysis of multicultural competencies and psychotherapy process and outcome. *Journal of Counseling Psychology*, *62*(3), 337–350. https://doi.org/10.1037/cou0000086

Tatum, B. D. (1997). Racial identity development and relational theory: The case of Black women in White communities. In J. V. Jordan (Ed.), *Women's growth in diversity: More writings from the Stone Center* (pp. 91–106). Guilford Press.

Terrell, F., Taylor, J., Menzise, J., & Barrett, R. K. (2009). Cultural mistrust: A core component of African American consciousness. In H. A. Neville, B. M. Tynes, & S. O. Utsey (Eds.), *Handbook of African American psychology* (pp. 299–309). Sage Publications, Inc.

Tolin, D. F., Frost, R. O., Steketee, G., & Muroff, J. (2015). Cognitive behavioral therapy for hoarding disorder: A meta-analysis. *Depression and Anxiety*, *32*(3), 158–166. https://doi.org/10.1002/da.22327

Turner, D. T., Burger, S., Smit, F., Valmaggia, L. R., & van der Gaag, M. (2020). What constitutes sufficient evidence for case formulation-driven CBT for psychosis? Cumulative meta-analysis of the effect on hallucinations and delusions. *Schizophrenia Bulletin*, *46*(5), 1072–1085. https://doi.org/10.1093/schbul/sbaa045

U.S. Census Bureau. (2021). *About the topic of race*. https://www.census.gov/topics/population/race/about.html

van der Kolk, B. A. (2014). *The body keeps the score: Brain, mind, and body in the healing of trauma*. Penguin Random House.

Vera, E. (2020). A prevention agenda for 2020 and beyond: Why environmental interventions matter now more than ever. *Journal of Prevention and Health Promotion*, *1*(1), 5–33. https://doi.org/10.1177/2632077020937690

Ward, E. C., & Brown, R. L. (2015). A culturally adapted depression intervention for African American adults experiencing depression: Oh Happy Day. *American Journal of Orthopsychiatry*, *85*(1), 11–22. https://doi.org/10.1037/ort0000027

Ward, L. M. (2004). Wading through the stereotypes: Positive and negative associations between media use and Black adolescents' conceptions of self. *Developmental Psychology*, *40*(2), 284–294. https://doi.org/10.1037/0012-1649.40.2.284

Watson-Singleton, N. N., Black, A. R., & Spivey, B. N. (2019). Recommendations for a culturally-responsive mindfulness-based intervention for African Americans. *Complementary Therapy in Clinical Practice*, *34*, 132–138. https://doi.org/10.1016/j.ctcp.2018.11.013

Watts-Jones, D. (2002). Healing internalized racism: The role of a within-group sanctuary among people of African descent. *Family Process*, *41*(4), 591–601. https://doi.org/10.1111/j.1545-5300.2002.00591.x

Wenzel, A. (2019). *Cognitive behavioral therapy for beginners*. Routledge.

Williams, D. R. (2018). Stress and the mental health of populations of color: Advancing our understanding of race-related stressors. *Journal of Health and Social Behavior*, *59*(4), 466–485. https://doi.org/10.1177/0022146518814251

Williams, M. T., Holmes, S., Zare, M., Haeny, A., & Faber, S. (2022). An evidence-based approach for treating stress and trauma due to racism. *Cognitive and Behavioral Practice*. Advance online publication. https://doi.org/10.1016/j.cbpra.2022.07.001

Williams, M. T., Printz, D. M. B., & DeLapp, R. C. T. (2018). Assessing racial trauma with the Trauma Symptoms of Discrimination Scale. *Psychology of Violence*, *8*(6), 735–747. https://doi.org/10.1037/vio0000212

Wolkin, J. (2016, June 15). *The science of trauma, mindfulness, and PTSD*. https://braincurves.com/2016/06/17/repost-the-science-of-trauma-mindfulness-and-ptsd/

Zhang, A., Borhneimer, L. A., Weaver, A., Franklin, C., Hai, A. H., et al. (2019). Cognitive behavioral therapy for primary care depression and anxiety: A secondary meta-analytic review using robust variance estimation in meta-regression. *Journal of Behavioral Medicine, 42*(6), 1117–1141. https://doi.org/10.1007/s10865-019-00046-z

Zigarelli, J. C., Jones, J. M., Palomino, C. I., & Kawamura, R. (2016). Culturally responsive cognitive behavioral therapy: Making the case for integrating cultural factors in evidence-based treatment. *Clinical Case Studies, 15*(6), 427–442. https://doi.org/10.1177/1534650116664984

Zimmerman, M. A. (1995). Psychological empowerment: Issues and illustrations. *American Journal of Community Psychology, 23*(5), 581–599. https://doi.org/10.1007/BF02506983

Chapter 2

Racism and African American Mental Health

African American mental health is a complex phenomenon, as deeply entrenched cultural views can make dealing with mental health concerns difficult, and at times, nearly impossible for some members of this group. For example, in their review of factors affecting psychological help-seeking among African Americans, Taylor and Kuo (2019) found that normative beliefs such as "Black people must be strong" and "Seeking professional help shows a lack of confidence in God" often contribute to the underutilization of mental health services in this community. Expounding on these findings, psychologist Rheeda Walker (2020) noted that some African Americans believe Black people simply do not have time to deal with mental health issues and that prayer and perseverance are enough to overcome any emotional problem that might arise throughout the course of a person's life. For individuals with this view, therapy is for "crazy people" and the need for mental health support is interpreted as a sign of weakness. Similarly, many African Americans are also influenced by cultural norms that disapprove of the airing of one's "dirty laundry" in public, which leads to secrecy around poor mental health and a shouldering of one's burdens alone. For these individuals, personal fortitude and reliance on prayer or the church when external help is needed are preferred methods of coping. Obtaining support outside of the church is often not an option, or a best a last resort, as doing so may be interpreted as a lack of faith in God.

Despite the myths and stigma surrounding mental health in the African American community, statistics indicate African Americans experience mental health challenges to a no lesser extent than the rest of the population. According to the 2019 National Survey on Drug Use and Health, 11.9 percent of the non-Hispanic Blacks who participated in the survey reported experiencing serious psychological distress within the past year, which was nearly equivalent to the 12.7 percent of non-Hispanic Whites who were also surveyed (SAMHSA, 2020). Yet, when it comes to receiving professional help, only 25 percent of African Americans seek treatment for a mental health issue, compared to 40 percent of White individuals. Cultural norms

DOI: 10.4324/9781003196303-2

are one factor in the help-seeking behaviors of African Americans; however, other factors also have a negative impact on the mental health utilization rates among this population. In particular, research indicates that a lack of cultural sensitivity in the mental health services provided to this community, exacerbated by the low numbers of mental health professionals who are also people of color, often dissuade African Americans from seeking therapy (Taylor & Kuo, 2019). When they do seek therapy, these same factors may also lead to premature termination or poor treatment outcomes (Kilmer et al., 2019).

In this chapter, I take a broader look at the psychosocial context of African American mental health, with particular attention to the impact of racism on the psychological well-being of this community. Accordingly, primary constructs such as *race, racial identity development,* and *racism* are explored and the relationship between racism and psychological distress experienced among African Americans is discussed. Societal factors and various psychological phenomena specific to the African American community are also reviewed, and clinical examples illustrating how these factors may affect issues discussed during therapy are presented.

Activity 2.1: Knowledge Check—Racism and African American Mental Health

Before taking a deeper look at the psychosocial context of racism and African American mental health, let's start with a quick assessment of your general knowledge on this topic. Throughout the mental health literature, culture-specific knowledge has long been highlighted as one of the key components of multicultural counseling competence (Sue et al., 1992). In CBT, this knowledge is also viewed as critical to culturally sensitive cognitive conceptualization and treatment planning (J. M. Steele, 2020; J. M. Steele & Newton, 2022). Below, you will find several statements reflecting key knowledge areas required to effectively address the psychological effects of racism with African American clients. Read each statement and then rate yourself as it relates to each statement onto following scale: 0 = *Strong Disagree* to 4 = *Strongly Agree.*

1.	I can define the term race.	0	1	2	3	4
2.	I can discuss the differences between biological and social constructions of race.	0	1	2	3	4
3.	I can define the term racism.	0	1	2	3	4
4.	I can describe different forms of racism.	0	1	2	3	4
5.	I can list some of the psychological impacts of racism.	0	1	2	3	4

6. I can identify societal factors that contribute to racism and its psychological effects.	0	1	2	3	4
7. I can define racialized trauma.	0	1	2	3	4
8. I can describe the physical, emotional, and mental impacts of racialized trauma.	0	1	2	3	4
9. I can describe how racism leads to racialized trauma.	0	1	2	3	4
10. I can integrate considerations for race and racism into case formulation and treatment planning.	0	1	2	3	4

Like all aspects of clinical practice, cultural competence requires experience and ongoing professional development. Ideally, you have considerable knowledge in each area of culturally competent clinical practice described above. If not, think about how you can obtain additional information and training in the areas in which you may need further development. Reading this book, for example, is a great start! Examples of other ways to grow in cultural competence include subscribing to journals that explore the mental health issues of African Americans such as the *Journal of Black Psychology* and the *Journal of Multicultural Counseling & Development*, attending webinars and conference presentations, and reading laypersons magazines such as *Black Mental Health Today*.

Defining Race

Due to its historical context, the concept of race can be difficult to define. In Chapter 1, *race* was broadly defined as groups of people who share physical characteristics such as skin color, facial features, and other hereditary traits (Cokley, 2007). Individuals with light skin, fine hair, narrow noses, and thin lips, for example, may be identified as "White," while individuals with dark skin, coarse hair, wide noses, and thick lips may be identified as "Black." Yet, in your own experience, you may have observed that the physical characteristics which typically define various races are often shared across racial groups. For example, some individuals with Creole ancestry in southern states such as Louisiana may appear White physically but are identified as Black or African American. This contradiction between the physical characteristics that typically define race and the lived racial experience of these individuals illustrates just one of the numerous complexities in defining this construct. A related issue highlighted in this example concerns the "one-drop rule," wherein individuals in the United States are considered Black if they have any identifiable African American ancestry despite the multidimensional nature of their racial heritage (Khanna, 2010). While it is beyond the scope of this book to explore all of these complexities, issues relevant to the impact of racism on African American mental health including the myth of race as a biological construct and pseudoscience leading to certain false beliefs about genetic differences among the races are discussed below.

Because members of various racial groups are identified by their physical characteristics, many individuals believe that race is a biological construct; that is, race is a result of genetic variations among various racial groups. However, advances in the study of genetics show that all human beings are 99.9 percent alike, leaving only a small amount, 0.1 percent, of genetic difference within the entire population (Smedley & Smedley, 2005). Moreover, as mentioned in Chapter 1, 94 percent of human genetic variation that does occur is found within members of the same race, while only 6 percent of this variation exists between races (Burns & Vaughn, 2021). This means that biologically, people from the same race differ more from each other than they do from people of other races. Two people of African descent, for example, may be more biologically similar to a person of European descent than they are to each other. Moreover, there are no gene variants that are present in all individuals of one racial group and in no individuals of another, which means that no sharp genetic boundaries can be drawn among the races (Bonham et al., 2005).

In some ways, the idea that race is not biologically determined may be difficult to grasp given that this idea is out of sync with how most of us were socialized to think about this concept. For example, you may have been exposed to beliefs which suggest that certain racial groups naturally succeed more at sports, excel more academically, are better dancers, or are more prone to violence due to their genetic ancestry. In fact, research conducted by Plous and Williams (1995) found that 58.9 percent of the participants in their study endorsed at least one stereotype concerning inborn ability. Moreover, members of the White race were ten times more likely to be viewed by participants as naturally superior in art and abstract thinking, while African Americans were ten times more likely to be viewed as superior in athleticism and rhythm. Beyond this, 49 percent of the study's participants even endorsed stereotypical differences in physical characteristics such as pain tolerance, skull thickness, and skin thickness. While these findings may have been obtained almost 30 years ago, results from more recent studies confirm these stereotypes among the general population today, with research conducted by Hughey and Goss (2015) showing that many individuals continue to endorse racist discourse around issues such as athletics and genetics, and research conducted by Hoffman et al. (2016) showing racial bias in pain management and treatment among White medical students.

At an even more basic level, notions of a biological basis for race can be difficult to dispel due to what we see with our eyes. When we look at members of various racial groups, we see similarities in phenotypes, which refer to physical characteristics typically found in high prevalence among groups that share a historically common gene pool (López et al., 2015). Yet, contemporary science tells us that the differences we see in skin color, hair texture, etc. are a result of gradual and continuous adaptations that occur in the human species as we move across geography and climate, rather than the result of discrete racial categorizations (Duello et al., 2021).

In summarizing the discussion on race thus far, we see that race may be defined as groups of people who share physical characteristics such as skin color, facial features, and other hereditary traits (Cokley, 2007). However, despite racial categories being based on these physical characteristics, genetic research shows there is no biological basis for race and people are more alike than they are different (Burns & Vaughn, 2021; Duello et al., 2021). As you ponder these ideas, you may be wondering what they have to do with everyday clinical practice with African American clients. First, notions of biological determinants of race contribute to the persistence of stereotypes that lead to racial bias in how therapists conceptualize and relate to their clients. For example, research shows that negative stereotypes lead to differences in perceptions of psychopathology and even likeability among African Americans clients, especially when compared to their White counterparts (Atkinson et al., 1996; Jenkins-Hall & Sacco, 1991; López, 1989). To illustrate this point, Rosenthal (2004) investigated the effects of client race on the clinical judgment of 98 practicing European American rehabilitation counselors. According to the results of this study, African American clients were judged more harshly in their (a) general evaluation, (b) perceived psychopathology, and (c) estimates of educational and vocational potential. Moreover, these judgments persisted even after subsequent information about the client was provided.

Beyond racial bias during therapy, biological determinism leading to deeply entrenched racial stereotypes in U.S. society has also influenced the production of scientific research within the mental health profession itself. Scholars such as Robert Guthrie, one of the fathers of Black psychology, have long decried the profession's history of racism. In his seminal book, *Even the Rat was White*, for example, Guthrie (1976) described how pseudo-scientific techniques were used within psychology to promote nativistic themes and beliefs about intelligence that ultimately contributed to the eugenics movement and other racist social policies. Only recently, however, have organizations within the mental health profession begun to formally acknowledge their part in perpetuating biased science used to further racist ideologies. In 2021, the American Psychological Association adopted a resolution which states:

> The American Psychological Association failed in its role leading the discipline of psychology, was complicit in contributing to systemic inequities, and hurt many through racism, racial discrimination, and denigration of people of color, thereby falling short on its mission to benefit society and improve lives. APA is profoundly sorry, accepts responsibility for, and owns the actions and inactions of APA itself, the discipline of psychology, and individual psychologists who stood as leaders for the organization and field.
>
> (American Psychological Association, 2021, para 1)

This resolution is significant in that it concedes to psychology's role in the denigration of people of color in ways that have (a) had a negative impact on the quality-of-care people of color receive and (b) contributed to the racist systems and ideologies that inflict harm on their communities (American Psychological Association, 2021). The resolution also identifies the need for pathways to promote greater cultural competency and antiracism in knowledge production, clinical training, and workforce development within the profession.

Finally, while researchers recognize there is no biological basis for race, the concept nevertheless remains significant in contemporary society as a social construct (Graves, 2015). The idea of race in which is it understood today was first developed in the late 16th century in order to create the human hierarchies needed to justify European expansion and slavery (Smedley, 1999). Since that time, while there have been some changes in race-based practices such as slavery and de jure segregation, racial hierarchies that result in disparate life experiences and the inequitable distribution of resources remain. For example, Black people historically have been negatively affected by racial prejudice and discrimination in the healthcare system and have less access to quality care (American Psychiatric Association, 2017). Beyond this, race continues to be a primary way that individuals self-identify and relate to others, and positive racial identity has been related to lower psychological distress (Franklin-Jackson & Carter, 2007), stereotype threat (Davis et al., 2006), and imposter syndrome when mediated by self-esteem (Lige et al., 2017). Therefore, race as a social construct, including as it relates to racial identity, remains a central factor in African American mental health.

Reflection 2.1: One of the primary ideas expressed in the section above is that there is no biological basis for race (Bonham et al., 2005; Burns & Vaughn, 2021; Duello et al., 2021; Smedley & Smedley, 2005). This idea is vastly different from what many of us were socialized into believing about race. When reflecting on your personal life experiences, what have you been socialized into believing about race? How have you been socialized to think about race in your professional community? How might these beliefs influence how you work with African American clients?

Racial Identity Development

The term *racial identity* refers to an individual's sense of belonging to a particular racial group, while *racial identity development* refers to the process through which individuals develop a healthy view of: (a) themselves, (b) members of their racial group, and (c) members of other racial groups (Constantine et al., 1998). Within the counseling and psychology literature, several theories have been developed to describe this process; however, for more than 50 years, Nigrescence theory (Cross, 1971) has been the primary framework through which African American racial identity is conceptualized (Worrell et al., 2001). Nigrescence theory is a model of Black racial identity development that, in its initial conception, consisted of five stages known as Pre-encounter, Encounter, Immersion-Emersion, Internalization, and Internalization-Commitment (Cross, 1971). Originally, these stages were considered developmental in nature, with individuals conceptualized as beginning at a phase of identity characterized by low or negative racial salience and successively moving through each stage of the model until arriving at an identity reflective of confidence in one's Blackness and a commitment to social activism (Cross, 1971). Later, the theory was revised and expanded into an attitudinal model, wherein the Internalization and Internalization-Commitment stages were combined and various identity clusters within each stage were identified (Cross & Vandiver, 2001). Table 2.1 presents these stages, the identities associated with each stage, and questions you may use to explore the experiences of clients at each stage of development.

Pre-encounter

Stage 1 of the Nigrescence model is known as *Pre-encounter* (Vandiver et al., 2001). At this stage, the individual's worldview is dominated by Eurocentric determinants and the concept of race holds either low or negative salience (Cross, 1971). *Salience* refers to the importance of race in a person's life. It can range from low to high and be positive or negative. Attitudinally, the Pre-encounter worldview results in three identity clusters: (1) Assimilation, (2) Self-Hatred, and (3) Miseducation. Among individuals with an *Assimilation* worldview, identity centers around being American and race holds little personal significance (Vandiver et al., 2001). Accordingly, race and Black culture are not engaged among individuals with this identity and these

Table 2.1 Exploring Black Racial Identity Development

Stage	Identities	Questions
Pre-encounter: When the individual's worldview is dominated by Eurocentric values and ideologies and race holds little importance or is viewed negatively.	• **Assimilation**: An identity organized around being an American and an individual. Race holds low and/or negative salience. • **Miseducation**: A person who adopts stereotypical views of Black culture; however, these views do not affect their personal self-image. • **Self-Hatred**: A person who has internalized anti-Black stereotypes to the point of self- and group hatred.	1. What are the most important aspects of your identity? 2. How important is race to your identity? 3. What are some of the stereotypes associated with your racial group? 4. How did you learn these stereotypes? 5. How did/do these stereotypes affect the way you see yourself? 6. How did/do these stereotypes affect the way you see people in your racial group?
Encounter: When an event or a series of events leads to increased awareness of the significance of being Black and a change in pre-encounter identities.		1. What moments in your life stand out in terms of their impact on how you view yourself racially? 2. What events have clarified your understanding of what it means to a Black person in the United States? 3. What have you been taught or learned about on your own that has influenced how you view being Black personally and generally? 4. To what extent do you engage in activism surrounding race and racism? 5. What role, if any, has activism played in how you view being Black?

(Continued)

Table 2.1 (Continued)

Stage	Identities	Questions
Immersion-Emersion: When the individual begins to embrace Black culture and seeks to learn more about Africa and African Americans.	• **Intense Black Involvement**: A person who is deeply and intensely immersed in Black culture and history. • **Anti-White**: A person who has developed negative attitudes toward White people, primarily for their historical and continued involvement in the oppression of Black people.	1. How would you describe your level of interest in Black culture and history? 2. What is your sense of the contributions your ancestors have made over the years? 3. How do you feel about African Americans who do not embrace Black culture? 4. What are your perceptions of White people?
Internalization: When the individual views their Blackness with positivity and has an overall sense of comfort with themselves as racial beings.	• **Afrocentricity**: A person who adopts an African-centered orientation toward self, other Black people, and broader society. • **Biculturalist**: A person who gives equal weight to being Black and another aspect of their marginalized identity. • **Multiculturalist Racial**: A person who finds value in Black culture as well as the cultures of other marginalized groups. • **Multicultural Inclusive**: A person who accepts and values all cultural groups.	1. How comfortable with your racial identity are you? 2. How do other aspects of your identity compare to your racial identity? 3. What values or cultural perspectives guide your current worldview? 4. To what extent do Afrocentric values guide your worldview? 5. How comfortable are you with members of other racial groups? 6. What bonds or similarities do you feel, if any, with members of other racial groups?

individuals may even work to eliminate programs designed to remedy racial inequities such as affirmative action or the Voting Rights Act (Cross & Vandiver, 2001). In contrast, race holds a greater level of significance for individuals with a *Self-Hatred* identity; however, this salience is negative in the sense that these individuals have decidedly anti-Black perspectives and endorse anti-Black stereotypes that have been internalized to the point of hatred for self and the broader Black community. Like individuals with an Assimilation identity, people with a Self-Hatred identity typically limit their engagement in Black problems and Black culture (Cross & Vandiver, 2001). Finally, the third, more recently identified identity, *Miseducation*, describes individuals who have accepted negative stereotypes about African Americans generally, but have not internalized these stereotypes to the point of self-hatred, personally.

Encounter

The next phase of Black racial identity development is known as the Encounter stage. This stage begins when an event or a series of events leads to increased awareness of the meaning of being Black and triggers a change in Pre-encounter identity (Vandiver et al., 2001). For many individuals, these events take place within the context of personal experiences and observations, education, or activism (Neville & Cross, 2017). *Personal experiences and observations* refer to direct or vicarious experiences with racism and discrimination, while *education* refers to formal or informal learning about the history and cultural experiences of various groups of Black people. Ways in which individuals typically engage in formal education include activities such as taking university courses or participating in community-based workshops. Informal education may consist of activities such as travel or independent reading. The third type of Encounter event, *activism*, refers to participation in activities such as advocating for changes in laws and unjust social policies, capturing social injustices on film or video, and protests. Typically, a main outcome of Encounter events, whether they occur in the form of experience, education, or activism, is the experience of a racial awakening wherein individuals gain greater awareness of racism and the fact that they are a member of a racial group targeted by racism (Neville & Cross, 2017). This awareness is significant in that it leads to the next stage of development, Immersion-Emersion.

Immersion-Emersion

After events resulting in an increased awareness of the significance of race, individuals experience a shift in worldview leading to a phase of Black racial identity development known as the *Immersion-Emersion* stage. This phase reflects a period of life wherein individuals begin to embrace Black culture and eagerly seek to learn more about Africa and African Americans (Vandiver et al., 2001). In the expanded Nigrescence model, this stage includes two identity clusters: (1) Intense Black Involvement and (2) Anti-White. The *Intense Black Involvement* identity describes what Vandiver et al. (2001) call "unbridled enthusiasm" for information about Africa and African Americans, characterized by a voracious consumption of Black art, literature, and history, as well as increased participation in historically Black organizations and social institutions (p. 177). While individuals at this stage of development may experience pride in their membership in the Black community, they also frequently experience feelings of rage and guilt as they gain greater awareness of the atrocities experienced by Black people. These feelings may lead to the other cluster at this stage, *Anti-White* identity attitudes (Vandiver et al., 2001). As stated, individuals with an Anti-White identity may experience a sense of rage as a result of the oppression inflicted upon Black people. This rage often manifests as hatred toward White people and White culture, as well as anger toward oneself for having previously ignored or downplayed the role of race in one's life. Eventually, however, these views are typically transformed into more egalitarian ideals as individuals move into the final stage of Black racial identity development, Internalization (Vandiver et al., 2001).

Internalization

At the final stage of Black racial identity development, *Internalization*, individuals begin to view their Blackness with positivity and experience an overall sense of comfort with themselves as racial beings (Vandiver et al., 2001). The specific identity attitudes at the Internalization stage include: (1) Afrocentricity, (2) Biculturalist, (3) Multiculturalist Racial, and (4) Multiculturalist Inclusive. According to Cross (1991), Afrocentricity may be defined as "a Black American interpretation of what it means to have an African perspective" (p. 222). More specifically, Belgrave and Allison (2019) defined Afrocentricity as "the values, beliefs, and behavior of the indigenous people of Africa and those in the Diaspora who share in this cultural heritage" (p. 31). These values, beliefs, and behaviors may include, spirituality, ancestral connection, interdependence, collectivism, respect for truths derived from cultural knowledge, respect for elders, and unity, for example. In Black racial identity development, individuals with an *Afrocentricity* identity have a worldview characterized by a prizing of these values, beliefs, and behaviors. Moreover, they stress the importance of engagement in

Black problems and culture (Cross & Vandiver, 2001). For others, identity attitudes at this stage may be more *Biculturalist* in nature, where being Black and having another marginalized identity such as being a woman holds salience. Finally, for yet others, identity at this stage may focus on accepting Black culture and the cultures of other marginalized groups in the *Multiculturalist Racial* identity or accepting and valuing all other cultural groups in what is considered the *Multiculturalist Inclusive* identity (Worrell et al., 2001).

Understanding where clients fall within the above stages of Black racial identity development offers insight into the client's worldview and lived experience as a racial being. Beyond this, knowledge of the client's level of racial identity development has other significant implications for clinical practice. First, studies show a statistically significant relationship between racial identity and mental health. A study conducted by Franklin-Jackson and Carter (2007), for example, found that high levels of Internalization attitudes reflected greater psychological well-being and moderated the effects of cultural racism. Conversely, Pre-encounter attitudes were related to higher levels of psychological distress and less awareness of cultural racism. Moreover, racial identity has been shown to be directly related to how individuals cope with racial discrimination and race-based stress. In a recent study, Carter et al. (2017) found that individuals with higher Internalization attitudes experienced less race-based stress, while individuals with Immersion-Emersion attitudes experienced more stress. Accordingly, from a clinical perspective, knowledge of the client's racial identity status can provide indications of protective factors or identify a need for interventions such as psychoeducation on the nature of racism and active coping strategies.

A second clinical implication for racial identity is potential for the construct to influence the quality of therapeutic dyad. Williams (2018), for example, suggested that attitudes reflected in the client's racial identity may affect both the therapeutic alliance, as well as retention. Moreover, clients at certain levels of racial identity development may answer questions more accurately when matched with a therapist from the same racial background; however, clients who are lower in racial identity may not work well with a therapist from their racial group due to fears of being judged (Williams, 2018). Therefore, in cross-racial therapeutic dyads, knowledge of the client's racial identity may aid in the development of a more effective therapeutic alliance by providing insight into the types of attitudes and concerns to broach in the intracounseling dynamics of the counseling relationship. Knowledge of the client's racial identity may also provide a greater understanding of the client's presenting concerns.

Case Illustration: Tiffany

Tiffany is a 25-year-old African American woman who is seeking therapy due to ongoing issues in the relationship with her romantic partner, Jackson. Tiffany and Jackson, who both recently graduated from college, met during their junior year. Since graduating, Jackson has expressed interest in marriage; however, Tiffany is concerned about the "lack of growth" she has observed in Jackson over the past three years. During sessions, Tiffany has explained that when she and Jackson first started dating, they were both young and learning who they are as individuals. Since that time, Jackson has experienced very little change in his overall outlook on life from Tiffany's perspective. She is especially concerned with what she perceives as his "selling out" to corporate America. She loves Jackson but worries they might not be compatible.

In the excerpt below, Tiffany and her therapist discuss the problems in her relationship with Jackson. As you read the excerpt, notice how the therapist uses the themes presented in Table 2.1 to explore Tiffany's racial identity and gain a fuller understanding of her presenting concern.

Therapist: Tiffany, I hear you're worried you and Jackson may not be compatible. Tell me more about that.

Tiffany: Okay. When Jackson and I first started dating, we were both young and figuring things out, like figuring out who we wanted to be. I feel like I took on this task wholeheartedly and really thought about the type of person I want to be for myself and my future children but he's just following what society says equates to success.

Therapist: And this concerns you.

Tiffany: Yes! I mean, think about it. All society teaches you to care about is climbing the corporate ladder and making lots of money. There's no concern for helping or giving back to the community.

Therapist: Tiffany, I can tell these are things you are really passionate about.

Tiffany: Exactly. My parents were very active in the community. I was always raised with the idea "each one should reach one." Then, when I was in my senior year of college, I took several Africana Studies classes, which just reinforced the importance of working to improve things for people who look like me.

Therapist: It sounds like the way your parents raised you and what you learned in your Africana Studies courses really influence how you see yourself today.

Tiffany: Yeah. I'm a proud Black woman and I want to be married to a proud Black man but it's like being Black doesn't mean anything to him.

Therapist: That's quite a statement, Tiffany. How do you feel about Black people who don't seem embrace Black culture?

Tiffany: I mean, I would never say this to Jackson, but it's like they're sellouts! You know what I'm saying? And I feel like it's already affecting our lives together. For example, last week we went shopping for holiday cards. I wanted to buy some Kwanzaa cards and he went on and on about how it's just a made-up holiday. Then he asked me why the "normal" holidays weren't good enough. I just ignored him because I didn't want to hurt his feelings but in the back of my mind I was thinking, "This is why I can't marry you." Even if it is a "made-up" holiday, the ideas it promotes are important. I want my kids to grow up thinking about things like unity and collective responsibility. Kwanzaa is a great way to do that.

Therapist: I see. It sounds like there are significant value differences between the two of you.

Tiffany: Yes. And that's just one example. The other day I was feeling anxious and a little bit depressed because I had gotten into a disagreement with my manager who told me that she had received complaints about my hair being "unprofessional." When I talked to Jackson about it, all he said was everybody has to make adjustments if they want to fit into corporate America. Well, I actually don't care about "fitting in"...

In the above dialogue, evidence is given as to how knowledge of Black racial identity development may inform the clinical interview and add to the conceptualization of client issues. Using basic counseling techniques, the therapist began the dialogue with probing statements and a reflection of feeling, which invited Tiffany to share more information about the concerns which led her to therapy. As a result, the therapist learned about childhood events and coursework that appear to have had a significant influence on Tiffany's sense of identity. Recall that personal experiences and education often lead to shifts in worldview that transition individuals into a stage of Black racial identity development characterized by "unbridled enthusiasm" for Black culture, a desire to learn more about Africa and African Americans, and in some instances, disapproval of African Americans who do not embrace Black culture; that is, the Immersion-Emersion stage (Neville & Cross, 2017; Vandiver et al., 2001, p. 177). Based on this understanding, the therapist acknowledged the connection between these events and Tiffany's sense of identity, which led to the revealing of additional information concerning the significance Tiffany assigns to her identity as a Black woman and provided further evidence of Immersion-Emersion identity attitudes. Tiffany's response to the therapist's question regarding her views toward African

Americans who do not embrace Black culture is yet another indication of these attitudes.

In terms of case conceptualization, it seems that much of the conflict in the relationship between Tiffany and Jackson stems from differences in their racial worldviews. As mentioned, Tiffany's identity attitudes tend to reflect those at the Immersion-Emersion stage, while Jackson's identity status appears to be consistent with a Pre-encounter Assimilation worldview. In particular, the lack of emphasis Jackson places on traditional Afrocentric values such as giving back to the community, his preference for American holidays, his desire for status and prestige, and his willingness to conform to Eurocentric standards suggest a worldview guided primarily by Eurocentric ideologies. Because Tiffany is at a stage of Black racial identity development dominated by intense involvement in Black culture, it is likely the lack of significance Jackson assigns to aspects of Black culture and his Assimilation identity would be a cause of concern for Tiffany. Moreover, due to Tiffany's stage of racial identity, it is also likely that the microaggressions and racial discrimination she is experiencing at work would result in significant psychological distress, suggesting a need for clinical intervention (Carter et al., 2017).

Racism and its Psychological Impact Among African Americans

As illustrated in the case of Tiffany, race has a multifaceted role in the lives of African Americans. For Tiffany, race was a source of pride and a significant aspect of her identity. However, matters of race such as the racial discrimination Tiffany experienced in her workplace are also a source of stress for many African Americans. In fact, one recent study found that as many as 92 percent of Black Americans believe discrimination against their community continues to be problematic in America today (NPR/*Robert Wood Johnson Foundation/Harvard T.H. Chan School* of *Public Health*, 2017). Given these statistics, recent research findings which indicate that 70.8 percent of counselors had worked with clients who reported experiences of race-based trauma (Hemmings & Evans, 2018) and 96.5 percent of counselors hear at least one report of discrimination from clients of color at least occasionally during counseling (Giordano et al., 2021) are no surprise. In my own clinical experience, race and racism have without exception been a source of psychological distress among all of the African American adults I've seen during therapy, and among many of the children and adolescents I treat as well. The process of helping these clients unpack the mental health impacts of racism has required a thorough understanding of the multifaceted nature of racism and its psychological ramifications. Accordingly, the paragraphs below define racism and explore its psychological consequences.

Case Illustration: Idris

Idris is a 42-year-old African American man who initiated therapy due to symptoms of depression including low mood, irritability, sleep disturbance, and generalized lethargy and inertia. During intake, Idris attributed his current difficulties to what he described as workplace discrimination. Idris is the head coach of a Division III men's baseball team. In his role as head coach, Idris has experienced significant success including leading his team to its first national championship appearance. Despite this success, Idris believes he is undercompensated and poorly recognized. For example, Idris reports that since joining his college ten years ago, several less experienced White coaches have been hired at salaries nearly equivalent to his current pay. Moreover, during staff meetings, Idris finds his decisions are constantly being challenged and members of staff frequently look to his assistant coach, who is White, for guidance rather than Idris. These issues, coupled with a lack of diversity in his program, have left Idris feeling isolated and without support. Idris reports that he has attempted to find a coaching position elsewhere but has not been able to garner interest from teams at his level of coaching. He attributes these difficulties to not being a part of the "good old boys" club and feels somewhat hopeless about his ability to advance in his career.

Given the complicated and multifaceted nature of racism, definitions of this construct abound. According to racial trauma expert Robert T. Carter (2007), the term *racism* can be broadly defined as "the transformation of racial prejudice into individual racism through the use of power directed against racial group(s) and their members, who are defined as inferior" (pp. 24–25). Inherent in this definition is the idea that racism reflects a system of social structures that provides or denies access, safety, resources, and power based on race categories, producing and reproducing race-based inequities. In the case of Idris, for example, we see race-based inequities reflected in his wages, the status and credibility he is afforded by his colleagues, and in his limited access to career advancement opportunities commensurate with his record of experience. While these and similar race-based inequities seen in other social structures such as healthcare, education, housing, incarceration, and immigration take a psychological toll on the lives of people of color, their ultimate purpose is for the unequal distribution of resources, power, and economic opportunity to those at the top of the racial hierarchy. Accordingly, addressing racism with African Americans not only necessitates competence in helping clients manage the psychological distress that occurs as a result of racism, but also it requires an ability to help clients develop the sense of empowerment needed to challenge the status quo.

Another significant aspect of the definition of racism provided above is the idea that this construct is rooted in notions of superiority and inferiority (Carter, 2007). These notions of superiority and inferiority are known as

White supremacy. According to DiAngelo (2018), White supremacy can be defined as "the all-encompassing centrality and assumed superiority of people defined and perceived as white and the practices based on this assumption" (p. 28). Essentially, White supremacy is a worldview that depicts White culture as the ideal for humanity and confers structural power and privileges to White people as a group. Encompassed within this worldview are several ideologies that are often unarticulated but nevertheless serve as part of the foundation of mindsets that rationalize racial disparities. These ideologies include individualism, objectivity, and meritocracy (DiAngelo, 2018). *Individualism* refers to an ideal that suggests each person is a unique individual and group membership has little to do with success. *Objectivity* is an ideal that suggests it is possible to be free of all bias. Finally, *meritocracy* refers to an ideal that suggests each person succeeds on the basis of his or her character and work ethic.

Through White supremacy and its supporting ideologies, members of the dominant racial group have freedom from the psychic weight of race, to move freely in most spaces, and to be reflected as the norm in nearly all aspects of social life (DiAngelo, 2018). More importantly, however, White supremacy limits these freedoms for people of color and has the effect of ascribing blame to the victims of inequitable social conditions. For example, inequities in crime, health, education, socioeconomic status, and other markers of quality of life among African Americans are often blamed on a lack of morality, lower intelligence, or laziness among this group rather than the systemic racism in the policies and practices leading to these inequities. This type of blame adds to the heaviness of racism for people of color and often results in a sense of powerlessness, helplessness, and hopelessness.

The definition of racism discussed above broadly states that racism can be defined as the transformation of racial prejudice into racial discrimination (Carter, 2007). More specific definitions of the term, however, offer insight into the situational contexts in which the racism occurs. As mentioned in Chapter 1, *interpersonal racism*, for example, refers to conscious or subconscious discrimination against a person or group because of race on an individual level, while *institutional racism* refers to racist policies and practices within various institutions like schools, government, and the media (Evans et al., 2021). These acts of racism may be expressed overtly, through actions such as the use of racial slurs, racial profiling, police brutality, and hate crimes, or covertly through things like implicit bias in hiring, banking, police protection, housing, networking opportunities, and customer service (Ni, 2021). While overt and covert racism at individual or institutional levels can both result in psychological distress, trauma due to covert racism may be more difficult to recognize due to its ambiguous and insidious nature.

Finally, in addition to terms such as interpersonal racism and institutional racism, McConahay et al. (1981) introduced the term *modern racism* into the literature to describe the form of prejudice African Americans experienced in the United States subsequent to the Civil Rights movement. Defined as "beliefs that racism is not a continuing problem [and] African Americans should put forth their own efforts to overcome their situation in society without special assistance," the term modern racism speaks directly to the ideologies that lead to the ambiguous and often unspoken aspects of racism described earlier (Henry, 2010, p. 575). Two closely related concepts that further explain this idea are colorblind racial attitudes and microaggressions. *Colorblind racial attitudes* refer to the belief that race should not and does not matter (Neville et al., 2001). The two dimensions of colorblind racial attitudes are known as color evasion and power evasion (Neville et al., 2013). *Color evasion* refers to attitudes that ignore race and deny a system of racial hierarchies, while *power evasion* refers to the idea that everyone has the same chance to succeed. Color and power evasion colorblind messages such as "I don't see race" and "Everyone has the same opportunity" suggest that African Americans and other oppressed groups experience poor social outcomes due to their own inadequacies, and discriminatory social systems have little or no part to play. Additionally, colorblind racial attitudes also ignore the role positive racial identity development has as a protective factor against racism.

The other type of modern racism, *microaggressions*, refers to subtle, often unintentional, put-downs that reflect prejudiced or discriminatory messages about minority groups (Sue et al., 2019). Originally coined by Chester Pierce (1974), Sue et al. (2019) later identified three types of microaggressions: Microinsults, microassaults, and microinvalidations. *Microinsults* refer to unintentional comments or behaviors that demean a person's heritage or social identity, while *microassaults* are comments, behaviors, or environmental cues that more overtly convey discriminatory messages. The other type of microaggressions, *microinvalidations*, refers to comments or behaviors that negate or dismiss the cognitive, affective, or experiential realities of individuals from marginalized backgrounds. Each of these three types of microaggressions can be verbal or delivered through an organization's physical environment and can even be the result of good intentions. For example, many African Americans are often confronted with slights such as "You speak so well," from well-meaning colleagues or admirers. While meant as a compliment, this microaggression reflects a societal perception of African Americans as being generally unintelligent or inarticulate and identifies the person to whom the compliment was directed as an exception (J. M. Steele, 2020).

Research on Racism and African American Mental Health

As mentioned above, racism occurs interpersonally and institutionally, and may be overt or covert in nature. Of relevance to the clinical setting, research suggests experiences of overt racism leads to several different types of negative mental health outcomes among African Americans. Broadly, a significant body of research has found a relationship between racism and generalized psychological distress among these clients (Williams & Williams-Morris, 2000). More specifically, however, studies have linked racial discrimination experienced by this population to mental health concerns such as anxiety, depression, internalized racism, negative affect, and ability to cope. A study conducted by Joseph et al. (2021), for example, found that personal and vicarious racial discrimination were associated with negative emotions and lower coping resources in daily-life moments among a sample of African American adults. Similarly, in other measures of the effects of daily racism, Johnson and Carter (2020) found that past year and lifetime experiences of racism were positively associated with internalized shame. Moreover, the findings of Johnson and Carter's (2020) study also indicated that this relationship also remains when racism is experienced vicariously. In terms of anxiety, research conducted by Graham et al. (2015) found that racist experiences and past year frequency of racist experiences were significantly and positively correlated with anxious arousal. Likewise, in terms of depression, a meta-analysis of 12 recent studies conducted by Britt-Spells et al. (2018) found a positive association between perceived discrimination and depression symptoms among Black men. These findings replicate previous research which suggests there is a statistically significant relationship between racial discrimination and depression among both African American men and women (Pieterse et al., 2012).

In terms of more covert forms of racism, research suggests colorblind racial attitudes and microaggressions also contribute to poor mental health outcomes among African Americans. A study conducted by Barr and Neville (2014), for example, found that higher levels of colorblind racial attitudes, combined with a higher frequency of mainstream socialization messages (provided by parents), resulted in negative mental health scores among young Black adults. Moreover, research conducted by Neville et al. (2005) found that greater endorsement of colorblind racial beliefs was related to higher levels of victim blame attributions of racial inequality, internalized oppression, and justification of social roles or social dominance orientation. This suggests that colorblind racial attitudes not only have an impact on mood and affect but on endorsement of legitimizing beliefs that serve to maintain racial inequalities as well. Concerning microaggressions, a recent study of Black university students found that racial microaggressions are positively associated with anxiety symptoms (Liao et al., 2016), while another study of Black, Latina/o, Asian, and multiracial participants found that a higher cumulative experience with racial microaggressions is a statistically significant predictor of depressive symptoms and of how positively or negatively one views the world (Nadal et al., 2014). Of note, this study also found that Black and Latina/o participants experienced more inferiority-related microaggressions than Asian participants, and Black participants experienced more criminality-related microaggressions than both Asian and Latina/o participants.

In sum, the research on racism and African American mental health provides substantial evidence of the deleterious effect of racism on the African American community. Unfortunately, with the advent of social media and the rising incidence of publicized social unrest, the impact of racism on the mental health of African Americans does not appear to be improving. A study conducted by Das et al. (2021), for example, found that the recent publicized police killings of unarmed African Americans resulted in an 11 percent increase in emergency department visits related to depression among African Americans in the concurrent month and three months following the exposure. Given the impact of social events on both the acute mental health of African Americans and their ongoing development and well-being, knowledge concerning various societal factors contributing to the experience of racism among this community is another key area of knowledge necessary for effective work with these clients. Some of these factors are discussed in the following paragraphs.

Societal Factors Contributing the Experience of Racism

As discussed in Chapter 1, treatment planning in CBT relies heavily on each client's individual cognitive conceptualization (Beck, 2020). Traditionally, cognitive conceptualization entails consideration of relevant early life experiences and their impact on the development of a client's intermediate cognitions. For marginalized individuals such as African Americans, however, societal factors linked to racism also have an impact on the development of these cognitions (Bailey et al., 2014). Recently, I developed a model cognitive developmental model of internalized racism that considers these factors (Steele, 2020). Some of these factors, which include the historical legacy of slavery, Black Codes, segregation, the media, and other social determinants of mental health are briefly discussed here for your review. The model itself is discussed in the Internalized Racism section below.

Slavery

African Americans have a rich cultural history. Part of this history includes a tradition of values, customs, foods, and even language patterns that find their roots in Senegal, Gambia, Ghana, Nigeria, and other countries along the west coast of Africa. Much of this tradition serves as the organizing structure of the Afrocentric worldview, as well as the foundation for many of the positive indigenous coping strategies found within the African

American community. Yet, another less positive aspect of history also has a significant influence on the lived experiences of African Americans. This historical influence is slavery. In particular, slavery represents a time in history during which many of the dehumanizing ideologies that continue to have an adverse impact on the self-concept of African Americans today were developed (DeGruy, 2017). Moreover, many of the contemporary social determinants that adversely affect the mental health of African Americans, factors such as poverty and incarceration, also find their roots in slavery (Gottlieb & Flynn, 2021). Accordingly, while the historical legacy of the African American community extends far beyond the introduction of African slave labor in the North American colonies, slavery nevertheless remains relevant as a source of cultural trauma within this population (Halloran, 2019).

Much of the African diaspora in the world's western hemisphere can be attributed to the era of slavery initiated by England, Spain, and Portugal during the early 16th century. In the British colonies, forced African labor can be traced all the way back to 1619, although formalized slavery was not institutionalized until the start of the 18th century (Smedley, 1999). During this time, English laws and statutes were gradually introduced into the colonies in order to deny Africans basic freedoms such as the right to bear arms, hold property, vote, buy, sell, congregate, travel without permission, receive education, serve in militias, or legally marry and parent (J. M. Steele, 2020). The effect of these laws was the creation of an established class of slave labor which provided not only the labor but also the financial means necessary for continued conquest and colonization of the western part of the globe. Yet, while slavery provided the English with the labor and economic resources necessary to build their empire, moral justification was also needed to legitimize the inhumane subjugation of African people. Accordingly, the English adopted an ideology of White supremacy that depicted African religion and customs as savagery, demonized African skin-color and phenotypes, and idealized White beauty, language, and cultural norms (Smedley, 1999). In essence, White supremacy provided moral and intellectual support for slavery by ascribing natural causes and personal blame to Africans for their state of oppression (Sidanius, 1993). It also portrayed Africans as ignorant and docile heathens, in need of saving by the White race.

While slavery was eventually abolished in the United States, its societal and psychological effects continue to be observed through ongoing asymmetric power relations and historical trauma experienced among current-day African Americans (Bailey et al., 2014). *Historical trauma* refers to psychological distress that has been experienced by a group of people over time and across generations (Mohatt et al., 2014). Recently, DeGruy (2017) introduced the concept of posttraumatic slave syndrome to conceptualize this trauma. According to DeGruy (2017), *posttraumatic slave syndrome* can be defined as "transgenerational adaptations associated with traumas, past and present, from slavery and ongoing oppression" (p. 8). In this definition, DeGruy (2017) conceptualized *trauma* as "a [physical, emotional, psychological, or spiritual] injury caused by an outside, usually violent force, event or experience" (p. 8). Among African Americans, according to DeGruy (2017), the impact of this injury has been the transgenerational transmission of distorted attitudes, beliefs, and behaviors. Expressed in different, perhaps somewhat less controversial terminology, Menakem (2017), who explored similar ideas in his work on racialized trauma, used the term *traumatic retentions* to describe this distortion of attitudes and behaviors. According to Menakem (2017), examples of traumatic retentions among African Americans include self-hate, internalized racism, a bias for light skin over dark skin, a preference for shopping in White-owned businesses, corporal punishment, use of the N-word, and denigration of other African Americans who have achieved success (p. 167).

Black Codes

On January 1, 1863, President Abraham Lincoln issued the Emancipation Proclamation, which freed all persons previously held as slaves. This proclamation should have ushered in an era of liberty among the formerly enslaved Africans; however, any hopes for true freedom were short lived. Soon after slavery ended, local and state municipalities began to issue laws known as Black Codes in order to limit access to voting, education, and equal treatment under the law (Bailey et al., 2014). For example, many Black Codes limited the types of property Black people could own, upheld strict vagrancy and labor contract rules, and implemented anti-enticement measures designed to punish individuals who offered higher wages to Black laborers already under contract (J. M. Steele, 2020). In Mississippi, one Black code even prevented White people from selling, lending, or giving Black or biracial individuals firearms, knives, ammunition, or liquor, punishable by a fine of $50 and 30 days of imprisonment.

Black Codes had the effect of producing labor conditions similar to those experienced during slavery. However, with the enactment of Black Codes, the country also saw the development of a new set of legitimizing myths that in some cases were actually in direct conflict with those previously expressed under the ideology of White supremacy. *Legitimizing myths* refer to "values, attitudes, beliefs, causal attributions and ideologies which provide moral and intellectual justification for increasing or decreasing levels of social inequality among social groups" (Sidanius et al., 1996, p. 386). Whereas Black people were previously portrayed as ignorant and docile, in need of saving by the White race, they were now primarily viewed as dangerous, hostile, and even criminal, legitimizing their restrictions. In spite of the obvious contradiction in these perspectives, both remained encompassed within the cosmology of beliefs that contribute to poor mental health among African Americans (Sidanius et al., 1996). For example, when conceptualized as part of a larger theoretical framework known as *social dominance orientation*, legitimizing beliefs such as African Americans are inherently inferior, African Americans are lazy, African Americans who attempt to assert their rights through protest are criminal rioters, and African Americans who do not get ahead have only themselves to blame have been proven to have an impact on psychological factors like internalized racism and colorblind racial attitudes (Neville et al., 2005; Sidanius et al., 1996). Moreover, research additionally shows that higher levels of social dominance orientation are also correlated with higher victim blaming, which may have implications for therapists who work with clients challenged by racism (Neville et al., 2005).

Segregation

Like Black Codes, codified segregation laws also have an impact on the social context framing racism and African American mental health today (J. M. Steele, 2020). *Segregation* refers to the legalized restriction of access to opportunities and services based on some aspect of one's social identity (Clark et al., 2004). In the United States, segregation became institutionalized as a result of the 1896 Supreme Court decision in the *Plessy v. Ferguson* case (Bailey et al., 2014). According to the details of the case, Homer Plessy, who described himself as "seven-eighths Caucasian and one-eighth African blood," was a train passenger who refused to leave the vacant seat he had taken in the "Whites only" section of the train. Upon his refusal, Plessy was arrested and convicted of violating a Louisiana state law requiring railroads to provide separate cars for Black passengers. In response, Plessy filed a petition claiming the law violated the Equal Protection Clause of the 14th Amendment, which brought him all the way to the Supreme Court where the doctrine of "separate but equal" was upheld (Bailey et al., 2014). As a result of this ruling, African Americans experienced segregation in nearly all aspects of public life including education, housing, transportation, healthcare, and use of public facilities for almost 60 years, which research shows contributed to disparate social outcomes such as high disease and mortality rates, poor housing, and substandard access to education (K. B. Clark et al., 2004).

In terms of African American mental health, one of the more significant outcomes of segregation was the profoundly negative affect it had on the psychosocial development of African American children. In particular, based on the famous doll studies conducted by psychologists Kenneth and Maime Clark, it was determined that segregation caused African American children to develop a sense of inferiority and personal humiliation that often led to self-hatred and rejection of other African Americans (K. B. Clark et al., 2004). According to K. B. Clark et al. (2004), these reactions often continued throughout childhood and into adulthood, resulting in a host of symptoms including aggression toward either members of their own group or members of the dominant group, withdrawal, rigid conformity to prevailing White middle-class values, defeatism, low aspirations, depression, and anxiety. Due to issues such as transgenerational trauma and current-day de facto segregation, these reactions remain a relevant concern.

Media

In contemporary society, the media plays a significant role in perpetuating the ideologies that contribute to racism, primarily through the proliferation of stereotypes that reinforce legitimizing myths and portray African Americans as undeserving and to blame for their social status (Prilleltensky & Gonick, 1996). *Stereotypes* are beliefs about the personal attributes of a group of people that are sometimes overgeneralized, inaccurate, and resistant to new information (Myers, 2005, p. 333). They may apply to all members of a particular social identity or they may be unique to the intersection of multiple social identities. African American women, for example, are often subjected to several common stereotypes in the media, namely: (a) the "mammy" stereotype, in which African American women are depicted as "the faithful, obedient domestic servant," (b) the "Jezebel" stereotype, which portrays African American women as sexually deviant, and (c) the "Sapphire" stereotype, in which Black women are viewed as hostile and nagging (Collins, 2009, p. 80). Not only do these stereotypes contribute to self-rejecting beliefs among African American women, but they also have the effect of helping to maintain oppressive societal structures. According to Collins (2009), this occurs by symbolizing the ideal relationship of Black women to White men, rationalizing widespread sexual assault by White men against Black women, and placing blame on the Black woman for emasculating her Black male partner and causing the economic and social turmoil in the Black family. African American men on the other hand are often subjected to the criminal stereotype in the media, which occurs through bias in news reporting, "reality-based" crime shows, and overrepresentation of the criminal stereotype in film and music (Rome, 2004). Other stereotypes of African American men include that of "the Brute," "the Buck," "the Tom," "the Coon," and more recently, "the Magic Negro" (N'cho, 2015). According to N'cho (2015), one effect of these stereotypes among African American men is a feeling of invisibility, which in some instances results in undermining of their masculinity, intelligence, and emotional needs.

In terms of research, studies show that the media not only has an impact on how African Americans are viewed by society, but it also affects how

African Americans view themselves. A study of African American high school students, for example, found that frequent music video viewing and stronger identification with popular White male characters were linked to lower performance self-esteem and lower social self-esteem, respectively (Ward, 2004). Conversely, strong identification with Black male characters predicted higher performance self-esteem, appearance self-esteem, and total self-esteem. These findings highlight the idea that within the context of African American mental health, identification with cultural White ideals may harm aspects of one's sense of self and diminish the protective value of positive in-group identification. Similarly, another study of the relationship between the media and mental health among African American adolescents also suggests that stereotypes have a harmful effect on this population, as 80 percent of the participants in the study believed that negative depictions of African Americans in the media have a "grave impact" (Smith, 2020). Of additional note, 27 percent of the participants also believed that the media is trauma inducing, 20 percent suggested the media affected adolescents' self-worth, and 13 percent believed that African American adolescents were desensitized by the saturation of negative depictions of African Americans.

Other Social Determinants

Finally, while slavery, Black Codes, and legal segregation have technically been abolished, their legacy lives on in other social determinants of mental health. This is evidenced in contemporary laws and policies that lead to issues such as mass incarceration and poverty among African Americans. Generally, a firmly established body of research suggests people of color are profiled, arrested, prosecuted, convicted, and sentenced more severely than their White counterparts (Alexander, 2010). More specific to African Americans, research shows that differences in sentencing laws result in racially disparate crime statistics wherein despite being a numeric minority in the overall population, 7.7 percent of Black men between the ages of 25 and 54 are imprisoned, compared to only 1.6 percent of White men (Nittle, 2019). Research additionally shows that more than 25 percent of Black men are incarcerated by the time they are in their mid-30s, and at any given time, nearly 2 percent of all Black individuals are imprisoned in either state or federal prisons (Gottlieb & Flynn, 2021).

According to historians, these statistics are closely related to arbitrary laws and policies adopted shortly after slavery in order to criminalize and then extract labor from Black people (Matos & Hodge, 2021). For example, Matos and Hodge (2021) discussed how laws such as being too close to a White person in public, walking "without purpose," walking next to railroad tracks, or assembling after dark criminalized Black people and created a pool of individuals that could then be leased for plantation work. A similar exploitation of prison labor for public works projects or "chain gangs" also took place during this time period and continued until the mid-1950s. And although it has been several decades since the 1950s, the through line from slavery to mass incarceration continues today, with research conducted by Gottlieb and Flynn (2021) finding that that a criminal charge in a county with high levels of slavery in 1860 increases the likelihood of pretrial detention, the probability of a sentence of incarceration, and the length of incarceration sentences. Furthermore, while these findings held true for both White and Black citizens, results also suggested that a 10-percentage-point increase in the share of the population that was enslaved was associated with a 5-percentage-point increase in the probability of being sentenced to incarceration for Black individuals and a 3-percentage-point increase for White individuals (Gottlieb & Flynn, 2021).

The racial disparities evidenced in research such as that conducted by Gottlieb and Flynn (2021) may be shocking, but they do not occur by chance. Analysis of this and other similar studies suggests that in addition to discrimination in specific criminal justice policies (e.g., "three strikes" laws and mandatory minimum prison sentences for felony drug convictions), disparity in the enforcement of race-neutral laws and bias at each stage of the criminal justice process also contribute to the disproportionate incarceration of Black people (Hinton et al., 2018). Beyond the obvious personal harms that result from discriminatory criminal justice practices, the mass incarceration of Black people has significant psychosocial consequences for their families and communities. In particular, Hinton et al. (2018) argued that individual impacts to employability, housing, and access to public services removes economic resources from the Black community and drives a cycle of poverty. Poverty, in turn, leads to higher levels of violent crime, particularly in poor urban neighborhoods. Exposure to violence increases the risk of having adverse childhood experiences or developing a mental health condition such as post-traumatic stress disorder, depression, and anxiety (Do et al., 2019; Myers et al., 2015).

Reflection 2.2: In CBT, understanding of environmental factors influencing the client's presenting concerns is not considered necessary for effective treatment. However, recognition of the client's early life experiences and social context can aid the therapist's cognitive conceptualization and provide insights for clients that lead to catharsis and motivation (Beck, 2020; J. M. Steele, 2020). After reading about some of the societal factors that contribute to psychological distress within the African American community, how has your awareness of the relationship between various social conditions and mental health changed? What role might these factors have in how you conceptualize issues among the African American clients you've seen?

Psychological Phenomena

At the beginning of this chapter, I emphasized the significance of cultural knowledge in understanding how racism may affect the mental health of African American clients. To this end, I discussed key concepts such as race, racial identity, and racism, as well as societal factors that contribute to the experience of racism among African Americans. In this final section, I additionally explore several psychological phenomena that prove relevant to racism and African American mental health—some unique to this community, others applicable to the broader population of marginalized groups in our society as a whole. These phenomena include stereotype threat, deservingness, John Henryism, strong Black woman schema, racial trauma, and internalized racism. The section ends with a case example that illustrates how culture-specific psychological phenomena may present during therapy.

Stereotype Threat

Stereotype threat is defined as the fear of conforming to negative stereotypes about one's social group (C. M. Steele & Aronson, 1995). As previously discussed, throughout U.S. history, African Americans have been stereotyped as lazy and unintelligent, and these stereotypes have served as legitimizing myths to justify disparities between African Americans and other social groups in nearly all facets of life (Green, n.d.). In response, some African Americans may worry about confirming these stereotypes during test situations, leading to worsened performance on both intellectual and nonacademic cognitive and sensorimotor tasks (David, 2009; Whaley, 2018). One study, for example, found that when primed for their identity as an athlete, academically engaged African American college students performed worse on difficult and easy items on a test of verbal reasoning (Stone et al., 2012). According to the study's authors, these results are consistent with theory which suggests that when confronted with cues that directly activate an imbalance between their group identity, personal performance goals, and a negative group stereotype, stigmatized individuals who are highly invested in a performance domain can experience a decline in the cognitive and emotional resources needed to demonstrate their true potential. In terms of cognitive formulation, understanding these relationships can provide important insights into the mental representations of self and perceived social costs that lead to anxiety and worsened performance in feared situations.

Working Twice as Hard/Black Tax

While growing up, many African Americans are taught that "As a Black person in White America, you've got to work twice as hard to get half as far"

(DeSante, 2013, p. 342). This idea of working twice as hard as others, particularly one's White counterparts, is colloquially known within the African American community as *Black tax*. According to Palmer and Walker (2020), "Black tax is the psychological weight or stressor that Black people experience from consciously or unconsciously thinking about how White Americans perceive the social construct of Blackness" (para 2). In essence, Black people, aware of negative race-related stereotypes and the deficit lens through which Black people are viewed, believe they must outperform their White counterparts in order to be seen as equal. Although seemingly innocuous, these beliefs lead to behaviors that create a psychological burden for Black people. Obvious examples include pressure to excel in sports, academics, or in the workplace. However, this pressure also extends to mundane, everyday tasks such as going to the grocery store, doctor's appointments, or the bank, where many Black people, especially those of an older generation, perceive a need to be dressed in business attire in order to be taken seriously or avoid being profiled.

While understood anecdotally within the African American community, the phenomenon of working twice as hard is also supported by research. A study conducted by DeSante (2013), for example, found that "work ethic matters differently for Blacks and Whites. Whites are rewarded more for the same level of work ethic, and Blacks are punished more for the same perceived level of "laziness"' (p. 352). Similarly, a study conducted by McGee et al. (2019) also revealed themes centered on working twice as hard. Specifically, this study of African American doctoral students in engineering and computing programs revealed that many of these students felt pressure to prove they were worthy of full and unbiased participation in their departments. For example, some of the students identified a need to maintain a constant presence in the research activities of the department and lab, sacrificing weekends and holidays to a greater extent than White or Asian students in the program. Moreover, these students also reported experiencing a significant amount of distress as a result of these efforts, leading to a sort of survival mode described as a signal to the body and brain that well-being may be at risk.

John Henryism

In the literature, the differential standards pertaining to work ethic applied to African Americans are closely related to another phenomenon known as John Henryism. Referring to the African American folk hero, *John Henryism* is defined as "a psychological construct that describes a predisposition to repeated high effort coping in the face of exposure to adversity, including psychosocial stress, violence, discrimination, financial strain, and so forth" (Kahsay & Mezuk, 2022, p. 722). Broadly, research suggests John Henryism shares a significant relationship with African American mental health; however, the direction of that relationship depends on various contextual factors. Bronder et al. (2014), for example, found a negative correlation between John Henryism and depressive symptomology among Black women, although, the women who scored high on the construct were also more likely to report greater social support. In another study, Kahsay and Mezuk (2022) found similar results, wherein high John Henryism resulted in lower odds of lifetime suicidal ideation and major depression among Black adolescents. In contrast, Hudson et al. (2016) found that greater levels of John Henryism were associated with increased odds of depression among African Americans, according to data from the National Survey of American Life Reinterview. Consequently, it appears that whether John Henryism acts as a protective or risk factor in the development of psychological distress among African Americans may be variable. Nevertheless, given existing research findings, John Henryism is clearly a salient factor affecting African American mental health (Kahsay & Mezuk, 2022).

Strong Black Woman Schema

The *Strong Black Woman Schema*, also known as the *Superwoman Image*, is a stereotype in which African American women are portrayed as capable of having and doing it all (Abrams et al., 2014). In this phenomenon, Black women are ascribed qualities such as unyielding strength, responsibility, and self-sacrifice, reflecting implicit obligations to (a) "suppress fear and weakness, showcase strength, resist being vulnerable or dependent…and succeed despite limited resources," (b) "assume multiple roles such as financial providers and caregivers and possess the ability to independently support their families," and (c) "suffer quietly as they work to meet the expectations of their families, jobs, and larger society" (Abrams et al., 2014, pp. 503–504). While in some ways this phenomenon serves as a source of resilience, the Strong Black Woman Schema also contributes to psychological distress and the underutilization of mental health services among African American women. A study conducted by Watson and Hunter (2015), for example, found that greater endorsement of the Strong Black Woman Schema resulted in less psychological openness and less willingness to utilize mental health services. Likewise, in their study, Nelson et al. (2020) identified three negative outcomes associated with the Strong Black Woman Schema and professional help seeking, which included masking or ignoring pain, an inability to ask for help, and lack of self-care. Accordingly, understanding of the Strong Black Woman Schema is valuable in that it alerts therapists to the need to be intentional in exploring the ways in which an appearance of strength may mask psychological symptoms among African American woman. Strong Black Woman Schema also suggests a need to be proactive in helping these clients adopt more positive coping strategies such as self-compassion and collective and spiritual coping (Liao et al., 2020).

Racial Trauma

Racial trauma refers to mental and emotional injury caused by encounters with racism (Carter, 2007). Expounding on this definition, Carter (2007) developed what is known as the *race-based traumatic stress injury model* to further conceptualize the process that leads to psychic pain due to racism. In this model, racism is operationally defined as racial harassment, racial discrimination, or discriminatory harassment. *Racial harassment* refers to physical, interpersonal, and verbal assaults, treatment as stereotype, and assumptions of criminality or dangerousness. *Racial discrimination*, on the other hand, refers to behaviors such as barring access, exclusion, withholding information, and use of deception on the basis of race. *Discriminatory harassment* refers to aversive behaviors such as "White flight," isolation at work, denial of promotions, and questioning of qualifications. According to the race-based traumatic stress injury model, when individuals experience their encounters with any of these three types of racism as negative, memorable, sudden, and uncontrollable they develop trauma reactions (i.e., reactions characterized by intrusion, avoidance, and arousal). These reactions, in turn, produce significant psychological distress and negative impacts to the individual's functioning (Carter et al., 2017).

While not included in the *DSM-5*, a preponderance of research documents the incidence of racial trauma within the African American community (Carter et al., 2017; Kirkinis et al., 2021; Pieterse et al., 2012). One key takeaway from this research is that racial trauma does in fact result in physical, psychological, and neuropsychological symptoms similar to other forms of trauma such as PTSD. For example, individuals with racial trauma fear for their safety and often become hypervigilant, or "on guard" for new or repeated threats to their safety (U. S. Clark et al. 2018; Fani et al., 2021; Harnett 2020). These individuals may also experience withdrawal from their friends and family, have difficulty trusting others, and experience distressing symptoms such as anxiety, depression, nightmares, flashbacks, and intrusive thoughts (Abdullah et al., 2021; Bird et al., 2021; Mekawi et al., 2021). Accordingly, in order to effectively address racial trauma, therapists must have a good understanding of the overall nature of trauma and treatment of both its cognitive and physiological impacts. This includes knowledge of (a) assessment tools specific to racial trauma, (b) adapted cognitive restructuring strategies to challenge maladaptive thinking, (c) embodied healing strategies to address the physiological symptoms of trauma, and (d) empowerment strategies consistent with coping practices indigenous to the African American community.

Internalized Racism

Finally, the last psychological phenomenon relevant to African American mental health discussed in this chapter is internalized racism. *Internalized racism* refers to a negative view of oneself based on the perceived inferiority of one's own culture or race. Broadly, these perceptions are derived as individuals (a) internalize messages about the superiority of White culture and (b) accept negative stereotypes about their own racial/ethnic group (Bailey et al., 2014). While internalized racism is a psychological state, it is differentiated from other similar constructs such as low self-esteem in that internalized racism results in ideas and behaviors that reinforce racial oppression (Bivens, 2005). People with internalized racism, for example, often feel so overwhelmed by their feelings of shame and alienation that they feel powerless to enact change in their environments. As a result, existing social inequities remain unchallenged and the status quo is allowed to continue (Bivens, 1995).

Within the mental health literature, several cognitive processes have been identified as the mechanisms through which internalized racism is developed and maintained. In Chapter 1, I discussed cognitive models of internalized racism developed by Watts-Jones's (2002) and Bailey et al. (2014), wherein maladaptive thinking such as shame associated with being of African descent, belief in a biased representation of history, and internalization of negative stereotypes about African Americans lead to negative psychological and behavioral responses that have a negative impact on overall well-being and health. Elsewhere, I developed a model of internalized racism that builds on these prior conceptualizations by describing cognitive processes that occur once internalized racist beliefs are activated, as well as contextual factors that influence the development and maintenance of these beliefs (J. M. Steele, 2020). The model is shown in Figure 2.1.

As depicted in Figure 2.1, societal influences, along with individual childhood experiences, affect the core beliefs African Americans develop about themselves, other people, and their world, as well as the assumptions and rules they establish to guide their behavior in consideration of these beliefs (J. M. Steele, 2020). Once developed, core beliefs and assumptions specific to the racially stereotyped messages received from society are reinforced through interpersonal interactions that strengthen the sense of inferiority, shame, and powerlessness experienced within this group. Resulting race-related beliefs and continued exposure to racist interpersonal interactions, in turn, act as an additional lens through which everyday situations are interpreted. The corresponding emotional, behavioral, and physiological reactions that develop as result of how these situations are interpreted then lead to the reinforcement of dominant societal beliefs, which, as previously mentioned, is a definitional aspect of internalized racism (Bivens, 1995).

Case Illustration: Sasha

Sasha is a 35-year-old African American woman who is in counseling with her 14-year-old son, Joshua. Sasha's husband passed away in a tragic car accident five years ago, leaving Sasha to raise their son on her own. Prior to his death, Sasha and her husband frequently discussed their plans for Joshua's education, which included enrollment in their city's best private schools, as well as private tutoring. Sasha and her husband saw that Joshua was academically talented at a very early age, and as a result, developed high expectations for Joshua's college and career plans. Now that Joshua is in high school, Sasha is concerned he is "hanging with the wrong crowd." Joshua has not experienced a decline in his grades, but he did recently receive an in-school suspension due to an altercation between Joshua and one of his peers. Sasha blames Joshua's behavior on the new friends he has made since entering high school and wants Joshua to find friends with more similar backgrounds to Joshua and her family.

Joshua disagrees with his mother's assessment of the situation. From his perspective, Sasha has a problem with the friends he has made during high school because many of them are "poor Black kids" who have scholarships to the school. Sasha finds this accusation insulting, but also states that Joshua's father worked hard to make it out of "the hood" and would not approve of Joshua's new friendships. Sasha and Joshua have frequent arguments about the issue, causing Sasha to be worried and irritable. Sasha additionally reports that her issues with Joshua are starting to affect her work performance, as she has low energy and is increasingly distracted. This upsets Sasha who, as the first African American CEO of her company, believes she already "doesn't fit in" and has to work "twice as hard" as her colleagues to be respected. Sasha feels alone in dealing with her problems, stating that her mother raised her to be "strong," so she should be able to deal with her problems on her own. She initiated counseling as a last resort to manage the stress she is experiencing and address the problems in her relationship with Joshua.

Like many clients, Sasha did not enter therapy identifying internalized racism as a presenting concern. Nevertheless, in reviewing her case, each element of the cognitive model of internalized racism shown in Figure 2.1 is apparent. First, like many young Black women, Sasha was raised to be "strong" and manage problems on her own. This personal aspect of her childhood reflects the Strong Black Woman Schema, wherein Sasha was taught to showcase her strength and suppress any signs of fear or weakness (Abrams et al., 2014). Throughout her life, Sasha has also been influenced by negative stereotypes that depict African Americans as delinquent and unintelligent, as well as an absence of African Americans in affluent social spaces. As a result of these experiences, Sasha developed the core belief

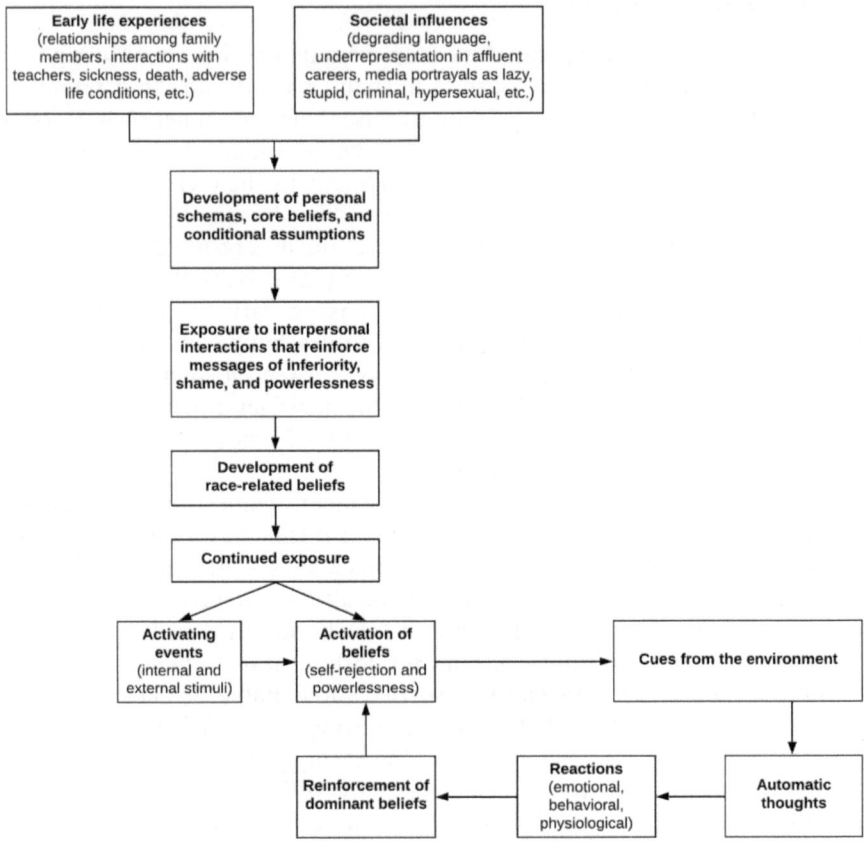

Figure 2.1 Cognitive Developmental Model of Internalized Racism.

Source: Steele, J. M. (2020). A CBT approach to internalized racism among African Americans. *International Journal for the Advancement of Counselling,* *42*(3), 217–233. https://doi.org/10.1007/s10447-020-09402-0

"I don't fit in" and the conditional assumption "If I work twice as hard, I'll be accepted," both of which reflect negative self-appraisals activated in her difficulties with Joshua and at her place of employment. Race-related beliefs reflecting negative assumptions about other members of her own racial group also appear to be activated in the situation with Joshua, alluding to other experiences and continued exposures that may have also reinforced negative race-related beliefs given their strength in the current situation.

Recall that in addition to internalized feelings of inferiority, a defining feature of internalized racism is the recapitulation of attitudes and behaviors that reinforce dominant societal beliefs and racial hierarchies (Bivens, 1995, 2005). This aspect of internalized racism is also evident in Sasha's response to her son's new friends. According to the model, Joshua's in-school suspension led to the thought "he's hanging with the wrong crowd," prompting reactions such as worry, irritability, and a doubling down of Sasha's negative race-related beliefs concerning African Americans from less affluent backgrounds. Rather than working to develop policies to ensure more equitable and enriching educational spaces for all children or engaging Joshua in positive racial socialization practices to affirm his identity as an African American man, Sasha is instead acting on negative stereotypes of African Americans and perhaps even contributing to the internalization of these stereotypes in her son.

Sasha may have little awareness of the ways in which her response to Joshua's situation reflects aspects of internalized racism. Given the sensitivity of issues related to race, examination of internalized racism requires a strong therapeutic alliance and careful broaching. These topics are explored in Chapters 4 and 5. Prior to that, strengths and potential sources of coping within the African American community are examined in Chapter 3, providing insight into adaptive ways of responding to the challenges described in this chapter.

References

Abdullah, T., Graham-LoPresti, J. R., Tahirkheli, N. N., Hughley, S. M., & Watson, L. T. J. (2021). Microaggressions and posttraumatic stress disorder symptom scores among Black Americans: Exploring the link. *Traumatology*, *27*(3), 244–253. https://doi.org/10.1037/trm0000259

Abrams, J. A., Maxwell, M., Pope, M., & Belgrave, F. Z. (2014). Carrying the world with the grace of a lady and the grit of a warrior: Deepening our understanding of the "Strong Black Woman" Schema. *Psychology of Women Quarterly*, *38*(4), 503–518. https://doi.org/10.1177/0361684314541418

Alexander, M. (2010). *The new Jim Crow: Mass incarceration in the age of colorblindness*. The New Press.

American Psychiatric Association. (2017). *Mental health disparities: African Americans*. https://www.psychiatry.org/File%20Library/Psychiatrists/Cultural-Competency/Mental-Health-Disparities/Mental-Health-Facts-for-African-Americans.pdf

American Psychological Association. (2021). *Apology to people of color for APA's role in promoting, perpetuating, and failing to challenge racism, racial discrimination, and human hierarchy in U.S.: Resolution adopted by the APA Council of Representatives on October 29, 2021.* https://www.apa.org/about/policy/racism-apology

Atkinson, D. R., Brown, M. T., Parham, T. A., Matthews, L. G., Landrum-Brown, J., & Kim, A. U. (1996). African American client skin tone and clinical judgments of African American and European American psychologists. *Professional Psychology: Research and Practice*, *27*(5), 500–505. https://doi.org/10.1037/0735-7028.27.5.500

Bailey, T.-K. M., Williams, W. S., & Favors, B. (2014). Internalized racial oppression in the African American community. In E. J. R. David (Ed.), *Internalized oppression: The psychology of marginalized groups* (pp. 137–162). Springer Publishing Company, Inc.

Barr, S. C., & Neville, H. A. (2014). Racial socialization, color-blind racial ideology, and mental health among Black college students: An examination of an ecological model. *Journal of Black Psychology, 40*(2), 138–165. https://doi.org/10.1177/0095798412475084

Beck, J. S. (2020). *Cognitive behavior therapy: Basics and beyond* (3rd ed.). Guilford Press.

Belgrave, F. Z., & Allison, K. W. (2019). *African American psychology: From Africa to America* (4th ed.). Sage Publications, Inc.

Bird, C. M., Webb, E. K., Schramm, A. T., Torres, L., Larson, C., & deRoon-Cassini, T. A. (2021). Racial discrimination is associated with acute posttraumatic stress symptoms and predicts future posttraumatic stress disorder symptom severity in trauma-exposed Black adults in the United States. *Journal of Traumatic Stress, 34*(5), 995–1004. https://doi.org/10.1002/jts.22670

Bivens, D. (1995). *Internalized racism: A definition*. https://www.racialequitytools.org/resourcefiles/bivens.pdf

Bivens, D. K. (2005). What is internalized racism? *Flipping the Script: White Privilege and Community Building, 1*, 43–51.

Bonham, V. L., Warshauer-Baker, E., & Collins, F. S. (2005). Race and ethnicity in the genome era: The complexity of the constructs. *The American Psychologist, 60*(1), 9–15. https://doi.org/10.1037/0003-066X.60.1.9

Britt-Spells, A. M., Slebodnik, M., Sands, L. P., & Rollock, D. (2018). Effects of perceived discrimination on depressive symptoms among Black men residing in the United States: A meta-analysis. *American Journal of Men's Health, 12*(1), 52–63. https://doi.org10.1177/1557988315624509

Bronder, E. C., Speight, S. L., Witherspoon, K. M., & Thomas, A. J. (2014). John Henryism, depression, and perceived social support in Black women. *Journal of Black Psychology, 40*(2), 115–137. https://doi.org/10.1177/0095798412474466

Burns, M. A., & Vaughn, K. R. (2021). Race metatheory: Toward a dissolution of a calamitous concept. *Professional Psychology: Research and Practice, 52*(5), 487–493. https://doi.org/10.1037/pro0000416

Carter, R. T. (2007). Racism and psychological and emotional injury: Recognizing and assessing race-based traumatic stress. *The Counseling Psychologist, 35*(1), 13–105. https://doi.org/10.1177/0011000006292033

Carter, R. T., Johnson, V. E., Roberson, K., Mazzula, S. L., Kirkinis, K., & Sant-Barket, S. (2017). Race-based traumatic stress, racial identity statuses, and psychological functioning: An exploratory investigation. *Professional Psychology: Research and Practice, 48*(1), 30–37. https://doi.org/10.1037/pro0000116

Clark, K. B., Chein, I., & Cook, S. W. (2004). The effects of segregation and the consequences of desegregation: A (September 1952) social science statement in the *Brown v. Board of Education of Topeka* supreme court case. *American Psychologist, 59*(6), 495–501. https://doi.org/10.1037/0003-066X.59.6.495

Clark, U. S., Miller, E. R., & Hegde, R. R. (2018). Experiences of discrimination are associated with greater resting amygdala activity and functional connectivity. *Biological Psychiatry. Cognitive Neuroscience and Neuroimaging, 3*(4), 367–378. https://doi.org/10.1016/j.bpsc.2017.11.011

Collins, P. H. (2009). *Black feminist thought*. Routledge.

Constantine, M. G., Richardson, T. Q., Benjamin, E. M., & Wilson, J. W. (1998). An overview of Black racial identity theories: Current limitations and considerations.

Applied and Preventive Psychology, 7(2), 95–99. https://doi.org/10.1016/S0962-1849 (05)80006-X

Cokley, K. (2007). Critical issues in the measurement of ethnic and racial identity: A referendum on the state of the field. *Journal of Counseling Psychology*, 54(3), 224–234. https://doi.org/10.1037/0022-0167.54.3.224

Cross, W. E., Jr. (1971). Toward a psychology of Black liberation: The Negro-to-Black conversion experience. *Black World*, 20(9), 13–27.

Cross, W. E. Jr. (1991). *Shades of Black*. Temple University Press.

Cross, W. E., Jr., & Vandiver, B. J. (2001). Nigrescence theory and measurement: Introducing the Cross Racial Identity Scale (CRIS). In J. G. Ponterotto, J. M. Casas, L. A. Suzuki, & C. M. Alexander (Eds.), *Handbook of multicultural counseling* (2nd ed., pp. 371–393). Sage.

Das, A., Singh, P., Kulkarni, A. K., & Bruckner, T. A. (2021). Emergency department visits for depression following police killings of unarmed African Americans. *Social Science & Medicine*, 269, 1–6. https://doi.org/10.1016/j.socscimed.2020.113561

David, E. J. R. (2009). Internalized oppression, psychopathology, and cognitive-behavioral therapy among historically oppressed groups. *Journal of Psychological Practice*, 15(1), 71–103.

Davis, C. III, Aronson, J., & Salinas, M. (2006). Shades of threat: Racial identity as a moderator of stereotype threat. *Journal of Black Psychology*, 32(4), 399–417. https://doi.org/10.1177/0095798406292464

DeGruy, J. D. (2017). *Post-traumatic slave syndrome: America's legacy of enduring injury and healing*. Uptown Press.

DeSante, C. D. (2013). Working twice as hard to get half as far: Race, work ethic, and America's deserving poor. *American Journal of Political Science*, 57(2), 342–356. https://doi.org/10.1111/ajps.12006

DiAngelo, R. (2018). *White fragility: Why it's so hard for White people to talk about racism*. Beacon Press.

Do, D. P., Locklar, L. R. B., & Florsheim, P. (2019). Triple jeopardy: The joint impact of racial segregation and neighborhood poverty on the mental health of Black Americans. *Social Psychiatry and Psychiatric Epidemiology*, 54(5), 533–541. https://doi.org/10.1007/s00127-019-01654-5

Duello, T. M., Rivedal, S., Wickland, C., & Weller, A. (2021). Race and genetics versus 'race' in genetics: A systematic review of the use of African ancestry in genetic studies. *Evolution, Medicine, and Public Health*, 9(1), 232–245. https://doi.org/10.1093/emph/eoab018

Evans, A. M., Hemmings, C., Ramsay-Seaner, K., & Barnett, J. (2021). Perceived racism and discrimination among people of color: An ethnographic content analysis. *Journal of Multicultural Counseling and Development*, 49(3), 152–164. https://doi.org/10.1002/jmcd.12221

Fani, N., Carter, S. E., Harnett, N. G., Ressler, K. J., & Bradley, B. (2021). Association of racial discrimination with neural response to threat in Black women in the US exposed to trauma. *JAMA Psychiatry*, 78(9), 1005–1012. https://doi.org/10.1001/jamapsychiatry.2021.1480

Franklin-Jackson, D., & Carter, R. T. (2007). The relationships between race-related stress, racial identity, and mental health for Black Americans. *Journal of Black Psychology*, 33(1), 5–26. https://doi.org/10.1177/0095798406295092

Giordano, A. L., Gorritz, F. B., Kilpatrick, E. P., Scoffone, C. M., & Lundeen, L. A. (2021). Examining secondary trauma as a result of clients' reports of discrimination. *International Journal for the Advancement of Counselling*, *43*(1), 19–30. https://doi.org/10.1007/s10447-020-09411-z

Gottlieb, A., & Flynn, K. (2021). The legacy of slavery and mass incarceration: Evidence from felony case outcomes. *Social Service Review*, *95*(1), 3–35. https://doi.org/10.1086/713922

Graham, J. R., Calloway, A., & Roemer, L. (2015). The buffering effects of emotion regulation in the relationship between experiences of racism and anxiety in a Black American sample. *Cognitive Therapy and Research*, *39*(5), 553–563. https://doi.org/10.1007/s10608-015-9682-8

Graves, J. L. III. (2015). Why the nonexistence of biological races does not mean the nonexistence of racism. *American Behavioral Scientist*, *59*(11), 1474–1495. https://doi.org/10.1177/0002764215588810

Green, L. (n.d.). Stereotypes: Negative racial stereotypes and their effect on attitudes toward African-Americans. https://www.ferris.edu/htmls/news/jimcrow/links/essays/vcu.htm

Guthrie, R. V. (1976). *Even the rat was White*. Harper & Row.

Halloran, M. J. (2019). African American health and posttraumatic slave syndrome: A terror management theory account. *Journal of Black Studies*, *50*(1), 45–65. https://doi.org/10.1177/0021934718880373

Harnett, N. G. (2020). Neurobiological consequences of racial disparities and environmental risks: A critical gap in understanding psychiatric disorders. *Neuropsychopharmacology*, *45*(8), 1247–1250. https://doi.org/10.1038/s41386-020-0681-4

Hemmings, C., & Evans, A. M. (2018). Identifying and treating race-based trauma in counseling. *Journal of Multicultural Counseling and Development*, *46*(1), 20–39. https://doi.org/10.1002/jmcd.12090

Henry, P. J. (2010). Modern racism. In J. M. Levine & M. A. Hogg (Eds.), *The encyclopedia of group processes and intergroup relations* (pp. 575–577). Sage Publications.

Hinton, E., Henderson, L., & Reed, C. (2018). *An unjust burden: The disparate treatment of Black Americans in the criminal justice system*. Vera Institute of Justice.

Hoffman, K. M., Trawalter, S., Axt, J. R., & Oliver, M. N. (2016). Racial bias in pain assessment and treatment recommendations, and false beliefs about biological differences between Blacks and Whites. *PNAS Proceedings of the National Academy of Sciences of the United States of America*, *113*(16), 4296–4301. https://doi.org/10.1073/pnas.1516047113

Hudson, D. L., Neighbors, H. W., Geronimus, A. T., & Jackson, J. S. (2016). Racial discrimination, John Henryism, and depression among African Americans. *Journal of Black Psychology*, *42*(3), 221–243. https://doi.org/10.1177/0095798414567757

Hughey, M. W., & Goss, D. R. (2015). A level playing field? Media constructions of athletics, genetics, and race. *Annals of the American Academy of Political and Social Science*, *661*(1), 182–211. https://doi.org/10.1177/0002716215588067

Jenkins-Hall, K., & Sacco, W. P. (1991). Effect of client race and depression on evaluations by White therapists. *Journal of Social and Clinical Psychology*, *10*(3), 322–333. https://doi.org/10.1521/jscp.1991.10.3.322

Johnson, V. E., & Carter, R. T. (2020). Black cultural strengths and psychosocial well-being: An empirical analysis with Black American adults. *Journal of Black Psychology*, *46*(1), 55–89. https://doi.org/10.1177/0095798419889752

Joseph, N. T., Peterson, L. M., Gordon, H., & Kamarck, T. W. (2021). The double burden of racial discrimination in daily-life moments: Increases in negative emotions and depletion of psychosocial resources among emerging adult African Americans. *Cultural Diversity and Ethnic Minority Psychology*, *27*(2), 234–244. https://doi.org/10.1037/cdp0000337

Kahsay, E., & Mezuk, B. (2022). The association between John Henryism and depression and suicidal ideation among African-American and Caribbean Black adolescents in the United States. *Journal of Adolescent Health*, *71*(6), 721–728. https://doi.org/10.1016/j.jadohealth.2022.07.006

Khanna, N. (2010). "If you're half black, you're just black": Reflected appraisals and the persistence of the one-drop rule. *The Sociological Quarterly*, *51*(1), 96–121. https://doi.org/10.1111/j.1533-8525.2009.01162.x

Kilmer, E. D., Villarreal, C., Janis, B. M., Callahan, J. L., Ruggero, C. J., Kilmer, J. N., Love, P. K., & Cox, R. J. (2019). Differential early termination is tied to client race/ethnicity status. *Practice Innovations*, *4*(2), 88–98. https://doi.org/10.1037/pri0000085

Kirkinis, K., Pieterse, A. L., Martin, C. Agiliga, A., & Brownell, A. (2021). Racism, racial discrimination, and trauma: A systematic review of the social science literature. *Ethnicity & Health*, *26*(3), 392–412. https://doi.org/10.1080/13557858.2018.1514453

Liao, K. Y., Weng, C. Y., & West, L. M. (2016). Social connectedness and intolerance of uncertainty as moderators between racial microaggressions and anxiety among Black individuals. *Journal of Counseling Psychology*, *63*(2), 240–246. https://doi.org/10.1037/cou0000123

Liao, K. Y.-H., Wei, M., & Yin, M. (2020). The misunderstood schema of the Strong Black Woman: Exploring its mental health consequences and coping responses among African American women. *Psychology of Women Quarterly*, *44*(1), 84–104. https://doi.org/10.1177/0361684319883198

Lige, Q. M., Peteet, B. J., & Brown, C. M. (2017). Racial identity, self-esteem, and the impostor phenomenon among African American college students. *Journal of Black Psychology*, *43*(4), 345–357. https://doi.org/10.1177/0095798416648787

López, I., Walker, L. H. M., & Spinel, M. Y. (2015). Understanding the association between phenotype and ethnic identity. In C. E. Santos & A. J. Umaña-Taylor (Eds.), *Studying ethnic identity: Methodological and conceptual approaches across disciplines* (pp. 119–148). American Psychological Association. https://doi.org/10.1037/14618-006

López, S. R. (1989). Patient variable biases in clinical judgment: Conceptual overview and methodological considerations. *Psychological Bulletin*, *106*(2), 184–203. https://doi.org/10.1037/0033-2909.106.2.184

Matos, K., & Hodge, J. (2021). *The chains of slavery still exist in mass incarceration*. Vera. https://www.vera.org/news/the-chains-of-slavery-still-exist-in-mass-incarceration

McConahay, J. B., Hardee, B. B., & Batts, V. (1981). Has racism declined in America? It depends on who is asking and what is asked. *Journal of Conflict Resolution, 25*(4), 563–579.

McGee, E. O., Griffith, D. M., & Houston, S. L. II. (2019). "I know I have to work twice as hard and hope that makes me good enough:" Exploring the stress and strain of Black doctoral students in engineering and computing. *Teachers College Record, 121*(4), 1–38. https://doi.org/10.1177/01614681191210040

Mekawi, Y., Carter, S., Brown, B., Martinez de Andino, A., Fani, N., Michopoulos, V., & Powers, A. (2021). Interpersonal trauma and posttraumatic stress disorder among Black women: Does racial discrimination matter? *Journal of Trauma & Dissociation, 22*(2), 154–169. https://doi.org/10.1080/15299732.2020.1869098

Menakem, R. (2017). *My grandmother's hands: Racialized trauma and the pathway to mending our hearts and bodies.* Central Recovery Press.

Mohatt, N. V., Thompson, A. B., Thai, N. D., & Tebes, J. K. (2014). Historical trauma as public narrative: A conceptual review of how history impacts present-day health. *Social Science & Medicine, 106,* 128–136. https://doi.org/10.1016/j.socscimed.2014.01.043

Myers, D. (2005). *Social psychology* (8th ed.). McGraw Hill.

Myers, H. F., Wyatt, G. E., Ullman, J. B., Loeb, T. B., Chin, D., Prause, N., Zhang, M., Williams, J. K., Slavich, G. M., & Liu, H. (2015). Cumulative burden of lifetime adversities: Trauma and mental health in low-SES African Americans and Latino/as. *Psychological Trauma: Theory, Research, Practice, and Policy, 7*(3), 243–251. https://doi.org/10.1037/a0039077

Nadal, K. L., Griffin, K. E., Wong, Y., Hamit, S., & Rasmus, M. (2014). The impact of racial microaggressions on mental health: Counseling implications for clients of color. *Journal of Counseling & Development, 92*(1), 57–66. https://doi.org/10.1002/j.1556-6676.2014.00130.x

N'cho, H. S. (2015). *Negotiating invisibility: A case study of African American men in a therapeutic support group* (Publication No. 3687728) [Doctoral dissertation, Boston College]. ProQuest Dissertations & Theses Global.

Nelson, T., Shahid, N. N., & Cardemil, E. V. (2020). Do I really need to go and see somebody? Black Women's perceptions of help-seeking for depression. *Journal of Black Psychology, 46*(4), 263–286. https://doi.org/10.1177/0095798420931644

Neville, H. A., Awad, G. H., Brooks, J. E., Flores, M. P., & Bluemel, J. (2013). Color-blind racial ideology: Theory, training, and measurement implications in psychology. *American Psychologist, 68*(6), 455–466. https://doi.org/10.1037/a0033282

Neville, H. A., Coleman, M. N., Falconer, J. W., & Holmes, D. (2005). Color-blind racial ideology and psychological false consciousness among African Americans. *Journal of Black Psychology, 31*(1), 27–45. https://doi.org/10.1177/0095798404268287

Neville, H. A., & Cross, W. E., Jr. (2017). Racial awakening: Epiphanies and encounters in Black racial identity. *Cultural Diversity and Ethnic Minority Psychology, 23*(1), 102–108. https://doi.org/10.1037/cdp0000105

Neville, H. A., Worthington, R., & Spanierman, L. B. (2001). Race, power, and multicultural counseling psychology: Understanding white privilege and color blind racial attitudes. In J. G. Ponterotto, J. M. Casas, L. A. Suzuki, & C. M. Alexander (Eds.), *Handbook of multicultural counseling* (2nd ed., pp. 257–288). Sage.

Ni, P. (2021). What are overt and covert types of racism? Characteristics of two types of racism. *Psychology Today*. https://www.psychologytoday.com/us/blog/communication-success/202111/what-are-overt-and-covert-types-of-racism

Nittle, N. K. (2019, February 18). The Black Codes and why they matter today: The Black Codes still impacting policing and prison in the 21st century. *ThoughtCo*. https://www.thoughtco.com/the-blackcodes-4125744

NPR/Robert Wood Johnson Foundation/Harvard T.H. Chan School of Public Health. (2017). *Discrimination in America: Experiences and views of African Americans*. https://www.rwjf.org/content/dam/farm/reports/reports/2017/rwjf441128

Palmer, R. T., & Walker, L. J. (2020, July 6). Proposing a concept of the Black tax to understand the experiences of Blacks in America. Diverse Issues in Higher Education. https://diverseeducation.com/article/182837/

Pierce, C. M. (1974). Psychiatric problems of the Black minority. In S. Arieti (Ed.), *American handbook of psychiatry* (pp. 512–523). Basic Books.

Pieterse, A. L., Todd, N. R., Neville, H. A., & Carter, R. T. (2012). Perceived racism and mental health among Black American adults: A meta-analytic review. *Journal of Counseling Psychology*, *59*(1), 1–9. https://doi.org/10.1037/a0026208

Plous, S., & Williams, T. (1995). Racial stereotypes from the days of American slavery: A continuing legacy. *Journal of Applied Social Psychology*, *25*(9), 795–817. https://doi.org/10.1111/j.1559-1816.1995.tb01776.x

Prilleltensky, I., & Gonick, L. (1996). Polities change, oppression remains: On the psychology and politics of oppression. *Political Psychology*, *17*(1), 127–148. https://doi.org/10.2307/3791946

Rome, D. (2004). *Black demons: The media's depiction of the African American male criminal stereotype*. Praeger.

Rosenthal, D. A. (2004). Effects of client race on clinical judgment of practicing European American vocational rehabilitation counselors. *Rehabilitation Counseling Bulletin*, *47*(3), 131–141. https://doi.org/10.1177/00343552040470030201

Sidanius, J. (1993). The psychology of group conflict and the dynamics of oppression: A social dominance perspective. In S. Iyengar & W. J. McGuire (Eds.), *Explorations in political psychology* (pp. 183–219). Duke University Press.

Sidanius, J., Levin, S., & Pratto, F. (1996). Consensual social dominance orientation and its correlates within the hierarchical structure of American society. *International Journal of Intercultural Relations*, *20*(3–4), 385–408. https://doi.org/10.1016/0147-1767(96)00025-9

Smedley, A. (1999). *Race in North America: Origin and evolution of a worldview* (2nd ed.). Westview Press.

Smedley, A., & Smedley, B. D. (2005). Race as biology is fiction, racism as a social problem is real: Anthropological and historical perspectives on the social construction of race. *American Psychologist*, *60*(1), 16–26. https://doi.org/10.1037/0003-066X.60.1.16

Smith, K. L. (2020). *The impact of media on African American adolescent mental health and behavior* (Publication No. 27740603) [Doctoral dissertation, Capella University]. ProQuest Dissertations & Theses Global.

Steele, C. M., & Aronson, J. (1995). Stereotype threat and the intellectual test performance of African-Americans. *Journal of Personality and Social Psychology*, *69*(5), 797–811. https://doi.org/10.1037/0022-3514.69.5.797

Steele, J. M. (2020). A CBT approach to internalized racism among African Americans. *International Journal for the Advancement of Counselling, 42*(3), 217–233. https://doi.org/10.1007/s10447-020-09402-0

Steele, J. M., & Newton, C. S. (2022). Culturally adapted cognitive behavior therapy as a model to address internalized racism among African American clients. *Journal of Mental Health Counseling, 44*(2), 98–116. https://doi.org/10.17744/mehc.44.2.01

Stone, J., Harrison, C., & Mottley, J. (2012). "Don't call me a student-athlete": The effect of identity priming on stereotype threat for academically engaged African American college athletes. *Basic and Applied Social Psychology, 34*(2), 99–106. https://doi.org/10.1080/01973533.2012.655624

Substance Abuse and Mental Health Services Administration. (2020). Mental and behavioral health - African Americans. https://minorityhealth.hhs.gov/mental-and-behavioral-health-african-americans

Sue, D. W., Arredondo, P., & McDavis, R. J. (1992). Multicultural counseling competencies and standards: A call to the profession. *Journal of Multicultural Counseling and Development, 20*(2), 64–88. https://doi.org/10.1002/j.2161-1912.1992.tb00563.x

Sue, D. W., Sue, D., Neville, H. A., & Smith, L. (2019). *Counseling the culturally diverse: Theory and practice* (8th ed.). John Wiley & Sons, Inc.

Taylor, R. E., & Kuo, B. C. H. (2019). Black American psychological help-seeking intention: An integrated literature review with recommendations for clinical practice. *Journal of Psychotherapy Integration, 29*(4), 325–337. https://doi.org/10.1037/int0000131

Vandiver, B. J., Fhagen-Smith, P. E., Cokley, K. O., Cross, W. E., Jr., & Worrell, F. C. (2001). Cross's Nigrescence model: From theory to scale to theory. *Journal of Multicultural Counseling and Development, 29*(3), 174–200. https://doi.org/10.1002/j.2161-1912.2001.tb00516.x

Walker, R. (2020). *The unapologetic guide to Black mental health: Navigate an unequal system, learn tools for emotional wellness, and get the help you deserve.* New Harbinger.

Ward, L. M. (2004). Wading through the stereotypes: Positive and negative associations between media use and Black adolescents' conceptions of self. *Developmental Psychology, 40*(2), 284–294. https://doi.org/10.1037/0012-1649.40.2.284

Watson, N. N., & Hunter, C. D. (2015). Anxiety and depression among African American women: The costs of strength and negative attitudes toward psychological help-seeking. *Cultural Diversity & Ethnic Minority Psychology, 21*(4), 604–612. https://doi.org/10.1037/cdp0000015

Watts-Jones, D. (2002). Healing internalized racism: The role of a within-group sanctuary among people of African descent. *Family Process, 41*(4), 591–601. https://doi.org/10.1111/j.1545-5300.2002.00591.x

Whaley, A. L. (2018). Advances in stereotype threat research on African Americans: Continuing challenges to the validity of its role in the achievement gap. *Social Psychology of Education: An International Journal, 21*(1), 111–137. https://doi.org/10.1007/s11218-017-9415-9

Williams, D. R., & Williams-Morris, R. (2000). Racism and mental health: The African American experience. *Ethnicity & Health, 5*(3–4), 243–268. https://doi.org/10.1080/713667453

Williams, M. T. (2018, March 20). Ethnic and racial identity and the therapeutic alliance. *Psychology Today*. https://www.psychologytoday.com/us/blog/culturally-speaking/201803/ethnic-and-racial-identity-and-the-therapeutic-alliance

Worrell, F. C., Cross, W. E., Jr., & Vandiver, B. J. (2001). Nigrescence theory: Current status and challenges for the future. *Journal of Multicultural Counseling and Development*, *29*(3), 201–213. https://doi.org/10.1002/j.2161-1912.2001.tb00517.x

Chapter 3

Strengths and Potential Sources of Coping Within the African American Community

African American lives are often viewed through the lens of racial trauma. However, being African American encompasses so much more than the pain of racial oppression. Within the African American community lies a rich tapestry of cultural traditions, communal bonds, and faith in a higher power that creates depth, forges ties, and offers hope in the face of adversity. When considered within the context of addressing the mental health needs of this community, these elements of African American culture additionally serve as strengths and protective factors beneficial to coping and resilience within this population.

While African American culture offers a deep well of resources valuable to the promotion of psychological health and wellbeing, the therapist's use of these resources to aid their clients in enhancing wellness can be difficult without requisite knowledge of what these resources are and how to use them in the therapeutic process. In CBT, identification of strengths and sources of coping can be guided through the implementation of CBT approaches focused on the promotion of resilience and other positive qualities. Padesky and Mooney's (2012) four-step strengths-based cognitive behavior therapy model, for example, describes methods therapists may use to bring a client's resilience and hidden strengths into the client's awareness. These methods, which are discussed in further detail later in this chapter, are advantageous to the process of empowering African American clients to heal from racism given their potential to help people face and manage negative life events. In the working phase of treatment, identification of strengths and sources of coping can also provide the foundation for strength-based cognitive conceptualization (J. S. Beck, 2020).

In this chapter, I describe specific strengths and sources of coping within the African American community with the goal of assisting therapists in gaining the knowledge and skills necessary to achieve the objectives described above. The chapter begins with a discussion of the African-centered worldview and how that worldview may be useful in challenging maladaptive beliefs and behaviors that develop in response to racism. Next, culture-specific strategies

DOI: 10.4324/9781003196303-3

for coping with racism are explored. The chapter concludes with a discussion of the strengths-based approach to CBT, how it may be utilized to increase the client's awareness of their strengths, and how the approach may be employed as a means to overcome the psychological effects of racism.

African-Centered Worldview

In discussing the African-centered worldview, it may be helpful to first define the term *worldview*. According to Kohl (2006), a "worldview constitutes our psychological orientation in life and determines how we think, behave, make decisions, and define events. It includes one's group and individual identities, beliefs, values, and language that construct a reality for perceiving life events" (p. 176). African American clients with a collectivist worldview, for example, may emphasize interdependence and family kinship ties, family values, and deference to authority over the competition and an individualism typically accentuated within a Eurocentric worldview (Hunter, 2008). In the therapeutic context, this is significant as most theories of psychotherapy focus on notions of self and emphasize personal achievement. Contextualizing theories of psychotherapy such as CBT to be more inclusive of alternative worldviews allows therapists and clients to view problems and strengths in ways that are culturally congruent and authentic. This, in turn, provides opportunities to validate the lens through which clients interpret and make meaning in their environment, which may increase self-efficacy and affirm the value of the client's cultural heritage.

Psychological literature which delineates the African-centered worldview is vast and expansive (e.g., Akbar, 1984; Asante, 1988, 1998; Baldwin, 1984; Diop, 1974; Grills, 2002; Hilliard, 1986; Kambon, 1992; Nobles, 1991). Nearly five decades ago, Vernon Dixon (1977) described the axiological (i.e., value), epistemological (i.e., knowledge), and logic (i.e., reasoning) tenets associated with an African-centered worldview, which he characterized as the man-to-person relationship, affect-symbolic imagery cognition, and diunital logic (Carroll, 2010). Within this characterization, the man-to-person relationship axiology describes a value-orientation based upon being, felt-time, communalism, and harmony with nature. In clarifying these concepts, Dixon (1977) described *being* as individuality expressed within the constrictions of the needs of the group. A contemporary articulation of African-centered being is illustrated in African American hashtags such as #MyBlackIsBeautiful, which expresses a prizing of individuality within the context of the shared strengths and beauty of African American culture, broadly. The second concept, *felt-time*, is described as an orientation to time based on one's phenomenological experience. Dixon (1977) illustrated this description with an example from the Liatuka people who call October "The Sun" because the sun is very hot in that month. The third aspect of the man-to-person relationship axiology, *communalism*, is illustrated through the proverb, "Whatever happens to the individual happens to the whole group and whatever happens to the whole group happens to the individual." This idea is also similar to the African-centered philosophy of *ubuntu*, or the idea that "I am because we are," which further emphasizes the idea that a person's humanity cannot be fully realized outside of communal connection (Turner et al., 2022). The final aspect, *harmony with nature*, is reflected in belief in the universal oneness between humanity and the phenomenal world. These characteristics of the African-centered worldview are all contrasted with Eurocentric worldview preferences for doing, future-time, individualism, and mastery over nature.

In terms of the ways in which an individual experiences or knows reality, Dixon (1977) described an African-centered epistemology as one in which feeling supersedes thinking and then knowing, what he called affect-symbolic imagery cognition. In this way of knowing, *affect* refers to the ways in which the feeling, emotive self is brought into the experiencing of one's environment, for example, dancing to acknowledge a touchdown, while *symbolic imagery* refers to the use of words, gestures, tones, rhythms, objects, etc. to convey meaning, for example, through use of a metaphor such as "No shade," which is meant to assuage the potential to darken another's reputation through one's forthcoming assertion. Reality in the African-centered worldview is constructed through the synthesizing of these two aspects of knowing. In a light illustration of this epistemology that combines the two previous examples, a football player who celebrates a touchdown with a dance in the endzone and who when questioned about it at a later press conference makes the statement, "No shade, but can't nobody touch me" might be understood to be expressing confidence in his ability while also remaining humble in an African-centered way. Again, Dixon (1977) compares this epistemology to the Eurocentric worldview, which he conceptualized as knowledge derived through a process of reflection, measurement, thinking, knowing, being, and then feeling.

Last, in examining logic in African-centered and Eurocentric worldviews, Dixon (1977) described reasoning within the African-centered worldview as a diunital, both/and approach wherein everything is understood to be "apart and united at the same time" (Carroll, 2010, p. 116). This is contrasted by a dichotomous Eurocentric worldview wherein perceptual space is understood as either/or. In an earlier paper, Dixon (1970) illustrated this concept with a discussion of Black economics, which he described as simultaneously being affected by the universal principles of economics as well as the unique qualities of the Black experience and culture. This illustration was to refute Eurocentric arguments that "economics is economics and there is no black economics" (Dixon, 1970, p. 425). Given that a primary premise of this text is that cultural factors such as race and racism have a unique impact on the mental health of African Americans, this aspect of the African-centered worldview is especially relevant to the clinician's understanding of effective treatment within this population.

In another discussion of the African-centered worldview, ways of knowing and being are rooted in seven principles known as the Nguzo Saba (Karenga, 1965, 1996). These seven principles include: (1) *umoja* (unity), (2) *kujichagulia* (self-determination), (3) *ujima* (collective work and responsibility), (4) *ujamaa* (cooperative economics), (5) *nia* (purpose), (6) *kuumba* (creativity), and (7) *imani* (faith). Together, these principles describe: (1) maintaining unity as a family, community, and race of people, (2) defining, naming, creating, and speaking for oneself, (3) building and maintaining the African American community and solving problems collectively in the community, (4) building and maintaining retail and helping businesses to profit in the African American community, (5) collectively building communities that will restore the greatness of African people, (6) finding new, innovative ways to leave communities of African descent in more beautiful and beneficial ways than the community inherited, and (7) belief that through God, family, heritage, and leaders in the struggle, victory will be experienced by all Africans, globally. Within the African American community, the Nguzo Saba provide the foundation of a cultural holiday known as Kwanzaa, which was first developed by Dr. Maulana Karenga in 1966 to unite and empower African Americans in the Los Angeles community who were dealing with the aftermath of the Watts riots. In the psychological literature, the Nguzo Saba also provide the theoretical foundation for several studies exploring the impact of African-centered principles on clinical intervention and treatment outcomes (e.g., Kwate, 2003; Lateef et al., 2022; Perry-Mitchell & Davis-Maye, 2017).

Ontological and epistemological elements across the descriptions put forth by both Dixon (1977) and Karenga (1965, 1996), as well as those put forth in other Afrocentric frameworks, suggest that an African-centered worldview is one that emphasizes spirituality, cooperation, interdependence, the collective responsibility of the individual to the group, harmony with other living things, and balance within one's own existence. According to Shipp (1983), even Black Americans who are estranged from African traditions exhibit parallel customs, evidenced for example in African American cultural norms around the role of extended family, respect for old age, and reverence toward God. The assertion that even African Americans who do not have known familial or cultural connections to African cultures retain aspects of the African-centered worldview is also empirically supported through research which suggests that African-centered interventions are broadly associated with positive outcomes in Black adults' self-concept, cultural identity, emotional coping skills, and reduction of depressive symptoms (Lateef et al., 2022). Moreover, knowledge of the African-centered worldview is also beneficial to the therapeutic relationship, as therapists who can adopt this worldview when working with African American clients may have a better understanding of the values, beliefs, frame of reference, and cultural characteristics affecting the client's presenting concerns, strengthening the bond between client and therapist (Todisco & Salomone, 1991).

To summarize, elements of the African-centered worldview that have been transferred across generations and throughout the African diaspora offer important potential resources for coping in the African American community. Application of this worldview in clinical settings, therefore, may assist therapists in formulating more culturally relevant and effective case conceptualizations and treatment approaches with this population. In the brief session excerpt that follows, the therapist draws on aspects of the African-centered worldview as she explores the concerns of Agozi, a 31-year-old Nigerian American man seeking counseling due to an ongoing history of depression. At intake, Agozi denied thoughts of suicide but endorsed several other symptoms of depression including feelings of sadness, worthlessness, hopelessness, and somatic complaints in the form of increased flareups of an autoimmune disorder he was diagnosed with two years prior to intake. As you read through the excerpt, notice how the therapist utilizes her knowledge of the African-centered worldview in guided discovery of cognitions associated with Agozi's situation. Then, complete the questions that follow the excerpt to identify additional considerations for guided discovery and cognitive restructuring with this client from an African-centered perspective.

Case Illustration: Agozi

Therapist: Okay, Agozi. The first thing we've identified for our agenda today concerns a situation with one of your sisters in Nigeria. Tell me more about that.

Agozi: Well, both of my sisters were young adults when my parents immigrated to the United States, so they stayed behind in Nigeria. I am the only sibling who was born here. Since my parents passed away, I've had to take responsibility for the care of my eldest sister.

Therapist: That sounds like quite a duty, especially across such a long distance.

Agozi: It is so stressful. Recently, it's become even more stressful. My sister has made poor choices for most of her life but now that she's gotten older the consequences of her choices are finally catching up with her. Unfortunately, I am the one who must deal with them.

Therapist: What are some of these consequences you must deal with?

Agozi: Well, my sister's romantic relationships have always been unstable. She's never settled down with someone who was reliable and could provide her with a home. Her current relationship is ending, and she doesn't have another place to live. She wants me to pay for an apartment in the city she lives in now. We have a family home she could return to, but she doesn't want to go there because she feels judged by the people in the community. To be honest, I understand how she feels to some extent.

Therapist: I see. By the sound of your voice and your body language, it seems as if you're feeling overwhelmed and frustrated by this situation.

Agozi: I am.

Therapist: Agozi, you also seem a little sad.

Agozi: That's true. I am sad about it.

Therapist: Can I ask, what is it about this situation that is most saddening for you?

Agozi: Well, I feel sad for my sister of course, but I feel sad for myself too. I'm not sure how I'm supposed to do all of this. How am I supposed to take care of myself, take care of my family home, and pay the rent on an apartment for my sister all at the same time? How am I supposed to handle all this responsibility?

Therapist: What are you telling yourself about your ability to handle this responsibility?

Agozi: I don't think I can do it. I don't even know if I want to do it.

Therapist: Let's say that both thoughts were true, that you can't do it and that you don't want to do it. What would that mean about you?

Agozi: I guess it would mean that I'm a failure.

Therapist: Who would think of you as a failure?

Agozi: My parents. I know I'm expected to handle this responsibility as the only male in the family, especially since I don't have my own family to take care of. Plus, I believe that my ancestors are looking to me to correct some of the mistakes that have occurred in our family over the past few generations. I don't have room to fail. But I have a right to live my life too.

Therapist: It sounds like you're in a war between two sets of needs, responsibility to your family and responsibility to yourself, is that right?

Agozi: Yes, that's a good way to put it.

Therapist: So, what would happen if either side won?

Agozi: I'd be unhappy either way.

Therapist: Agozi, with thoughts about being unhappy no matter what, I can see why you're feeling sad and depressed. These types of thoughts about self, the world, and the future lead to feelings of depression often. Perhaps we can work on brokering a peace between the two sides in this war. Does that sound okay?

Agozi: Yes.

The case of Agozi offers unique considerations for application of the African-centered worldview in the clinical context. In the session excerpt above, evidence of the African-centered worldview is apparent in the client's presenting problem, as well as the therapist's identification of a cognitive target (Waltman et al., 2021). First, African-centered values are evident in Agozi's concern for his sister and his sense of responsibility to his family. As previously mentioned, the African-centered worldview places value on interpersonal relationships and an intergenerational family structure (Thabede, 2008). Whereas family structure within a Eurocentric framework is typically conceptualized according to the nuclear family unit of mother, father, and children, with primary responsibility for children ending once they enter adulthood (Katz, 1985; Simões & Alberto, 2015), family structures within African communities are often more expansive and inclusive of extended family members and fictive kin, with responsibility for care lasting into adulthood depending on the social needs of the individual. For example, in many African communities, men have an obligation to care for the widows and orphans of a deceased relative (Mafumbate, 2019). In African American families, many aspects of the African-centered family structure have been retained, as extended family members and fictive kin often play a role in the socialization and care of children and other family members, including the provision of social and financial support (Causey et al., 2015). Agozi is a first-generation child of Nigerian immigrants and thus may have experienced some level of acculturation contributing to changes in his cultural beliefs; nevertheless, given the transportability of the African-centered worldview among Black people living in the United States, Agozi has likely retained many African-centered family values. He may, however, be experiencing some difficulty balancing these values with those of the prevailing U.S. culture, leading to what he endorsed as the "war" between value systems.

A second closely related issue of potential relevance to the African-centered worldview, and Agozi's chief complaint, concerns African-centered beliefs around the relationship between the absence of a harmonious relationship with members of the supernatural world and illness (Caroline et al., 2015). Specifically, Caroline and her colleagues (2015) explain that in the African-centered worldview, both psychopathology and physical illness result when disharmony exists between people and the ancestors. Agozi is experiencing a decline in mood as well as flareups of an autoimmune disorder that coincide with the onset of his current episode of depression. Within an African-centered framework, Agozi may relate these difficulties to his belief that his ancestors expect him to correct some of the mistakes that have occurred in his family over time. As the therapist continues to develop her case formulation and approach, treatment should be holistic in nature, emphasizing psychological, spiritual, and physical healing (Caroline et al., 2015). Continued guided discovery, therefore, may include gaining a phenomenological understanding (Waltman et al., 2021) of Agozi's views on the spiritual aspects of his mental distress and physical illnesses.

At this point in the session, guided discovery has focused on targeting Agozi's most central cognitions and their emotional impacts. Accordingly, the therapist has concentrated on fleshing out the underlying meanings Agozi associates with his most distressing thoughts, as targeting these emotionally significant meanings allows the therapist and client to work at a deeper level (Waltman et al., 2021). To do so, the therapist implemented a classic strategy, the downward arrow technique, with the African-centered worldview as a conceptual frame. The therapist began by first asking clarifying questions such as "Can I ask, what is it about this situation that is most saddening for you?" and "What are you telling yourself about your ability to handle this responsibility?" to identify distressing thoughts occurring in the situation with his sister. Upon learning that Agozi does not think he can or even wants to handle the responsibility of caring for his sister, the therapist then implements the downward arrow technique, asking the client "What would that mean about you?" Agozi's response to this question was significant, with Agozi indicating that his thoughts in the situation mean "I'm a failure." While this language is consistent with what CBT therapists typically conceptualize as a core belief, knowledge of the African-centered man-to-person axiology (Dixon, 1977) led the therapist to continue her query, exploring aspects of being and communalism with the question, "Who would think of you as a failure?" As a result of this line of inquiry, the therapist and Agozi were able to gain a clearer understanding of what to target to bring about meaningful change in the client's life; that is, his belief "I'll be unhappy either way." Throughout the guided discovery, the therapist further drew upon the African-centered worldview through her use of imagery to describe Agozi's problem as a "war between two sets of values."

Activity 3.1: Continuing the Case of Agozi

Imagine you are the therapist in the case of Agozi. Consider his presenting concerns and the African-centered worldview. Then, respond to the following questions.

1. Based on the African-centered worldview, what questions might you ask Agozi to develop a shared definition of happiness?
2. Based on the African-centered worldview, what questions might you ask Agozi to further understand the emotional experience associated with his belief "I'll be unhappy either way"?

Assessment of an African-Centered Worldview

In the case illustration above, Agozi was a first-generation son of Nigerian immigrants. This aspect of his identity may have uniquely influenced the immediacy of African-centered values in his life. Like Agozi, individuals throughout the African American community vary in the extent to which they endorse an African-centered consciousness according to factors such as acculturation, racial identity development, and racial and gender socialization. Accordingly, therapists should work to appreciate the ways in which these attributes of self and identity may influence individual expressions of an African-centered worldview (Belgrave & Allison, 2019). Sue (2001) developed one of the most popular identity frameworks, which he organized according to universal, group, and individual levels of personal identity. In this framework, *universal* aspects of personal identity refer to commonalties shared among all human beings, including "(a) biological and physical similarities, (b) common life experiences (birth, death, love, sadness, and others), (c) self-awareness, and (d) ability to use symbols such as language" (Sue, 2001, p. 793). *Group* aspects of personal identity refer to shared cultural values and beliefs with specific reference groups. These groups may be fixed, such as race, gender, ability, and age, or nonfixed such as education, socioeconomic status, marital status, and geographic location. Finally, *individual* aspects of identity refer to characteristics that are unique to an individual's personal history, interests, and abilities. Given the diversity that exists within the African American community, direct assessment of an African-centered worldview can provide information necessary to determine how these various dimensions of self and identity influence an individual client's psychological orientation (Belgrave & Allison, 2019).

Within the literature, there are several scales designed to assist therapists with the task of assessing aspects of the African-centered worldview (e.g., Baldwin, 1984; Kambon, 1992). The Africentrism Scale, for example, was developed to assess an African-centered worldview according to the principles of the Nguzo Saba (Grills & Longshore, 1996). This assessment, therefore, explores the extent to which individuals are Africentrically oriented based on the values of unity, self-determination, collective work and responsibility, cooperative economics, purpose, creativity, and faith. Example items on the Africentrism Scale include "Black people should make their community better than it was when they found it," "I owe something to Black people who suffered before me," "The problems of other Black people are their problems, not mine," and "The success I have had is mainly because of me, not anyone else." According to research conducted by Kwate (2003), these items load onto two factors labeled *General Africentrism* and *Individualism-Communalism*.

Use of instruments such as the Africentrism Scale (Grills & Longshore, 1996) provides valuable assessment information, as they help to clarify the lens through which clients interpret situations and make meaning. These scales additionally provide a way to measure the effectiveness of interventions designed to increase African-centered consciousness. As discussed in Chapter 1, a considerable amount of healing from the effects of racism involves consciousness-raising and claiming one's voice and power in a system of oppression. Furthermore, increasing consciousness of the African-centered worldview in particular is thought to bring healing to the lives of people of African descent by restoring a sense of self that is authentic to the individual's being and supportive of the cultural and intellectual autonomy of people of African descent (Caroline et al., 2015). Accordingly, therapeutic interventions when working with African Americans may be enhanced by assisting clients with reaching greater African self-consciousness in terms of addressing psychopathology, which within an African-centered framework occurs because of disharmony between an individual and God, family, the community, or the ancestors (Caroline et al., 2015; Kwate, 2003). For example, returning to the case of Agozi, cognitive restructuring informed by J. S. Beck's (2020) information processing theory with this client may focus on helping him to acknowledge ways in which he is already living consistently with his values, as well as looking to the cultural insights of his ancestors for wisdom, performing body-centric interventions rooted in African healing and movement, and drawing on spirituality to enrich self-compassion and loving-kindness (Byrdsong et al., 2013).

Reflection 3.1: Comparing Afrocentric and Eurocentric Worldviews

Table 3.1 provides a comparison of values associated with Afrocentric and Eurocentric worldviews. As suggested from the table, one of the most significant differences between these worldviews is collectivist versus an individualistic orientation. What are the implications of these differences for diagnosis, case conceptualization, and treatment planning? For example,

Table 3.1 Comparison of Afrocentric and Eurocentric Values

Afrocentric Values	Eurocentric Values
Collective work and responsibility	Competition
Cooperative economics	Each person pulls themselves up by their own bootstraps
Interdependence	Independence
The group is the primary unit	The individual is the primary unit
Everyone is valuable	Value is hierarchical
Spiritualism	Dualism
Flexible time schedules	Rigid time schedules

how might a focus on one's inner experience, as well as goals and interventions that are ultimately reflective of what is best for the individual, be out of sync with African-centered values that prioritize the group and interdependence? How can you, as a clinician, be more sensitive to these differences?

Positive Racial Socialization

So far in this chapter, I've discussed the African-centered worldview and have illustrated ways in which this worldview may be relevant to treatment. As stated, individuals may vary in the extent to which they endorse an African-centered worldview due to factors such as parental upbringing and acculturation. Another factor that influences endorsement of an African-centered worldview while also serving as a source of protection and coping in itself is racial socialization. *Racial socialization* can be defined as "behaviors, communications, and interactions that address how African Americans ought to feel about their cultural heritage and how they should respond to the racial hostility or confusion in American society" (Brown, 2008, p. 33). A recent meta-analytic review of research shows that positive racial socialization has broadly been found to benefit mental health and wellbeing including decreases in internalizing symptoms such as anxiety, depression, and low self-esteem, as well as reductions in externalizing behaviors such as aggression, going to jail, and anti-social traits (Reynolds & Gonzales-Backen, 2017). Likewise, other studies substantiate additional associations between positive racial socialization and academic performance (Del Toro & Wang, 2021), the ability to identify Black stereotypes in the media (Adams-Bass et al., 2014), and planning and active coping (Womack & Sloan, 2017).

More specific to the healing of racial trauma, research has also shown that positive racial socialization may mitigate the effects of covert and overt forms of racial discrimination. Recent research conducted by Su et al. (2021), for example, found that experiences of racist events and racial microaggressions were associated with higher levels of alcohol consumption and more alcohol problems; however, positive racial socialization by friends moderated these associations. Similarly, according to research conducted by Brown and Tylka (2011), African Americans who receive more positive racial socialization messages from their parents or caregivers as teenagers have greater resilience when confronted with racial discrimination. Moreover, according to this research, racial socialization messages that emphasize one's cultural legacy have an especially significant impact on resilience in the face of discrimination, suggesting that messages which focus on one's cultural legacy "may be more helpful than messages that simply instruct children to be proud of being an African American without providing a foundation for why they should be proud (e.g., the history and legacy of civil rights)" (Brown & Tylka, 2011, p. 276).

In sum, African Americans with stronger racial socialization tend to have better overall mental health and are better equipped to handle the psychological fallout of racial prejudice, discrimination, or harassment more specifically. According to Okeke-Adeyanju et al. (2014), the primary themes of racial socialization include cultural pride, preparation for bias, egalitarianism, self-worth, and responding appropriately to negative messages. Racial socialization through *cultural pride* involves communicating messages that highlight the history, strengths, and accomplishments of African Americans. *Preparation for bias* involves gaining the skills necessary to handle and cope with negative race-based encounters. *Egalitarianism* involves working toward racial equality, while *self-worth* focuses on one's view of self. Last, *responding appropriately to negative messages* refers to the development of strategies to challenge and eliminate stereotyped views of African Americans in one's thinking (Okeke-Adeyanju et al., 2014).

Given its psychosocial benefits, CBT therapists can expand their proverbial "toolbox" by encouraging clients to adopt cognitive and behavioral strategies that support positive racial socialization. Many of the aspects of racial socialization described above such as cultural pride, preparation for bias, self-worth, and responding appropriately to negative messages can be facilitated through interventions that also assist with positive racial identity development. For example, parents and caregivers who provide their children with racial pride messages to encourage positive racial identity development also provide positive racial socialization because these messages promote feelings of self- and collective-worth and teach about racial inequalities and strategies for coping with racial adversity (Neblett et al., 2009). For therapists, this implies that integrating strategies such as the use of affirmations, learning about Black history, and participation in Black cultural events and institutions in both family and individual contexts into the client's treatment plan may support positive racial socialization and have a positive effect on clients' ability to cope with racial discrimination.

Another way African Americans can experience positive racial socialization, particularly egalitarianism, is through participation in Black social movements. In the past, many of these social movements have focused on an appreciation for Black aesthetics and culture. The Black is Beautiful movement, for example, began in the 1960s with the goal of counteracting the harmful psychological impacts of negative messages about Black beauty and culture. This movement, as described by journalist Lilly Workneh (2022), initially started behind the camera of Kwame Brathwaite, a Harlem photographer who sought to overthrow the conventional Black aesthetic at the time, which was preferential toward White hair textures and styles, in favor of natural hair and African designs. More recently, the beauty of Black people and Black culture has been widely embraced through social media movements such as #BlackGirlMagic, #BlackBoyJoy, and #BlackExcellence.

The appreciation for Black beauty and culture evident in these movements often provides a framework for responding to minoritized experiences in the contemporary moment, particularly among Black women (Q. Williams et al., 2022). Participation in other social movements in the African American community that emphasize equal treatment in society can further bolster these effects. For example, high levels of support for, and to a lesser extent, action in the Black Lives Matter movement, which initially started in 2013 in response to the murder of Trayvon Martin, a 17-year-old African American boy who was killed by a neighbor while walking home from a convenience store, has been found to be protective again depressive symptoms in the context of discrimination (Watson-Singleton et al., 2021).

To summarize, positive racial socialization provides several psychosocial benefits, especially enhanced ability to cope with racial discrimination (Brown, 2008; Brown & Tylka, 2011; Reynolds & Gonzales-Backen, 2017; Su et al., 2021; Womack & Sloan, 2017). Therefore, CBT therapists should consider drawing upon activities that foster positive racial socialization to promote healing and empowerment among African American clients. Table 3.2 provides examples of specific activities CBT therapists may consider utilizing to support positive racial socialization (Steele & Newton, 2023).

Religion and Spirituality

As indicated previously, religion and spirituality are key aspects of the African-centered worldview that remain salient for many African Americans, including those who are estranged from more traditional African practices (Shipp, 1983). In fact, statistics indicate that 83 percent of polled Black Americans have an absolute belief in God, while an additional 11 percent have a fairly certain belief (Pew Research Center, 2014). Moreover, 75 percent of Black Americans state that religion is very important to their lives, with another 16 percent endorsing religion as somewhat important. Accordingly, many African Americans view religion and spirituality as significant sources of hope and meaning when faced with obstacles, making these factors crucial to understanding wellness and coping within this community (Avent Harris et al., 2021). Consider the case of Sheryl and notice the integration of religious and spiritual themes in her discussion of her current methods of coping at intake.

Case Illustration: Sheryl

Sheryl is a 35-year-old CEO of a large financial consulting firm in Chicago, Illinois. Sheryl, who is originally from a small rural town in the southern part of the state, initiated counseling due to symptoms of depression

Table 3.2 Cognitive and Behavioral Activities that Support Positive Racial Socialization

Cognitive Activities

Activity	Description
Affirmation Cards	Clients create affirmation cards reflecting thoughtful first-person statements that encourage positive thinking and good self-esteem. These cards may focus on developing new narratives about oneself and challenging internalized racism and self-hate.
Naming Internalized Racism	Clients conduct a historical review of negative core beliefs and schemas, especially those reflecting internalized racism, identifying the stereotypes and negative thoughts, feelings, and behaviors associated with various life events.
Recalling Experiences with Racism and Responding to Self with Compassion	Clients use the cognitive model to identify maladaptive thoughts, feelings, and behaviors that develop in response to racism and practice cognitive restructuring emphasizing self-compassion.
Responding to a Friend	Clients externalize their problems and develop solutions or cognitive reframes by pretending to give advice to a friend in a similar situation.
Identifying Proud Family Moments	Clients modify negative core beliefs and schemas by looking to achievements made by family members or individuals they admire as data to support the development of new more positive beliefs.
Creating a Catchphrase	Clients create a catchphrase or saying they can use to boost themselves during times of adversity. Examples include "I come from survivors, I am a survivor" and "What we won't do is give up."

Behavioral Activities

Activity	Description
Self-Compassion/ Lovingkindness Meditation	Clients engage in meditation, focusing on being non-judgmental, loving, kind, accepting, and compassionate toward oneself in response to racism and racial trauma.
Conducting Interviews	Clients interview others who have experienced racism and/or racial trauma, focusing on identifying common reactions and problem-solving approaches.
Participating in Black Cultural Events	Clients participate in Black cultural events such as annual Juneteenth or Kwanzaa celebrations.
Attending Black Cultural Institutions	Clients attend cultural institutions, i.e., places that document, interpret, and facilitate engagement with one's cultural heritage such as the Smithsonian National Museum of African American History and Culture in Washington, DC or a local organization.

Source: Steele, J. M., & Newton, C. S. (2023). *Black lives are beautiful: 50 tools to heal from trauma and promote positive racial identity*. Routledge.

including low mood, poor sleep, headaches, and feelings of hopelessness. Precipitating events leading to the current episode of depression included racial hostility at her place of employment, as well as concern for her 14-year-old daughter who was also experiencing racial hostility in her freshman year of high school. Sheryl explained that upon entering high school, her daughter, Mariah, enrolled into a predominantly White college preparatory academy where she has been isolated from her peers and frequently targeted with negative racial stereotypes by both students and teachers. While Sheryl empathizes with her daughter, the difficulties Mariah is experiencing at school are causing tension in their relationship. Mariah has become increasingly anxious, progressing to school refusal. Sheryl acknowledges the pain Mariah is in, but also believes that racism is part of the Black experience and should not prevent Mariah from going to school and succeeding. Sheryl uses herself as an example, noting her success as one of the few African American students in her hometown and the fact that she continues to excel at work despite experiencing racial microaggressions such as being labeled as too aggressive and paid less than White colleagues she outperforms. Sheryl does admit, however, that although she excels at work, the racial hostility she experiences has taken a psychological toll, with Sheryl stating, "I struggle to see God's plan in this, but I trust his purpose for my life" and "I don't know what I would do without prayer."

As illustrated in the case of Sheryl, religion and spirituality are one means through which African Americans derive a sense of purpose, direction, and coping when challenged by racism. This makes sense given the statistics presented earlier which indicate that 75 percent of Black Americans believe religion is very important to their lives (Pew Research Center, 2014). Adding additional context to this statistic, not only do a vast majority of African Americans consider religion and spirituality to be very important to their lives, 47 percent attend religious services at least once a week, 36 percent attend once or twice a month, and only 17 percent seldomly or never attend religious services. The religious group most identified with among African Americans is historically Black protestant (Pew Research Center, 2014). Therefore, given the centrality of religion and spirituality among African Americans, as well as the number of African Americans who identify as historically Black protestant, knowledge of values rooted in what is known as the Black church is critical to understanding mental health and strategies for healing from racism within this population (Plunkett, 2014).

According to Plunkett (2014), the *Black church* may be defined as "any specific institution in which the congregation is predominantly African American even though the religious denomination itself is predominantly White" (p. 209). Within this definition, the primary historically Black traditions include the African Methodist Episcopal Church, the African Methodist Episcopal Zion Church, the Christian Methodist Episcopal Church, the National Baptist Convention, U.S.A., Incorporated, the National Baptist Convention of America, Unincorporated, the Progressive National Baptist Convention, and the Church of God in Christ. An extensive amount of psychological research has documented the axiological tenets of these traditions that make them beneficial to coping with racism (Constantine et al., 2000; Taylor & Chatters, 2010). Broadly, the Black church is connected to a greater African-centered worldview wherein all aspects of life are dependent upon one's relationship with God. This relationship, in turn, is characterized by the core values of love, inclusiveness, justice, and freedom (Plunkett, 2014). Within this context, many African Americans view their relationship with God as one central to coping with problems, including racism, because it provides hope that a just and loving God will answer the prayers of anyone who comes to him in faith. Referring to the case illustration of Sheryl, this point is exhibited in Sheryl's belief that through prayer and her relationship with God, an explanation for how to survive and thrive despite her difficulties will eventually be revealed.

In further consideration of the role of religion and spirituality in coping among African Americans, therapists should keep in mind that while values associated with the Black church provide sources of coping, they also inform negative attitudes toward professional help-seeking among African Americans. Plunkett (2014) noted that African Americans with strong ties to the Black church may view seeking professional counseling as a lack of faith. They may also think God will not intervene where there is a lack of faith and, therefore, engage in alternatives to professional help-seeking such as increased individual prayer, communal prayer, and church attendance. Therapists may assuage some of these concerns and increase the cultural relevance of the services they provide by encouraging clients to think about how the tenets of CBT align with their spiritual beliefs. For example, many African Americans find hope in scriptures that promise success by meditating on the word of God and being transformed by the renewing of the mind, which is consistent with CBT principles associated with cognitive restructuring and mindfulness. Additionally, therapists may further draw parallels between spiritual coping and CBT by acknowledging the value of activities such as individual prayer, communal prayer, and church attendance in behavioral activation and mindfulness practices.

Finally, in concluding the discussion on the role of religion and spirituality in coping with racism, it is important to note that while a vast majority of African Americans endorse Black protestant beliefs, some subscribe to different religious traditions. For example, approximately three percent of Black American adults identify with a non-Christian faith such as Islam (Mohamed et al., 2021). Another three percent of Black American adults identify as atheist or agnostic. Therefore, when exploring potential religious or spiritual coping, therapists should broach this topic broadly, for example, using a question such as "Do you have any spiritual or religious beliefs that are important to how you see the world or cope with problems?" Moreover, therapists should also be sensitive to the potential for religious trauma among African Americans, particularly as it relates to sexual orientation and abuse. In these cases, it may be more helpful to focus on coping derived from one's personal sense of spirituality or relationship with God, rather than benefits associated with membership in a specific religion or church body.

Cultural Healing Practices

Within the psychological literature, an increasing number of clinical models advocate for the inclusion of cultural healing practices in the treatment of raced-based trauma and clinical concerns. According to Chioneso et al. (2020), *cultural healing practices* refer to "specific rituals, drumming, dancing, singing, and storytelling" (p. 99). From an African-centered perspective, these practices foster healing by connecting individuals with each other, the ancestors, and the spiritual realm. In their community healing framework pertaining to racial trauma, for example, Chioneso et al. (2020) utilized storytelling as a tool for resisting oppression, fostering healing, promoting spiritual communion, restoring cultural identities, building community, and developing counterhegemonic stories. Specifically, the authors described a variety of interventions including testimony therapy, sociotherapy, digital storytelling, documentaries, public community reflection events, and developing new community narratives, which they found promoted social bonding and commitments, enhanced the wellbeing of others, increased connectedness, enhanced collective memory, and fostered critical consciousness. From a CBT perspective, these types of interventions also have the potential to offer creative and culturally congruent approaches to cognitive and behavioral change, including weakening maladaptive schemas and strengthening more adaptive schemas.

The Telling One's Story exercise illustrated in Chapter 8 is one example of how storytelling may be used to help clients tell their personal stories, find meaning in their stories, and tell themselves new stories, with, from a CBT perspective, the intent of helping clients review and modify maladaptive core and intermediate beliefs. Another storytelling exercise titled, Your Family Story, draws upon elements of positive racial socialization discussed earlier in this chapter such as cultural pride, preparation for bias, egalitarianism, self-worth, and responding appropriately to negative messages, with a similar goal of challenging maladaptive beliefs about one's ability to surmount discrimination and other racial stressors (Steele & Newton, 2023). In this exercise, clients are encouraged to find the oldest living member of their family and engage them in an interview using the questions below with the goal of learning how family members have overcome racism in the past.

The interview can be completed in one setting, over several weeks, or across several months.

- When and where were you born?
- How did our family come to live there?
- What is your earliest childhood memory?
- How did our family deal with hard times and setbacks?
- Do you remember experiencing any discrimination or prejudice? If so, how did you handle it?
- What family traditions you remember?
- What are some of the stories that have come down to you about your parents, grandparents, or maybe even more distant ancestors?
- What things bring you a sense of pride concerning our family heritage?
- What are struggles you have had to overcome as a person of color? How have you overcome those struggles?
- Of all the things you learned from your parents, what do you feel was the most valuable?

Once the client has completed the interview, data obtained from the relative's story can be used to help develop counternarratives to the stories of bondage, servitude, and oppression that at times seem to define the Black community and often lead to maladaptive race-related beliefs or internalized racism (Steele, 2020). For example, returning to the earlier case of Sheryl, over the course of therapy, Sheryl was able to identify the belief, "Talking about my pain makes me weak," which was maladaptive because it led to loneliness and depression, and placed a strain on the relationship with her daughter, Mariah. As part of the Your Family Story exercise, Sheryl learned about how her grandmother had been one of only a few Black registered nurses in the Bay Area of California during the 1960s. During this time, Sheryl's grandmother often encountered racism from patients who were verbally abusive, questioned her competence, or outright refused to receive care from a Black nurse. In response to this racial hostility, Sheryl's grandmother recalled gathering with the other Black nurses in her community for weekly prayer meetings. At these meetings, the nurses would pray, but they would also share their feelings and concerns, receive affirmation and support, and develop plans to alert hospital administration to the treatment they were receiving. Sheryl's grandmother reported that as a result, she and the other women were able to see changes in the hospital system, although they took time. More important, the women were able to receive the emotional support they needed to maintain the psychological strength and fortitude necessary to handle the challenges of integration.

Through her completion of the Your Family Story exercise, Sheryl was able to decrease the believability of "Talking about my pain makes me weak" from 99 percent to 5 percent. She additionally developed the alternative belief, "Talking about my pain gives me the strength and support I need to keep going." To strengthen the new belief, Sheryl and her therapist completed an advantages/disadvantages analysis of the old belief, examining the advantages and disadvantages of continuing to hold the old belief, as well as the advantages and disadvantages of changing the old belief (J. S. Beck, 2020). Sheryl then kept a positive data log, documenting evidence to support her new belief, "Talking about my pain gives me the strength and support I need to keep going," as she tested sharing more of her thoughts and feelings with friends and family (Padesky, 1994).

Activity 3.2: Your Family Story

Try the Your Family Story exercise for yourself. Schedule a time to interview an elder family member, using the questions provided previously as a guide. Then, reflect on this process and the information you learned using the reflection questions that follow.

Reflection Questions

1. To what extent did this exercise help you to identify and challenge any maladaptive core beliefs or schemas in your life? How so?
2. Based on your own experience, what considerations should you make when implementing this exercise with clients? For example, might it be helpful to encourage clients to journal their thoughts after the experience or develop their own set of reflection questions?

Beyond storytelling, dance movement therapy is another popular form of healing within the African American community (Farr, 1997). Within the African-centered worldview, dance and movement may be considered one expression of Afrocentric values such as spirituality, community, and harmony with God and nature. Psychologically, dance and movement also provide the benefit of creating a sense of empowerment and belongingness with those whom dance is shared (Young & Goldstein, 2023). Williams et al. (1999), for example, described the use of dance among other cultural practices as a tool for developing a self-loving spiritual being in a therapy group for African American women. According to these authors, the women who participated in the group reported significant personal benefit from the group, including safety, belonging, and culturally congruent processing of life experiences. Similarly, Campbell (2019) also advocated for the use of dance movement therapy in educational programming with African American youth in Chicago's Roseland community. Elements of the programming, titled Healing in Motion, included opening rituals for each module with body-based components to help increase awareness and promote grounding, as well as additional activities designed to utilize movement as a form of connection and expression. Relevant to healing from racism, these elements of the program not only have the potential to increase awareness and promote grounding, connection, and emotional expression, but also to facilitate healing from transgenerational trauma, according to Campbell (2019).

Given the emotional, spiritual, and psychological benefits of dance and movement, CBT therapists may consider incorporating this strategy into approaches that draw on use of the body to promote mindfulness or enhance mood. For example, when engaging clients in activity scheduling or behavioral activation, therapists may encourage clients to consider dance as an activity that brings about a sense of pleasure and/or accomplishment. Likewise, mindful dance may also be used to decrease cognitive fusion and cultivate present-moment and somatic awareness when experiencing symptoms associated with racial discrimination or hostility.

Strengths-based CBT

Finally, the sources of coping discussed throughout this chapter may be integrated into CBT using approaches that allow therapists to focus on client strengths rather than their problems. One specific tool that assists therapists with gathering information about client strengths is the strengths-based cognitive conceptualization diagram (J. S. Beck, 2020). Like the traditional problem-focused cognitive conceptualization diagram, the strengths-based cognitive conceptualization diagram organizes the client's patterns of cognitions and behaviors. Its specific components include: (a) important life events and personal assets, (b) adaptive core beliefs, (c) adaptive intermediate beliefs, (d) adaptive coping strategies, and (e) situations, adaptive automatic thoughts, and adaptive behaviors. With this positive data, therapists can more intentionally focus on how clients successfully overcome challenges, while also identifying ways to strengthen positive beliefs and coping strategies (J. S. Beck, 2020).

To obtain this data from clients, J. S. Beck (2020) suggested posing questions that explore a client's adaptive core and intermediate beliefs such as, "What are the clients most central adaptive beliefs about themselves? Others? The world?" and "What general assumptions, rules, attitudes, and values does the client have?" Padesky and Mooney (2012), however, provide more specific guidance on the exploration of client strengths. Their framework, known as the strengths-based CBT model, consists of the following four steps: (1) search for strengths, (2) construct a personal model of resilience, (3) apply the personal model of resilience to life difficulties, and (4) practice resilience. Step 1, search for strengths, consists of working with clients to identify strategies, beliefs, and personal assets that can promote positive qualities. This is done by working with clients to search for "hidden strengths" in everyday experiences. Step 2 consists of creating a list of the strategies to implement the strengths identified at step 1 (i.e., a personal model of resilience) that can be generalized to a variety of situations, as well as images or metaphors to make these strategies memorable. Step 3 consists of helping the client think about how these strengths can be applied to a specific obstacle. In step 4, the client and therapist devise behavioral experiments to apply the personal model of resilience (Padesky & Mooney, 2012).

The paragraphs that follow illustrate how strengths-based CBT (Padesky & Mooney, 2012) and the strengths-based cognitive conceptualization diagram (J. S. Beck, 2020) was utilized with a case example, Alicia. The case is presented, followed by session excerpts illustrating guided discovery at each step of strengths-based CBT, emphasizing the sources of coping discussed throughout this chapter. The case is concluded with a completed strengths-based cognitive conceptualization diagram, drawing from the data obtained throughout the guided discovery.

Case Illustration: Alicia

Alicia is a 19-year-old African American woman seeking counseling due to difficulties in her transition to college. Her primary symptoms include irritability, social isolation, and depressed mood. At intake, Alicia reported poor interactions with instructors and peers. Explaining these difficulties, Alicia described frequent microaggressions in her environment, for example, the absence of BIPOC perspectives in her courses and being excluded from social events by her roommates. In discussing her concerns further, Alicia expressed regret about her decision to accept a scholarship to the predominantly White university she is currently enrolled at rather than attending one of the historically Black colleges her parents went to. According to Alicia, she was raised in a home that emphasized racial pride and she looked forward to experiencing new racial awakenings similar to what her parents say they experienced as a result of their time at college. Instead, Alicia reports feeling devalued and, at times, demeaned because of her race at her current university. While exploring this issue at her third session, Alicia states, "I've made the biggest mistake of my life. I just can't handle this." In response, the therapist utilized Padesky and Mooney's (2012) strengths-based CBT model to help Alicia more accurately perceive strengths and resources that might allow her to solve her problems and manage her emotions more effectively. The dialogue that follows is taken from the therapist's implementation of the model at each step. As you read through the dialogue, notice the therapist's intentional inclusion of African-centered sources of coping as she works with Alicia to increase awareness of unacknowledged strengths.

Step 1: Search for Strengths

Therapist:	Alicia, thank you for trusting me enough to share something that's clearly causing you a great deal of pain. It sounds like you're feeling overwhelmed and hopeless about your future at the university. Am I understanding that correctly?
Alicia:	Yes, that's exactly right.
Therapist:	Sometimes, exploring your strengths can be helpful when trying to figure out how to cope with or overcome challenges in your life. Could we spend some time working on that today?
Alicia:	Sure.
Therapist:	Great. In previous sessions, you've talked a lot about being raised in a home that emphasized racial pride. I understand that for many Black families, this includes not only instilling pride in your cultural heritage and traditions, but also preparing you for experiences with discrimination. This is often done by talking about the history of racism in this country and teaching you how to respond. Did your family have conversations like this while you were growing up?
Alicia:	Yes.
Therapist:	What were these conversations like?
Alicia:	Well, education was always important to my parents for a lot of reasons. To them, education is one of the few strategies Black people have for achieving upward socioeconomic mobility and equality. So, they talked to me a lot about the importance of education as a Black person. I was really supported by my parents with my schoolwork, and I always tried to do my best in my classes.
Therapist:	So, it sounds like you're saying you took your parents' advice to heart and have been successful academically, is that correct?
Alicia:	Yes.
Therapist:	And, did you say there were other reasons education was important to your parents as well?
Alicia:	Yes. They often talked to me about how education was at the center of the Civil Rights Movement and desegregation. Unfortunately, even though it was a long time ago, not much has changed.
Therapist:	How do you think they got through it back then?
Alicia:	Well, I know community was important. And standing on your principles.
Therapist:	Okay, Alicia. I hear a few personal qualities that may serve as strengths as you attempt to deal with the microaggressions you experience at school. First, you're very knowledgeable about Black history, and second, you're a good student. I also hear quite a few strengths you can draw upon from your ancestors

and members of your community, things like community bonds
and principled action.

Alicia: That's true.

Therapist: Let's see what other strengths you can come up with.

Alicia: Sounds good. [The therapist and Alicia continue to identify
strengths from Alicia's personal qualities and cultural heritage,
creating a list.]

Step 2: Construct a Personal Model of Resilience

Therapist: Now that we've created a list of strengths, let's talk about how
you've put these strengths into action in the past. Which would
you like to start with?

Alicia: Let's talk about community first.

Therapist: Okay. Tell me about how you've used community to help with
problems before.

Alicia: Well, when I was in high school, I noticed that my little sister's
school library didn't have many books with diverse characters
or authors. In response, some of my friends and I started a community fundraiser and were able to donate over 100 books not
only to my sister's school, but to other grade schools as well.

Therapist: Wow, that's pretty impressive! What were some of the specific
steps you took to accomplish all of that?

Alicia: Umm, well, first I had to see that there was a problem. Because
the dominant racial group is considered the norm, sometimes
people don't even notice what's missing. Then, I had to convince people that this was an important issue and that we
needed to do something about it. After that, I had to organize
volunteers and communicate the need to the community to get
their support.

Therapist: So, it sounds like it took a lot of skills for you to be able to
mobilize the community for this project. You were a critical
thinker, you were a motivator, and you were an organizer.

Alicia: I guess I never thought about it that way.

Therapist: Were there any there any unhelpful thoughts or difficult emotions you had to deal with?

Alicia: Yes.

Therapist: What were they?

Alicia: I was really worried that nobody would help.

Therapist: What did you tell yourself to deal with that worry?

Alicia: I just focused on having faith and trusting that God would
make everything work out.

Therapist: Okay. So, another way you utilized your strengths was by focusing on faith and trusting in God. Alicia, I think you're coming

up with a lot of strategies that may be useful in dealing with the microaggressions you experience at your university. Let's talk about how you've used some of the other strengths on your list and then think about how you can apply the strategies you identify to your current situation. We'll call this your personal model of resilience.

Alicia: Okay. [The therapist and Alicia continue to identify strategies to include in the personal model of resilience.]

Step 3: Apply the Personal Model of Resilience

Therapist: Alicia, so far, you've said you believe that attending a PWI was a mistake, which has led to you feeling overwhelmed and hopeless.

Alicia: Yes.

Therapist: Ideally, how would you like to respond to this situation instead?

Alicia: Well, I'd like to feel hopeful and empowered.

Therapist: How can some of the strategies in your personal model of resilience help you to do that?

Alicia: The first thing I can do is focus on my faith. I know that God has a purpose for everything and that he can make all these problems work out for my good.

Therapist: Okay, focus on your faith. What else can you do?

Alicia: I guess I can also draw on my community and advocacy skills. There aren't very many Black students on campus but there are some. I'm sure I'm not the only one going through this. I can seek support from them or from some of our allies. I could even get people together to advocate for changes if I wanted to.

Therapist: These sound like good ideas, Alicia. Is there an image you can hold in your mind that could help you remember these strategies?

Alicia: I guess I could think about it like being a sojourner in a foreign land. I'm there to learn and maybe even build relationships and help others, but I always have a home to return to.

Therapist: That's beautiful, Alicia! Usually, a next step would be for us to develop some kind of experiment for you to test these strategies out; however, given that the microaggressions you experience at the university are ongoing, I'm thinking you will naturally have opportunities to implement what you've talked about today.

Alicia: Probably so.

Therapist: With that said, why don't you take note of how well the strategies in your personal model of resilience work for you over the week, and at our next session, we can talk about any adjustments that might be necessary.

Alicia: Okay.

Step 4: Practice Resilience

Therapist: Alicia, how did use of your personal model of resilience go over the week?
Alicia: It was kind of rocky, but I'd say that it went well overall.
Therapist: Tell me more about it.
Alicia: This week, we had an assignment where we had to write an opinion paper on the book *The Alchemist*. I wrote about limitations in the book in terms of the potential for its themes to communicate that people don't achieve their goals because they simply don't desire them enough, which essentially minimizes or invalidates the experiences of BIPOC and other marginalized populations. I shared this opinion during our class discussion and a couple of the other Black students in course agreed with me. I thought about community in my personal model of resilience and decided to introduce myself when class was over. We're getting together on Tuesday. So, I guess you could say that over the past week I was a sojourner using her community building and critical thinking skills.
Therapist: I like that, Alicia! It sounds like you're feeling a little bit more in control of the situation.
Alicia: I am. I'm still disappointed but I also think there are some good opportunities to help make things better for African Americans who come after me, which has always been important to me.
Therapist: That's awesome, Alicia!

In the case of Alicia, culturally responsive exploration of strengths is illustrated through the therapist's acknowledgment of racial pride as a potential source of coping. Broadly, parental socialization messages emphasizing appreciation of Black history and aesthetics tend to be positively associated with college student academic engagement (Banerjee et al., 2017). More directly related to the case of Alicia, extant research also suggests parental racial socialization messages in the form of preparation for bias may reduce the impact of academic inferiority microaggressions among African American undergraduates (McGee & Kruger, 2022). The therapist in the case utilized an integrated style (Day-Vines et al., 2007) to broach this potential source of coping with Alicia, which then served as a launching point for exploration of additional strengths. While doing so, the therapist was also careful to avoid stereotyping the client by not assuming that all African Americans receive parental racial socialization messages in the form of preparation for bias. This is significant, as research shows that this specific type of messaging is less common than broader cultural socialization messages (Osborne et al., 2021).

One of the benefits of strengths-based CBT also illustrated in the case of Alicia is that it helps clients focus on staying resilient rather than solving problems (Padesky & Mooney, 2012). Through the application of aspects of her personal model of resilience focused on faith, critical thinking, and community, Alicia's feelings of overwhelm and hopelessness were diminished, while her sense of control was increased. A focus on staying resilient as opposed to problem-solving can help clients feel less discouraged (Padesky & Mooney, 2012); however, research shows that directly or indirectly confronting racism can also provide emotional relief when dealing with racial oppression by increasing the client's sense of empowerment (Sue et al., 2019). Therefore, therapists who utilize a strengths-based approach to CBT when dealing with racial discrimination should seek to maintain an appropriate balance between resilience and empowered action. Use of a strengths-based cognitive conceptualization diagram, as shown in Figure 3.1, may help with this process. While working to complete the diagram with clients, therapists should emphasize the importance of drawing on personal strengths without

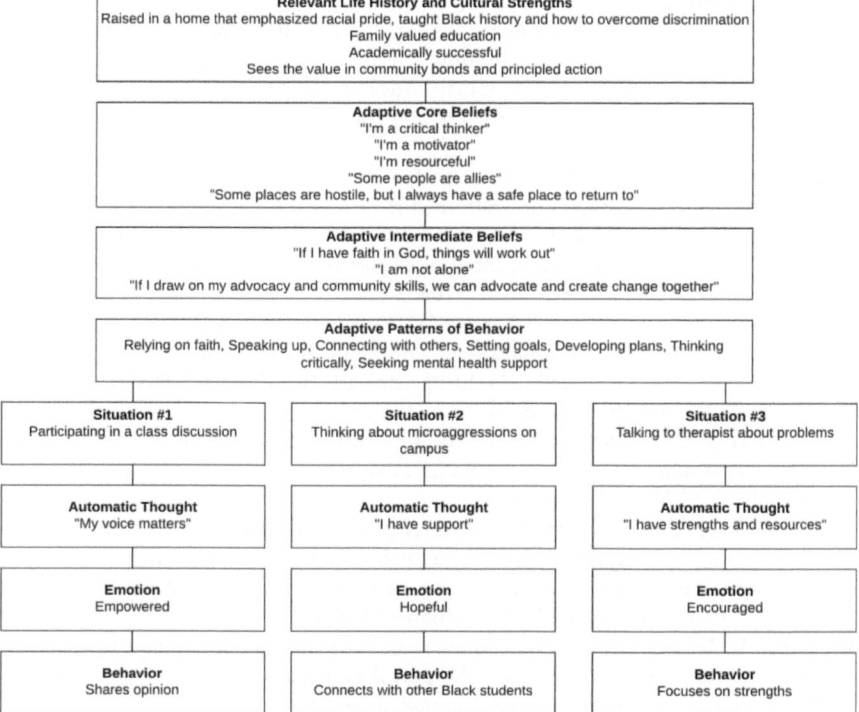

Figure 3.1 Alicia's Strengths-Based Cognitive Conceptualization Diagram. Adapted from Beck, J. S. (2020). *Cognitive behavior therapy: Basics and beyond* (3rd ed.). Guilford Press.

foregoing one's mental health needs and while also holding people in positions of power accountable.

References

Adams-Bass, V. N., Stevenson, H. C., & Kotzin, D. S. (2014). Measuring the meaning of Black media stereotypes and their relationship to the racial identity, Black history knowledge, and racial socialization of African American youth. *Journal of Black Studies, 45*(5), 367–395. https://doi.org/e10.1177/0021934714530396

Akbar, N. (1984). Afrocentric social services for liberation. *Journal of Black Studies, 14*(4), 395–413. https://doi.org/10.1177/002193478401400401

Asante, M. K. (1988). *Afrocentricity*. Africa World Press.

Asante, M. K. (1998). *The Afrocentric idea* (Rev. ed.). Temple University Press.

Avent Harris, J. R., Haskins, N., Parker, J., & Lee, A. (2021). Womanist theology and relational cultural theory: Counseling religious Black women. *Journal of Creativity in Mental Health*, 1–19. https://doi.org/10.1080/15401383.2021.1999359

Baldwin, J. A. (1984). African self-consciousness and the mental health of African-Americans. *Journal of Black Studies, 15*(2), 177–194. https://doi.org/10.1177/002193478401500203

Banerjee, M., Rivas-Drake, D., & Smalls-Glover, C. (2017). Racial-ethnic socialization and achievement: The mediating role of academic engagement. *Journal of Black Psychology, 43*(5), 451–463. https://doi.org/10.1177/0095798416687705

Beck, J. S. (2020). *Cognitive behavior therapy: Basics and beyond* (3rd ed.). Guilford Press.

Belgrave, F. Z., & Allison, K. W. (2019). *African American psychology: From Africa to America* (4th ed.). Sage Publications, Inc.

Brown, D. L. (2008). African American resiliency: Examining racial socialization and social support as protective factors. *Journal of Black Psychology, 34*(1), 32–48. https://doi.org/10.1177/0095798407310538

Brown, D. L., & Tylka, T. L. (2011). Racial discrimination and resilience in African American young adults: Examining racial socialization as a moderator. *Journal of Black Psychology, 37*(3), 259–285. https://doi.org/10.1177/0095798410390689

Byrdsong, T. R., Mitchell, A. B., & Yamatani, H. (2013). Afrocentric intervention paradigm: An overview of successful application by a grassroots organization. *Journal of Human Behavior in the Social Environment, 23*, 931–937. https://doi.org/10.1080/10911359.2013.831298

Campbell, B. (2019). Past, present, future: A program development project exploring post traumatic slave syndrome (PTSS) using experiential education and dance/movement therapy informed approaches. *American Journal of Dance Therapy, 41*, 214–233. https://doi.org/10.1007/s10465-019-09320-8

Caroline, A., Niceta, I., Irene, K., Mathenge, J., Muriithi, J., & Rose, O. (2015). African worldview: An integrated psychological perspective. *International Journal of Humanities Social Sciences and Education, 2*(5), 53–61.

Carroll, K. K. (2010). A genealogical analysis of the worldview framework in African centered psychology. *Journal of Pan African Studies, 3*, 109–134. https://www.jpanafrican.org/docs/vol3no8/3.8AGenealogical.pdf

Causey, S. T., Livingston, J., & High, B. (2015). Family structure, racial socialization, perceived parental involvement, and social support as predictors of self-esteem in African American college students. *Journal of Black Studies, 46*(7), 655–677. https://doi.org/10.1177/0021934715592601

Chioneso, N. A., Hunter, C. D., Gobin, R. L., McNeil Smith, S., Mendenhall, R., & Neville, H. A. (2020). Community healing and resistance through storytelling: A framework to address racial trauma in Africana communities. *Journal of Black Psychology, 46*(2–3), 95–121. https://doi.org/10.1177/0095798420929468

Constantine, M. G., Lewis, E. L., Conner, L. C., & Sanchez, D. (2000). Addressing spiritual and religious issues in counseling African Americans: Implications for counselor training and practice. *Counseling and Values, 45*(1), 28–39. https://doi.org/10.1002/j.2161-007X.2000.tb00180.x

Day-Vines, N.L., Wood, S. M., Grothaus, T., Craigen, L., Holman, A., Dotson-Blake, K., & Douglass, M. J. (2007). Broaching the subjects of race, ethnicity, and culture during the counseling process. *Journal of Counseling & Development, 85*(4), 401–409. https://doi.org/10.1002/jcad.12069

Del Toro, J., & Wang, M. T. (2021). School cultural socialization and academic performance: Examining ethnic-racial identity development as a mediator among African American adolescents. *Child Development, 92*(4), 1458–1475. https://doi.org/10.1111/cdev.13467

Diop, C. A. (1974). *The African origins of civilization: Myth or reality*. Lawrence Hill.

Dixon, V. J. (1970). The di-unital approach to "Black economics". *The American Economic Review, 60*(2), 424–429. https://www.jstor.org/stable/1815840

Dixon, V. J. (1977). African-oriented and Euro-American-oriented world views: Research methodologies and economics. *The Review of Black Political Economy, 7*, 119–156. https://doi.org/10.1007/BF02689392

Farr, M. (1997). The role of dance/movement therapy in treating at-risk African American adolescents. *The Arts in Psychotherapy, 24*(2), 183–191. https://doi.org/10.1016/S0197-4556(97)00004-X

Grills, C. (2002). African-centered psychology: Basic principles. In T. A. Parham (Ed.), *Counseling persons of African descent: Raising the bar of practitioner competence* (pp. 10–24). Sage.

Grills, C., & Longshore, D. (1996). Africentrism: Psychometric analyses of a self-report measure. *Journal of Black Psychology, 22*(1), 86–106. https://doi.org/10.1177/00957984960221007

Hilliard, A. G., III. (1986). The wisdom of Kemetic governance. In M. Karenga & J. Carruthers (Eds.), *Kemet and the African worldview* (pp. 131–148). University of Sankore Press.

Hunter, C. D. (2008). Individualistic and collectivistic worldviews: Implications for understanding perceptions of racial discrimination in African Americans and British Caribbean Americans. *Journal of Counseling Psychology, 55*(3), 321–332. https://doi.org/10.1037/0022-0167.55.3.321

Kambon, K. K. K. (1992). *The African personality in America: An African-centered framework*. Nubian Nation.

Karenga, M. (1965). *Kwanzaa: Origin, concepts and practice*. Kawaida Publications.

Karenga, M. (1996). The Nguzo Saba (the seven principles): Their meaning and message. In M. K. Asante & A. S. Abarry (Eds.), *African intellectual heritage* (pp. 543–554). Temple University Press.

Katz, J. H. (1985). The sociopolitical nature of counseling. *The Counseling Psychologist, 13*(4), 615–624. https://doi.org/10.1177/0011000085134005

Kohl, B. G. Jr. (2006). Can you feel me now? Worldview, empathy, and racial identity in a therapy dyad. *Journal of Emotional Abuse*, 6(2/3), 173–196.

Kwate, N. O. (2003). Cross-validation of the Africentrism Scale. *Journal of Black Psychology, 29*(3), 308–324. https://doi.org/10.1177/0095798403254215

Lateef, H., Nartey, P. B., Amoako, E. O., & Lateef, J. S. (2022). A systematic review of African-centered therapeutic interventions with Black American adults. *Clinical Social Work Journal, 50*, 256–264. https://doi.org/10.1007/s10615-021-00825-9

Mafumbate, R. (2019). The undiluted African community: Values, the family, orphanage and wellness in traditional Africa. *Information and Knowledge Management, 9*(8), 7–13. https://doi.org/10.7176/IKM

McGee, T., & Kruger, A. C. (2022). Racial microaggressions and African American undergraduates' academic experiences: Preparation for bias messages as a protective resource. *Journal of Black Psychology, 48*(6), 726–750. https://doi.org/10.1177/00957984211067628

Mohamed, B., Cox, K., Schiller, A., & Beveridge, K. (2021). *Faith among Black Americans.* Pew Research Center. https://www.pewresearch.org/religion/2021/02/16/religious-beliefs-among-black-americans/

Neblett, E. W., Jr., Smalls, C. P., Ford, K. R., Nguyên, H. X., & Sellers, R. M. (2009). Racial socialization and racial identity: African American parents' messages about race as precursors to identity. *Journal of Youth and Adolescence, 38*(2), 189–203. https://doi.org/10.1007/s10964-008-9359-7

Nobles, W. (1991). Extended self: Rethinking the so-called Negro self-concept. In R. Jones (Ed.), *Black psychology* (3rd ed., pp. 295–305). Cobb & Henry.

Okeke-Adeyanju, N., Taylor, L. C., Craig, A. B., Smith, R. E., Thomas, A., Boyle, A. E., & DeRosier, M. E. (2014). Celebrating the strengths of Black youth: Increasing self-esteem and implications for prevention. *The Journal of Primary Prevention, 35*(5), 357–369. https://doi.org/10.1007/s10935-014-0356-1

Osborne, K. R., Caughy, M. O., Oshri, A., Smith, E. P., & Owen, M. T. (2021). Racism and preparation for bias within African American families. *Cultural Diversity and Ethnic Minority Psychology, 27*(2), 269–279. https://doi.org/10.1037/cdp0000339

Padesky, C. A. (1994). Schema change processes in cognitive therapy. *Clinical Psychology and Psychotherapy, 1*(5), 267–278.

Padesky, C. A., & Mooney, K. A. (2012). Strengths-based cognitive-behavioural therapy: A four-step model to build resilience. *Clinical Psychology & Psychotherapy, 19*(4), 283–290. https://doi.org/10.1002/cpp.1795

Perry-Mitchell, T., & Davis-Maye, D. (2017). Evidence-based African-centered HIV/AIDS prevention interventions: Best practices and opportunities. *Journal of Human Behavior in the Social Environment, 27*(1–2), 110–131. https://doi.org/10.1080/10911359.2016.1266861

Pew Research Center. (2014). *Religious landscape study: Race and ethnic composition.* https://www.pewresearch.org/religion/religious-landscape-study/racial-and-ethnic-composition/

Plunkett, D. P. (2014). The Black church, values, and secular counseling: Implications for counselor education and practice. *Counseling and Values*, *59*(2), 208–221. https://doi.org/10.1002/j.2161-007X.2014.00052.x

Reynolds, J. E., & Gonzales-Backen, M. A. (2017). Ethnic-racial socialization and the mental health of African Americans: A critical review. *Journal of Family Theory & Review*, *9*(2), 182–200. https://doi.org/10.1111/jftr.12192

Shipp, P. L. (1983). Counseling Blacks: A group approach. *The Personnel and Guidance Journal*, *62*, 108–111.

Simões, T. A., & Alberto, I. M. (2015). "But … we are Africans!" Family life cycle structuring and functioning in southern Angola. *Journal of Psychology in Africa*, *25*(6), 504–511. https://doi.org/10.1080/14330237.2015.1124602

Steele, J. M. (2020). A CBT approach to internalized racism among African Americans. *International Journal for the Advancement of Counselling*, *42*(3), 217–233. https://doi.org/10.1007/s10447-020-09402-0

Steele, J. M., & Newton, C. S. (2023). *Black lives are beautiful: 50 tools to heal from trauma and promote positive racial identity*. Routledge.

Su, J., Seaton, E. K., Williams, C. D., Spit for Science Working Group, & Dick, D. M. (2021). Racial discrimination, depressive symptoms, ethnic-racial identity, and alcohol use among Black American college students. *Psychology of Addictive Behaviors: Journal of the Society of Psychologists in Addictive Behaviors*, *35*(5), 523–535. https://doi.org/10.1037/adb0000717

Sue, D. W. (2001). Multidimensional facets of cultural competence. *The Counseling Psychologist*, *29*(6), 790–821. https://doi.org/10.1177/0011000001296002

Sue, D. W., Alsaidi, S., Awad, M. N., Glaeser, E., Calle, C. Z., & Mendez, N. (2019). Disarming racial microaggressions: Microintervention strategies for targets, White allies, and bystanders. *American Psychologist*, *74*(1), 128–142. https://doi.org/10.1037/amp0000296

Taylor, R. J., & Chatters, L. M. (2010). Importance of religion and spirituality in the lives of African Americans, Caribbean Blacks and non-Hispanic Whites. *Journal of Negro Education*, *79*(3), 280–294.

Thabede, D. (2008). The African worldview as the basis of practice in the helping professions. *Social Work/Maatskaplike Werk*, *44*(3), 233–245. https://doi.org/10.15270/44-3-237

Todisco, M., & Salomone, P. R. (1991). Facilitating effective cross-cultural relationships: The White counselor and the Black client. *Journal of Multicultural Counseling and Development*, *19*(4), 146–157. https://doi.org/10.1002/j.2161-1912.1991.tb00551.x

Turner, E. A., Harrell, S. P., & Bryant-Davis, T. (2022). Black Love, Activism, and Community (BLAC): The BLAC model of healing and resilience. *Journal of Black Psychology*, *48*(3–4), 547–568. https://doi.org/10.1177/00957984211018364

Waltman, S., Codd, R., III, McFarr, L., & Moore, B. (2021). *Socratic questioning for therapists and counselors: Learn how to think and intervene like a cognitive behavior therapist*. Routledge. https://doi.org/10.4324/9780429320392

Watson-Singleton, N. N., Mekawi, Y., Wilkins, K. V., & Jatta, I. F. (2021). Racism's effect on depressive symptoms: Examining perseverative cognition and Black Lives Matter activism as moderators. *Journal of Counseling Psychology*, *68*(1), 27–37. https://doi.org/10.1037/cou0000436

Williams, C. B., Frame, M. W., & Green, E. (1999). Counseling groups for African American women: A focus on spirituality. *Journal for Specialists in Group Work*, *24*(3), 260–273. https://doi.org/10.1080/01933929908411435

Williams, Q., Williams, B. M., & Brown, L. C. (2022). Exploring Black girl magic: Identity development of Black first-gen college women. *Journal of Diversity in Higher Education*, *15*(4), 466–479. https://doi.org/10.1037/dhe0000294

Womack, V. Y., & Sloan, L. R. (2017). The association of mindfulness and racial socialization messages on approach-oriented coping strategies among African Americans. *Journal of Black Studies*, *48*(4), 408–426. https://doi.org/10.1177/0021934717696789

Workneh, L. (2022, January/February). The rise of the Black is Beautiful revolution. *Essence*, 80–83.

Young, D. L., & Goldstein, T. R. (2023). Racial-ethnic minority participants in the marching arts: Intergroup experiences, perceptions of inclusion, and well-being. *Psychology of Aesthetics, Creativity, and the Arts*. Advance online publication. https://doi.org/10.1037/aca0000614

Chapter 4

Developing a Multicultural Orientation

Traditionally, cultural sensitivity in the therapeutic process has been defined according to the multicultural counseling competencies, which identify knowledge, attitudes, and skills in three primary areas: (1) awareness of one's own cultural values and biases, (2) understanding the worldview of culturally diverse clients, and (3) developing culturally appropriate interventions (Arredondo et al., 1996). While the multicultural counseling competencies have been credited with operationalizing multicultural values in the mental health profession, one major limitation of the competencies has been low empirical validation of their impact on therapeutic outcomes (Davis et al., 2018). In addition to low empirical validation, other limitations associated with the multicultural counseling competencies include language which implies that one achieves a final level of cultural competence, as well as limited consideration for the role of intersectionality in clients' cultural identities (Davis et al., 2018).

In response to the limitations of the multicultural counseling competencies, Owen et al. (2011) introduced multicultural orientation as a way to: (a) be more consistent with the process-oriented language typical of counseling, (b) clarify ways to understand the cultural identities of clients, and (c) increase the empirical basis from which cultural competence is conceptualized in the counseling process. This orientation, which consists of cultural humility, cultural opportunities, and cultural comfort, has been found to aid in the establishment of a strong working therapeutic alliance and a sense of safety for racial/ethnic minority clients (Davis et al., 2018). Research additionally suggests this orientation reduces premature termination and improves therapeutic outcomes. Accordingly, scholars who specialize in addressing race and racism with African American clients during therapy have increasingly recognized the utility of multicultural orientation in developing the dispositions and ways of being necessary for effective work with this population (Johnson & Melton, 2021).

In this chapter, you will be introduced to the various aspects of multicultural orientation and engage in several exercise to facilitate development of

DOI: 10.4324/9781003196303-4

this way of being with African American clients during therapy. Reflection questions are also included throughout the chapter to further assist in exploration of the deeply personal, and sometimes painful, subject matter characteristic of a multicultural orientation. The specific areas of reflection encouraged throughout this chapter include exploration of your personal values, biases, and level of racial identity. Activities designed to help you increase contact with members of the African American community and broach the topic of race during therapy are also discussed in the chapter.

Cultural Humility

Within the multicultural orientation paradigm, cultural humility is considered the foundational concept upon which all other aspects of the model are built upon (Hook et al., 2017). *Cultural humility* is defined as a way of being that seeks to understand how culture influences the worldviews of both the counselor and the client, as well as dynamics within the counseling relationship. According to Davis et al. (2018), this way of being consists of both intrapersonal and interpersonal characteristics that support both the development of the therapeutic alliance and the attainment of positive therapeutic outcomes when working with racially diverse clients. Intrapersonally, cultural humility involves having an accurate perception of one's worldview and limitations and being open to feedback. This includes recognition of one's personal values and biases, as well as the ability to manage instances of emotional defensiveness that arise when personal values and biases are elicited or challenged. Interpersonally, cultural humility involves being other rather than self-oriented, as one seeks to understand the cultural nuances of the client's values and worldview without being presumptuous or arrogant (Hook et al., 2017). Given the role of factors such as values and biases in the intra- and interpersonal aspects of cultural humility, the development of this pillar of multicultural orientation requires ongoing examination of these factors and their impact on the therapeutic process. Accordingly, the sections below take a closer look at the role of values and biases in the therapeutic context and present several activities and clinical examples to help you examine how they function during therapy with African American clients.

Values

In the past, the therapeutic process was characterized as being objective in nature. Today, most of us realize that therapy is largely a subjective venture, heavily influenced by our individual values (Jadaszewski, 2017). For example, because of how they are socialized into the profession, many therapists operate from a preference for values such as autonomy, self-expression, and self-development in their work with clients, which reflects the individualistic culture in which the mental health profession was developed (Christopher, 1996). However, when working with African American clients who embrace the collectivist/Afrocentric values described in Chapter 3, an assumed prioritizing of individualistic values such as autonomy may conflict with other important values such as interdependence and responsibility of the individual to the group (Shipp, 1983). Consider Justin, a 41-year-old African American man who entered therapy due to anxiety around career decision making. A traditional approach reflecting a value preference for self-fulfillment may focus on making a career decision that aligns with Justin's individual interests and goals, while a more Afrocentric approach may have a greater emphasis on making a decision that is in the best interest of the family (Belgrave & Allison, 2018). Therefore, when thinking about cultural humility and the role of values in our work with African American clients, it is important that we take a broader look at the type of values reflected in our clinical approach and seek to operate from the client's value perspective as much as possible.

Beyond awareness of the individualistic values inherent in most Western theories of counseling, including CBT, it is also important that therapists be aware of how their individual values may also influence the therapeutic process. A definition of *values* I like to keep in mind is, "A conception, explicit or implicit, distinctive of an individual or characteristic of a group, of the desirable which influences the selection from available modes, means and ends of action" (Kluckhohn, 1951, p. 395). This means that a value is not something that you simply think is a good idea but is something that guides what you do. In the therapeutic context, this suggests that a therapist's values have an impact on their approach to assessment, case conceptualization, and treatment planning. It is important to note, however, that because values may be explicit or implicit, therapists may not always be aware of the ways in which their personal values influence their approach to these clinical tasks. Continuing with the case of Justin, a therapist who does not take into account the role of interdependence in Justin's decision making may mistakenly conceptualize his anxiety as stemming from maladaptive fear of judgment from his family members rather than a lack in the skills necessary to balance his own interests with the needs of his family unit.

Fortunately, there are ways therapists can increase awareness of their values in order to avoid inadvertent values imposition in their work with clients. These strategies include engaging in thoughtful, ethical reflection and undergoing an explicit values clarification process (Tjeltveit, 2015). *Values clarification*, which can be defined as the process of exploring values that hold personal meaning, is a common strategy used in third-wave CBT approaches such as acceptance and commitment therapy. Activity 4.1, Mind Reading Machine (Harris, 2019), is an adaptation of an acceptance and commitment therapy values clarification technique that is designed to help you identify values that may have particular relevance to the therapeutic process. Complete the activity, which is found below, and then reflect on the similarities and differences between the values you identified, and the traditional Afrocentric values discussed in Chapter 3.

Activity 4.1: Mind Reading Machine

Imagine I place a mind reading machine on your head, and I tune it into the mind of a colleague or perhaps a clinical supervisor who knows you very well. You can now hear their every thought. As you tune in, they are thinking about YOU—about your view of what is considered psychologically healthy, how problems are developed, how clients change, and how therapists, in their professional roles, can help clients change. In the IDEAL world, where you have lived your life as the therapist you want to be, what would you hear them thinking? Write it down in a notebook. Then, consider the values that are reflected in what you've written. For example, perhaps your ideas are consistent with values commonly expressed in mental health such as autonomy, beneficence, fidelity, veracity, self-actualization, rationality, and independence. Reflect on the values you identified and then compare your values to the Afrocentric values described in Chapter 3. What are the implications of the similarities and differences you identified for your work with African American clients?

Implicit Bias

According to Banaji and Greenwald (2016), *implicit bias*, also known as *unconscious bias*, can be most simply defined as a hidden preference for one identity over another. In this definition, *preferences* refer to what we favor or reject, while *identity* typically refers to shared cultural values and beliefs within specific reference groups (e.g., race, gender, ability, age, etc.). Most people think of implicit biases as negative beliefs about certain cultural groups; however, in reality, these biases may be negative or positive and are based mostly on the stereotypes we have been socialized into believing about these groups. For example, consider Brianna, an African American woman who comes to her weekly therapy session immediately after ending her shift at a local retail store. Due to rush hour traffic, Brianna is usually five to ten minutes late for her appointment. A therapist who unconsciously subscribes to negative stereotypes about African Americans being late, lazy, or generally untrustworthy may view Brianna's behavior as a failure to take full responsibility for her mental health and may even be less respectful or pleasant to Brianna during their interpersonal interactions (Hall et al., 2015).

Conversely, the same therapist in a similar situation with a White client may view and respond to identical behavior with greater sympathy and compassion if that therapist holds more positive stereotypes about White women being vulnerable and in need of protection (Phipps, 2021).

We call the preferences that make up one's implicit bias "hidden" because they are governed by parts of the brain that operate automatically and outside of our awareness. The amygdala is an especially key region of the brain involved in the development of implicit bias. This part of the brain is an almond-shaped set of neurons located deep in the temporal lobe that is important in the acquisition and expression of a range of learned emotional responses, including fear and both positive and negative affect (Chekroud et al., 2014). It processes billions of stimuli per day and must quickly choose what to focus on, relying on schemas and patterns of information to do so. Unfortunately, the stereotypes we pick up over time from the environment around us (e.g., our family, our school, our community, the media) often act as the primary schemas that provide data for the amygdala in decision making, leading to the formation of bias and unconsciously influencing our behavior.

Bias is fundamental to the way human beings process the world—it does not necessarily reflect intentional bigotry or prejudice. Nevertheless, implicit biases are important to the therapeutic context because they affect our understanding, actions, and decisions in an unconscious way, making them difficult to control. This means that not all counseling responses are intentional, and explicit and implicit attitudes may diverge. For example, most individuals reject overt racism; yet research suggests counselors and counselors-in-training demonstrate implicit bias even when they rate themselves as multiculturally competent (Abreu, 1999; Boysen & Vogel, 2008; Castillo et al., 2007). A study conducted by Gushue (2004) illustrates this point. In this study, 158 White master's level counseling and clinical psychology students were given a fictitious counseling center intake report that differed only in terms of the race listed for the client. Half of the participants were given an intake form that listed the client's race as White, while the other half of the participants received a form that listed the client's race as Black. Results of this study showed that the Black client was perceived as significantly less symptomatic when compared to the White client in spite of the fact that all of the information presented in the intake outside of race was identical. According to Gushue (2004), this finding is consistent with previous research indicating that individuals from negatively stereotyped, low-status groups are judged differently than individuals from positively stereotyped, high-status groups. During therapy, these types of judgments, or implicit biases, have the potential to cause clients harm, as therapists who operate out of implicit bias may unconsciously assume, dismiss, or be insensitive to how aspects of a client's identity influence their perceptions of clients and their view of the client's presenting concerns (Gushue, 2004).

Case Illustration: Jeremiah

To illustrate how implicit bias may operate during therapy with African American clients, let's look at a clinical example, the case of Jeremiah. Jeremiah was a 24-year-old African American man referred to therapy by his probation officer. At intake, Jeremiah, who was on probation for assault, admitted to frequent outbursts of anger and irritability, which he attributed to his frustration with "the world being against me." In discussing the incident leading to his assault charge, Jeremiah explained that he had an argument with his parents early in the day and went to a bar to "let off some steam" with friends later the same evening. While at the bar, one of Jeremiah's friends noticed he was in a sad mood and made several jokes challenging Jeremiah's manhood given his public display of emotion. A verbal argument between the two friends ensued and escalated into a physical altercation, leading to Jeremiah's arrest and subsequent probation. As part of his probation requirements, Jeremiah attends a weekly anger management group; however, he continues to report feelings of anger and irritability and now endorses somatic complaints such as heart palpitations and tightness of the chest. Based on his current presentation of symptoms and his report of frequent outbursts over the past 12 months, the therapist diagnosed Jeremiah with intermittent explosive disorder and developed a treatment plan focused on emotional regulation and social skills training. Jeremiah has experienced little progress toward his therapy goals, however, causing his therapist to question his motivation for change and willingness to fully engage therapy.

As mentioned above, when operating out of implicit bias, therapists may unconsciously assume or dismiss details of the client's presenting concerns, leading to negative consequences in diagnosis and treatment outcomes (Gushue, 2004). Payne (2014), for example, cited research indicating that African American men with major depressive disorder are frequently mis- or underdiagnosed. One explanation for these research findings has been that clinicians often attribute depression symptoms in this population to behavioral or personality disorders rather than mood disorders, which may be related to implicit bias. A common stereotype about African Americans is that they are aggressive and hostile. Therapists who have been repeatedly exposed to this stereotype over many years and from many sources may come to unconsciously and automatically associate the concepts African American and aggressive/hostile with each other (Boysen, 2010), resulting, as Payne (2014) suggests, in the overdiagnosis of behavior disorders and the underdiagnosis of depressive disorders within this population. This may explain the lack of success therapists have had with Jeremiah so far. Specifically, given that features of intermittent explosive disorder such as anger, irritability, and physiological complaints are also common in depression, it is possible that negative stereotypes may have influenced the assessment process and that a more appropriate diagnosis of major depressive disorder may have been missed due to implicit bias. Moreover, a general lack of cultural competence in the assessment of depression in African American clients may have exacerbated the effect of implicit bias during therapy with Jeremiah, as the therapist may not have considered how social determinants such as socioeconomic status, racial and masculine identity, kinship and social support, self-esteem/mastery, and access to high-quality healthcare affect Jeremiah's symptom presentation (Watkins & Neighbors, 2013). For example, many African American men are socialized to refrain from expressing helplessness and vulnerability (Payne, 2014), which may have caused Jeremiah to deny or at least omit discussion of symptoms more commonly associated with depression such as crying or saddened affect at intake. Had the therapist been aware of the potential influence of implicit bias in her work with Jeremiah, she could have been more intentional in minimizing its impact by spending extra time establishing rapport with him and integrating an understanding of how symptoms may be culturally influenced among African Americans into her diagnostic procedures (Payne, 2014).

Cases like Jeremiah's illustrate the idea that while implicit bias may be evident to an outsider, the one holding this bias may not be aware of their attitudes due to the nature of how the brain processes and categorizes information. Accordingly, a primary professional goal of therapists should be to increase awareness of one's implicit biases in order to reduce their effect on the therapeutic process. In their book, *The Leader's Guide to Unconscious Bias*, Fuller et al. (2020) identified a multi-step model for making unconscious bias more explicit, which I have found particularly useful in the therapeutic context. The steps of this model, known as the Bias Progress Model, are: (1) identify bias, (2) cultivate connection, and (3) choose courage. The sections below describe these steps, along with activities to help you engage in each area.

Identify Bias

According to Fuller et al. (2020), identifying implicit biases requires individuals to (a) understand the relationship between their biases and their identities and (b) know when they are susceptible to bias. This task can prove difficult, however, given that implicit biases stem from unconscious thoughts that are automatic and outside of our awareness. Traditionally, professional development around culture and diversity in the mental health professions is approached through a process of deliberation and self-reflection; however, implicit biases cannot be adequately measured through conventional reflection tools such as self-report scales, journaling, or group discussion alone, as these tools rely heavily on explicit knowledge of oneself (Boysen, 2010). Instead, researchers have discovered that implicit biases are best uncovered through tools that use response latency, or timed groupings of words and images into certain categories. One of the most popular and widely researched response latency tests is known as the Implicit Association Test (IAT) (Banaji & Greenwald, 2016). Activity 4.2 below provides directions for taking the IAT, along with reflection questions to help you process your results. In Activity 4.3: My Story, you will use your IAT results along with your responses to the reflection questions to explore the relationship between your identity and your uncovered bias. Ideally, this combination of activities will help you discover more about your biases and how your identity has shaped and has been shaped by these biases.

Activity 4.2: The Implicit Association Test (IAT)

The Implicit Association Test (IAT) is a measure of attitudes and beliefs people may be unwilling or unable to report (https://implicit.harvard.edu/implicit/education.html). According to the test's website, the IAT does this by measuring the strength of associations between certain groups of people such as Black people and evaluations like good or bad, or stereotypes like athletic or clumsy (https://implicit.harvard.edu/implicit/iatdetails.html). Several versions of the IAT are available. For example, you can take tests to learn more about your implicit biases toward gender, religion, sexuality, or weight. For this activity, you will take the Race IAT, which explores attitudes toward Black and White racial groups. Your results will reveal a preference for one racial group over another, or possibly no preference at all. After completing the Race IAT, summarize your results in a journal or notebook. Then, respond to the subsequent reflection questions. To take the Race IAT, visit https://implicit.harvard.edu/implicit/selectatest.html.

Reflection Questions

- How can having a better understanding of your implicit biases help you in your work with African American clients?
- What feelings or reactions did you have upon learning your IAT results?
- How can you overcome any defensiveness that may arise when reviewing your results?

Activity 4.3: My Story

As mentioned above, implicit biases may be the opposite of one's explicit beliefs and values. For this reason, some individuals may experience disbelief and have difficulty accepting their results when the outcome is different than expected. Reflecting on life experiences that may have influenced your results can help you to remember that implicit biases do not necessarily reflect poor character on your part, but instead may be the result of how you were socialized by your family, the media, or broader society. Think about any life experiences that may have influenced your IAT results. Consider your childhood and family upbringing, the schools you went to, the neighborhoods you lived in, media messages, etc. and write about how they affected your perceptions of African Americans in your journal or notebook. Be sure to consider how your experiences may influence your comfort when working with African American clients and how you view their problems.

Cultivate Connection

Some people believe that once they become aware of their implicit biases, they can fix these biases on their own (Fuller et al., 2020). Yet, Fuller et al. (2020) argue that cultivating meaningful connections is the only way one can truly begin to see past their biases. According to Fuller et al. (2020), cultivating connection involves engaging with others to learn more about their experiences and points of view. As mentioned earlier, implicit biases develop primarily as the result of stereotypes we have been exposed to repeatedly and over time. Yet, while stereotypes are automatically activated when encountering members of another group, there are corrective processes we can engage in to moderate their influence and reduce implicit bias (Rivers et al., 2020). These corrective processes, however, are not as automatic as the activation of stereotypes and therefore require intentionality on our part as therapists (Devine, 1989; Fazio, 1990; Fazio et al., 1995). One simple strategy for dealing with implicit bias is known as stereotype replacement (Devine et al., 2012). This strategy involves recognizing when a response has been based on a stereotype, labeling the response as a stereotype, reflecting on why the response occurred, and replacing it with an unbiased response in the future. Two other more experiential strategies include increasing contact and counter-stereotypic imagining (Devine et al., 2012). These strategies are described in Activities 4.4 and 4.5 below. As you complete these activities, be aware of any defenses that may arise and seek to approach each experience with curiosity and openness.

Activity 4.4: Cultural Immersion Project

Increased contact with members of various cultural groups in their cultural context, or what is frequently referred to as *immersion*, is a common professional development activity in the fields of counseling, psychology, and social work (Shannonhouse et al., 2018). While the complexity of these experiences vary in terms of duration and frequency, the contact theory of intergroup relations states that three factors must be present during an immersion experience to result in a reduction of prejudice: (1) there must be enough time across repeated interactions for individuals to develop genuine closeness and meaningful relationships across group boundaries, (2) contact should take place as much as possible among participants of equal status, and (3) contact should be based on cooperation and mutual dependence (DeRicco & Sciarra, 2005). Moreover, this contact should also consist of pre-immersion planning/training beforehand and reflection afterward (Pope-Davis et al., 1997). With this in mind, the purpose of this project is to help you increase contact with members of the African American community in ways that feel genuine to you and authentic to your sense of community. To begin the Cultural Immersion Project, follow the steps below. Keep in mind that this activity will require both time and emotional commitments and should only be engaged when you feel ready to honor these commitments.

1. First, identify ways to engage with members of the African American community. This could include attendance at local holiday or community events such as Kwanzaa or MLK celebrations, volunteer experiences like joining the Boys & Girls Club or Big Brothers Big Sisters organization, or participation in a cultural institution like attending a church service or joining a racially diverse group focused on supporting the African American community such as the NAACP.
2. After selecting your specific immersion experience, take some time to reflect on any thoughts and feelings you might be having before the immersion experience. Note any fears or defensive reactions and seek the support of a trusted friend or cultural ally to work through these reactions as much as possible before beginning your experience.
3. Continue your reflection process by maintaining a journal of your thoughts and feelings during your immersion experience. Be sure to focus on aspects of the experience such as similarities between African American culture and your cultural/racial background, growth in your understanding of the African American experience, and changes in your level of comfort around members of the African American community.

4. Finally, once your immersion experience is complete, reflect on what you learned from the experience, noting any implicit biases you may have previously been unaware of and identifying how the experience will influence your future relationships with African American clients.

Activity 4.5: Counter-stereotypic Imagining

Counter-stereotypic imagining involves imagining counter-stereotypic images of individuals belonging to various social identities (Devine et al., 2012). According to Devine et al. (2012), whether these individuals are famous or not famous isn't important—what matters is that the exemplars are numerous and salient enough to challenge a stereotype's validity. An easy way to find these exemplars is to identify African Americans you personally know and admire. Another approach is to become more familiar with African Americans who have contributed to how you live your life on a daily basis. For example, History.com has an interesting list of eight African American inventors who made daily life easier. These individuals were responsible for inventions such as the three-way traffic light, the home security system, automatic elevator doors, and the carbon lightbulb filament. While this list focuses on inventors, African Americans have been influential in all spheres of life, including politics, education, science, sports, and entertainment. For this activity, write down stereotypes about African Americans to which you have been previously exposed. Then, identify the names of at least two exemplars to counter each stereotype.

Choose Courage

The last of the three steps I want to highlight in Fuller et al.'s (2020) Bias Progress Model is Choose Courage. This step is based on the idea that it is not enough for us to recognize and confront implicit bias in our lives—we must actively confront and seek to create spaces where all are valued (Fuller et al., 2020). According to Fuller et al. (2020), *courage* can be defined as "the mental or moral strength to strive and persevere in the face of uncertainty, fear, and difficulty" (p. 141). In a way, reading this book is an act of courage. On a personal level, it takes courage to recognize a need for growth in your ability to help your clients heal from racism. It also takes courage to sit with feelings of apathy, guilt, and vulnerability that commonly arise while discussing race. Yet, because we belong to a professional community that relies on the trust and respect of society-at-large, it is also important that we have the courage to speak out and advocate when we see implicit bias at play in our various work settings. Sometimes this courage requires us to be bold, or to demand immediate change (Fuller et al., 2020). At other times, we may have to exhibit careful courage, especially when there is significant risk to ourselves professionally or personally. Nevertheless, there are certain strategies we can use to notice when bias is happening, deal with bias, help others with bias, and address bias. Fuller et al. (2020) describe these strategies as: (1) the courage to identify, (2) the courage to cope, (3) the courage to ally, and (4) the courage to advocate. While a full discussion of these strategies is beyond the scope of this book, you can begin to reflect on how you might begin to implement each of these four aspects of courage in your professional role by imagining yourself in the scenario presented in Activity 4.6 and responding to the questions below.

Activity 4.6: Meet Maria

Maria is a 35-year-old African American single mother of two children, Jonathan, age 10, and James, age 11. She was referred to therapy by the children's school counselor for parent education training after her eldest child, James, received several school suspensions and was on the verge of expulsion. James, who had been a good student in previous years, was falling behind in his schoolwork and exhibiting disruptive behavior in his classes. In her referral, the school counselor expressed concern that Maria had not been to any parent-teacher conferences that year and that James was coming to school tired due to staying up late to complete chores and then homework. In discussing the issue with the therapist, Maria explained that she had to take on a second job after a car accident led to the unexpected death of her husband. Since his father's death, James has taken on more responsibility in the home and Maria cannot financially afford to take time off work to attend parent-teacher conferences. Maria is also concerned about James's behavior and is willing to follow the recommendations of the therapist and school counselor.

Reflection Questions

- What assumptions or biases might be reflected in this scenario?
- How might these biases affect the perceptions of the school counselor and the therapist?
- How might you address these biases in your interactions with the school counselor and in your own decision-making process as the therapist while acting as an ally or as an advocate?
- Whose support can you enlist as you attempt to address bias in this situation?

Cultural Opportunities

Cultural opportunities refer to markers that indicate an opportunity to explore topics related to culture and identity with a client (Owen et al., 2011). For example, cultural opportunities arise when clients directly mention some aspect of their cultural heritage or when you as the therapist recognize a potential impact of culture on the client's presenting concern (Hook et al., 2017). During therapy, cultural opportunities may be one of the more significant aspects of multicultural orientation, as research shows that failure to acknowledge race is a reason many people of color prematurely terminate or do not enter therapy (Cooper & Conklin, 2015). The broaching strategies described below clarify how counselors might approach or even create cultural opportunities to bring up the subject of race during therapy with clients. As you learn about broaching, think about your own clients and ways you can begin to take advantage of or initiate cultural opportunities during therapy.

Broaching

The concept of *broaching* was developed by Day-Vines et al. (2007) to define the process by which a counselor makes a deliberate effort to explore racial/ethnic and cultural (REC) concerns that may impact clients' presenting issues or the therapeutic relationship. Within the broaching framework, there are five broaching styles that include: (1) avoidant, (2) isolating, (3) continuing/incongruent, (4) integrated/congruent, and (5) infusing. The first style, *avoidant*, describes a therapist who views broaching as unnecessary and refuses to do so. According to Day-Vines et al. (2007), therapists with this broaching style typically maintain a race-neutral perspective and generally believe racial differences warrant little attention. At the next level of broaching, the *isolating* style, therapists may broach REC dimensions, but in a simple and superficial manner. These therapists often address culture using a single statement or question out of perceived obligation and with little connection to other aspects of the client's lived experiences. The third style, *continuing/incongruent*, reflects a desire to address culture, but with limited ability to explore these issues skillfully. For example, therapists at this level of broaching may maintain a healthy attitude toward the role of race in the client's presenting concerns but lack the cultural knowledge to adequately integrate culture into assessment and case conceptualization. At a more advanced level, therapists with an *integrated/congruent* style are effective at integrating culture into the various aspects of the therapeutic process and regularly implement culturally appropriate interventions. These therapists can also differentiate culture-specific behaviors from unhealthy human functioning and understand heterogeneity and the intersectional nature of identity. Finally, the last broaching style, *infusing*, describes the approach of therapists who not only view broaching as integral to therapy but are also committed to social justice outside of their professional work (Day-Vines et al., 2007).

Broaching statements may address REC issues in the client's presenting concerns or in the therapeutic relationship itself. Accordingly, these statements may be exhibited across four REC dimensions (i.e., intracounseling, intraindividual, intra-REC, and inter-REC) during counseling (Day-Vines et al., 2020). The *intracounseling dimension* focuses on identifying differences between the therapist and the client in order to acknowledge potential differences in worldview that may affect interpretations of the content discussed during therapy and to signal to the client that it is safe to explore race and other cultural concerns within the context of the therapeutic relationship. For example, in a cross-racial therapy dyad, the therapist may make a broaching statement as simple as, "Based on our outward appearances, there may be differences in how we see the world or understand issues due to our racial backgrounds. I hope that you feel comfortable discussing these differences with me whenever you think it's important, and I will do the same." Or you may consider also integrating a more standardized approach to broaching into therapy, for example, during your intake process. This similarly primes clients to have discussions about race and other aspects of culture at the outset of therapy and helps establish the therapeutic relationship as a safe environment to explore these topics in the future. Below is an example of how I broach race and culture during the intake process with my clients. After reading the example, complete Activity 4.7: Introducing Race Into the Therapeutic Process to develop your own broaching script.

To help you understand me and my approach to therapy a little better, I'd like talk to you some about my cultural background. Culture is an important part of the counseling process for many reasons. First, our cultural identities influence the way we see and experience the world. I identify as a heterosexual, African American woman, and this may affect how I understand your problems. However, it's really important that I understand the issues you discuss with me during therapy from your cultural worldview as much as possible. How do you identify your race/ethnicity? Sex? Gender? Sexual orientation? Religious or spiritual background? What are the most important aspects of your background or identity? At times, I may ask you how aspects of your culture influence the problems you experience. Additionally, many people experience discrimination because of their cultural identities, which may also contribute to their difficulties. In these cases, we may also explore strategies to help you achieve a greater sense of empowerment. Do you have any questions?

Activity 4.7: Introducing Race Into the Therapeutic Process

Now that you have read the broaching script example provided above, develop your own broaching script. Here are some questions to help you get started:

1. How does culture influence the relationship between the client and the therapist?
2. How would you invite clients to share about their own cultural identities?
3. What are your most salient cultural identities?
4. Broadly, in what ways does culture influence clients' presenting concerns?
5. How would you invite clients to explore how culture influences their presenting concerns, specifically?
6. How would you inform your clients of your intent to explore culture throughout therapy?

While the intracounseling dimension of Day-Vines et al.'s (2020) model focuses on broaching REC concerns within the therapeutic relationship, the domains outside of the intracounseling dimension explore the role of REC in the client's presenting concerns and lived experiences. The *intra-individual dimension*, for example, uses the concept of intersectionality to explore how the client's various identities (e.g., race, gender, ability, sexual orientation, religion, etc.), as well past and present experiences of oppression influence their worldview and presenting concerns. In contrast, the *intra-REC dimension* explores within-group difference between clients and others of the same REC group, as clients may have REC values, behaviors, and beliefs that vary from other members with the same identity. Last, the *inter-REC dimension* acknowledges the role of racism, discrimination, and oppression in the lives of clients. Therapists working within this dimension assist clients in addressing these forces psychologically and through advocacy using some of the strategies discussed later in Chapter 8.

Developing the ability to skillfully broach race and racism takes practice. Below, you will find a couple of brief client/therapist interactions to help you practice inviting clients to explore the impact of race and racism on their concerns. Here are some tips to consider as you decide how you might probe race and racism in these scenarios:

- Validate the client's experience
- Avoid imposing your personal values and beliefs onto client
- Seek to learn about the client's racial worldview from the client him/herself

- Acknowledge the impact of racism and other forms of discrimination on the client's life
- Look for ways to affirm the client's racial identity
- Avoid reducing the client's identity to race only
- Be direct

Activity 4.8: Broaching Race and Racism

The Case of Carmen

Carmen is a 20-year-old cisgender, African American woman who is seeking counseling due to social anxiety and difficulties transitioning into adulthood. Carmen, who is in her junior year of college, reports excessive worry about choosing "the right" major and having a successful career after graduation. She has changed her major three times since enrolling in college and continues to be uncertain about her current selection. Carmen often compares herself to her peers on social media and reports feelings of embarrassment, believing that her friends are more focused and successful than she is. Carmen is becoming increasingly isolated, as she finds it "easier to be alone than to deal with everyone judging me."

Therapist:	Carmen, what I hear you saying is that you don't believe you measure up when you compare yourself to your friends, is that correct?
Carmen:	I suppose it is. And it's so unfair. My friends don't have to deal with half of the stuff I do. Everyone has all of these expectations of me. I have to help take care of my younger brothers, go to school, and work. My family expects me to be strong and handle all of this. My older brother never had to do any of this.
Therapist Response:	Carmen, from what I understand, this idea of having to "be strong" is something many Black women have to deal with and can be pretty overwhelming at times.

Now You Try: The Case of Michael

Michael is a 15-year-old bi-racial client who identifies as non-binary and uses they/them pronouns. Michael's mother, Jennifer, made the referral to counseling, expressing concern about Michael's gender identity. Jennifer is African American and believes Michael has been negatively influenced by peers at the predominantly White performing arts high school they attend.

Michael is angry and frustrated with Jennifer. Jennifer and Michael constantly argue, and Michael "wants nothing to do with her."

Therapist:	Michael, I understand that your mother referred you to counseling because she has concerns about your gender identity, is that correct?
Michael:	Yes. She thinks I have a problem, but really, she's the one with the problem.
Therapist:	I imagine things are pretty difficult between you and your mother right now. Individuals with non-binary gender identities don't always receive the support they'd like from their families right away.
Michael:	It's hard enough dealing with my grandparents. I shouldn't have to deal with this from my mother too. It's like that whole side of the family has a problem.

Your Response:

Cultural Comfort

Cultural comfort refers to the level of comfort one has while discussing issues related to diversity, power, and oppression during therapy (Owen et al., 2011). When therapists are comfortable discussing these issues during therapy, they experience the emotional state of feeling at ease, open, calm, and relaxed (Hook et al., 2017). Conversely, therapists who are low in cultural comfort may feel awkward or tense when having these discussions. According to Hook et al. (2017), cultural comfort is a significant factor when working with clients from diverse racial/ethnic backgrounds for several reasons. First, therapists who are higher in cultural comfort are more likely to broach race or respond to cultural opportunities during therapy with their clients. Moreover, therapists with higher levels of cultural comfort have clients who are more likely to discuss cultural topics because the therapist has established a safe therapeutic environment. In my work with supervisees and counselors-in-training, I have discovered that one factor that appears to be particularly related to cultural comfort is the level of racial identity development evidenced in the therapist. Most models of racial identity development indicate that individuals at higher levels of racial identity development are curious about the impact of race on one's life experience and are committed to taking action against racism (Helms, 2014; Sue et al., 2019). Accordingly, in this final section of the chapter, I discuss racial identity development models for individuals with White racial backgrounds and people of color and the relationship of racial identity to the therapeutic context. The section ends with a few reflection questions to help you explore your own racial identity.

Racial Identity

Broadly, *racial identity* is defined as an individual's "psychological orientation to their own race and to other racial groups in the context of racial socialization in the United States" (Gushue & Constantine, 2007, p. 321). In Chapter 2, I discussed Black racial identity development and its relationship to various mental health factors among African Americans. In Chapter 3, I further discussed racial identity as a protective factor against racialized trauma in African Americans. Specifically, I noted how African Americans with a well-developed and affirming sense of racial identity not only have a more positive view of themselves as racial beings but also embrace other racial groups and have a commitment to social change and civil rights (Sue et al., 2019). Within the therapeutic relationship, the racial identity of the therapist has also been correlated to the therapist's ability to connect with individuals outside of their racial group, particularly as it relates to the development of multicultural counseling competence and the therapeutic alliance (Burkard et al., 1999). When thinking about cultural comfort then, learning more about racial identity development and exploring ways to advance one's own racial identity development can be a fruitful endeavor.

White Racial Identity Development

Recall that *racial identity development* refers to the process through which individuals develop a healthy view of: (a) themselves, (b) members within their racial group, and (c) members of other racial groups (Constantine et al., 1998). Within the mental health literature, Helms's (1995) White Racial Identity Development (WRID) model is one of the more frequently researched and applied theories of White racial identity (Malott et al., 2015). WRID was initially developed to describe the process by which White individuals become more self-aware and humanistic toward REM clients (Helms, 2014). Through decades of research and validation, Helms's (2014) WRID model has been refined to consist of six progressive statuses that describe "the dynamic cognitive, emotional, and behavioral processes that govern a person's interpretation of racial information in her or his interpersonal environments" (Helms, 1995, p. 184). The first three statuses, *contact, disintegration*, and *reintegration* reflect a racial worldview characterized by internalized White superiority, privilege, and racism.

Within the contact status, individuals are satisfied with the status quo and give little thought to the benefits of racism. With increased interaction among people of color, however, these individuals typically move into the disintegration status, at which point they begin to experience confusion or ambivalence about their racial group, maintaining attitudes such as "There is nothing I can do to prevent racism" (Helms, 2014, p. 15). At the reintegration status, however, individuals revert to a worldview characterized by idealization of the White race and intolerance for other racial groups. Beliefs at this status reflect a self-enhancing distortion of information, for example, reverse racism and White replacement conspiracy theories.

In contrast to the first three statuses of Helms's (2014) WRID model, the remaining three statuses, *pseudo-independence*, *immersion/emersion*, and *autonomy*, reflect an evolving non-racist identity. At the pseudo-independence status, individuals have a deceptive tolerance for other racial groups wherein the White racial group is viewed as the standard for acceptability. Individuals at this status may have colorblind racial attitudes and beliefs such as "White people should help Black people become equal to Whites" (Helms, 2014, p. 15). At the immersion/emersion status, however, individuals begin to more actively seek to understand how they benefit from White privilege, while they simultaneously take responsibility for racism by adopting an anti-racist stance and immersing themselves in communities of color. At the final status, individuals begin to enact anti-racist behavior within their own spheres of influence, having adopted a positive racial identity based on an internal set of standards and commitment to relinquish the privileges of racism (Helms, 2014). These individuals are receptive to feedback from people of color and have a true value for diversity.

Among White clinicians, research shows that more advanced levels of racial identity correlate to greater perceived multicultural competence and better therapeutic outcomes among racially diverse clients (Constantine, 2002; Johnson & Jackson Williams, 2015; Middleton et al., 2005, 2011; Ottavi et al., 1994; Vinson & Neimeyer, 2003). Johnson and Jackson Williams (2015), for example, found that advanced stages of White racial identity were correlated to higher levels of self-perceived multicultural counseling knowledge, awareness, and skills among a sample of graduate-level psychology students. Similarly, Middleton et al. (2011) also found advanced levels of White racial identity to be a statistically significant contributor to self-perceived multicultural counseling competence among clinical psychologists and professional counselors. Burkard et al. (1999) found that at its lower levels (i.e., disintegration and reintegration), White racial identity negatively affected ratings of the working alliance in same-racial and cross-racial vicarious counseling analogues, while higher levels of White racial identity (i.e., pseudo-independence and autonomy) had a positive effect on the working alliance. In sum, these studies suggest White racial identity not only has the potential to affect perceived levels of multicultural counseling competence among therapists, but in the therapeutic dyad as well.

The Racial/Cultural Identity Development Model

As mentioned in Chapter 2, the Nigrescence model of Black racial identity development (Vandiver et al., 2001) was the first and perhaps most influential model of its kind. Since its initial development in the 1970s, several models of racial identity development relevant to other communities such as Asian American and Latinx racial/ethnic groups have also been developed (Sue et al., 2019). In 1989, Atkinson and his colleagues developed the Racial/Cultural Identity Development Model (R/CID), which integrates the most common features across the various models of ethnic identity development. This model consists of five stages that explore an individual's attitude toward: (a) self, (b) others of the same group, (c) others of a different marginalized group, and (d) the dominant group. The stages in the R/CID model are known as: (1) conformity, (2) dissonance, (3) resistance and immersion, (4) introspection, and (5) integrative awareness. Like other models of racial identity development, the R/CID model provides important insights into attitudes and behaviors that define the process through which individuals develop a healthy view of themselves, members within their racial group, and members of other racial groups, as well as implications for the therapeutic context (Constantine et al., 1998).

In the R/CID model, conformity and dissonance represent lower levels of racial identity development. *Conformity* is defined as a preference for dominant cultural values over those belonging to one's own racial group. Accordingly, attitudes toward self and others of the same racial group at this stage of development are characterized by internalized racism, including a negative view of the physical and cultural attributes of one's own racial group and belief in a just world. Attitudes toward members of different marginalized groups are also viewed negatively, or at best, neutrally depending on how they are viewed within the dominant racial hierarchy. For example, Asian Americans may be viewed more positively than Latinx Americans (Sue et al., 2019). Conversely, attitudes toward members of the dominant group are characterized by White superiority and the belief that White cultural norms and values are to be admired and emulated. At the *dissonance* stage, the preferential view of the dominant group begins to be challenged as individuals have more counter-stereotypic encounters with members of various racial and ethnic groups. Accordingly, individuals at this stage of racial identity have a growing awareness that racism does exist and aspects of their own cultural norms and values are, in fact, positive in nature (Sue et al., 2019). Moreover, individuals at the dissonance stage also have a growing sense of camaraderie with members of other marginalized groups and a weakening sense of trust for members of the dominant group.

As the burgeoning of greater acceptance of one's own cultural group begins to occur at the dissonance stage, increased feelings of guilt, shame, and anger also begin to develop as individuals enter the *resistance and immersion stage* (Sue et al., 2019). However, individuals at the resistance and immersion stage are also developing a growing sense of pride and identification with their racial/cultural group, as well as a sense of empathy for members of other marginalized groups. In contrast, attitudes towards members of the dominant group are now characterized by distrust and even dislike. At the *introspection stage*, the characteristics of the resistance and immersion stage shift from a reactive stance against racism to a focus on positive self-definition (Sue et al., 2019). Accordingly, individuals at the introspection stage are becoming more open and less culture-centric in their attitudes toward self, others of the same racial group, and members of other marginalized groups; however, these individuals may also begin to experience some confusion as they realize some elements of dominant culture may be functional and desirable. Finally, as conflicts at the introspection stage are resolved, individuals enter the *integrative awareness stage*, which is characterized by appreciation for their own culture as well as positive aspects of the dominant culture.

While research concerning the racial identity of therapists of color and cultural sensitivity in the therapeutic context is somewhat limited, a study conducted by Matthews et al. (2018) has explored the relationship between multicultural counseling competence, ethnic identity, and multicultural self-efficacy. In the study, the researchers explored the relationship between these variables among 172 racially mixed professional counselors (i.e., Caucasian/White (68%), African American/Black (16.3%), Hispanic/Latino (8.1%), Asian (3.5%), Native American (0.6%) and others). Results of the study indicated positive and statistically significant correlations between multicultural counseling competence and ethnic identity, as well as ethnic identity and multicultural self-efficacy using a non-specific measure of ethnic identity development (i.e., the Multigroup Ethnic Identity Measure-Revised, Phinney & Ong, 2007). While these results are not specific to people of color only, they do lend some credibility to the idea that higher levels of racial/ethnic identity also have the potential to affect perceived levels of multicultural counseling competence among therapists belonging to racial/ethnic minority groups as well.

Reflection 4.1: Exploring Your Racial Identity

The sections above describe models of racial identity development for people of color and individuals belonging to White racial groups, and present research indicating that individuals with higher levels of racial identity may also have greater multicultural counseling competence. Yet, a question remains as to how we, as therapists, achieve a positive sense of belonging to our respective racial groups. A first step can be to locate yourself on the appropriate continuum of racial identity development presented above. If you are at lower levels of racial identity development, deliberate and thoughtful reflection on the experiences that have contributed to your view of race and your emotions around it can be beneficial. Engaging in activities to increase critical consciousness and contact with members from various racial groups can also be helpful. If you are at more advanced levels of racial identity, deliberate and thoughtful reflection can be beneficial for you too, as attitudes toward race can be deeply engrained and even unconscious, as described in the section on implicit bias. Accordingly, I encourage everyone to complete the reflection questions below and then commit to identifying ways to continue evolving as a racial being that are genuine and authentic for you.

1. When did you first become aware of yourself as a racial being?
2. What messages did you receive about your race early in life? What messages did you receive about other races?
3. In what ways do the racial identity development models presented above match your own racial development? Describe an experience to illustrate what you were like at each stage of the racial identity development model. If you have not reached certain stages, describe how you would like to see yourself at these stages in the future.
4. What can you do to continue growing in your racial identity? Are there beliefs you need to modify? New experiences to obtain?

References

Abreu, J. M. (1999). Conscious and nonconscious African American stereotypes: Impact on first impression and diagnostic ratings by therapists. *Journal of Consulting and Clinical Psychology, 67*(3), 387–393. https://doi.org/10.1037/0022-006X.67.3.387

Arredondo, P., Toporek, R., Brown, S. P., Jones, J., Locke, D. C., Sanchez, J., & Stadler, H. (1996). Operationalization of the multicultural counseling competencies. *Journal of Multicultural Counseling and Development, 24*(1), 42–78. https://doi.org/10.1002/j.2161-1912.1996.tb00288.x

Banaji, M. R., & Greenwald, A. G. (2016). *Blindspot: Hidden biases of good people.* Bantam Books.

Belgrave, F. Z., & Allison, K. W. (2018). *African American psychology: From Africa to America* (4th ed.). Sage Publications, Inc.

Boysen, G. A. (2010). Integrating implicit bias into counselor education. *Counselor Education and Supervision, 49*(4), 210–227. https://doi.org/10.1002/j.1556-6978. 2010.tb00099.x

Boysen, G. A., & Vogel, D. L. (2008). The relationship between level of training, implicit bias, and multicultural competency among counselor trainees. *Training and Education in Professional Psychology, 2*(2), 103–110. https://doi.org/10.1037/1 931-3918.2.2.103

Burkard, A. W., Ponterotto, J. G., Reynolds, A. L., & Alfonso, V. C. (1999). White counselor trainees' racial identity and working alliance perceptions. *Journal of Counseling & Development, 77*(3), 324–329. https://doi.org/10.1002/j.1556-6676. 1999.tb02455.x

Castillo, L. G., Brossart, D. F., Reyes, G. J., Gonoley, G. W., & Phoummarath, M. J. (2007). The influence of multicultural training on perceived multicultural counseling competencies and implicit racial prejudice. *Journal of Multicultural Counseling and Development, 35*, 243–254. https://doi.org/10.1002/j.2161-1912.2007.tb00064.x

Chekroud, A. M., Everett, J. A., Bridge, H., & Hewstone, M. (2014). A review of neuroimaging studies of race-related prejudice: Does amygdala response reflect threat? *Frontiers in Human Neuroscience, 8*, 179. https://doi.org/10.3389/fnhum. 2014.00179

Christopher, J. C. (1996). Counseling's inescapable moral visions. *Journal of Counseling & Development, 75*(1), 17–25. https://doi.org/10.1002/j.1556-6676.1996.tb02310.x

Constantine, M. G. (2002). Racism attitudes, White racial identity attitudes, and multicultural counseling competence in school counselor trainees. *Counselor Education and Supervision, 41*(3), 162–174. https://doi.org/10.1002/j.1556-6978.2002. tb01281.x

Constantine, M. G., Richardson, T. Q., Benjamin, E. M., & Wilson, J. W. (1998). An overview of Black racial identity theories: Current limitations and considerations. *Applied and Preventive Psychology, 7*(2), 95–99. https://doi.org/10.1016/S0962-1849 (05)80006-X

Cooper, A. A., & Conklin, L. R. (2015). Dropout from individual psychotherapy for major depression: A meta-analysis of randomized clinical trials. *Clinical Psychology Review, 40*, 57–65. https://doi.org/10.1016/j.cpr.2015.05.001

Davis, D. E., DeBlaere, C., Owen, J., Hook, J. N., Rivera, D. P., Choe, E., Van Tongeren, D. R., Worthington, E. L., Jr., & Placeres, V. (2018). The multicultural orientation framework: A narrative review. *Psychotherapy, 55*(1), 89–100. https://doi. org/10.1037/pst0000160

Day-Vines, N. L., Cluxton-Keller, F., Agorsor, C., Gubara, S., & Otabil, N. A. A. (2020). The multidimensional model or broaching behavior. *Journal of Counseling & Development, 98*(1), 107–118. https://doi.org/10.1002/jcad.12304

Day-Vines, N.L., Wood, S. M., Grothaus, T., Craigen, L., Holman, A., Dotson-Blake, K., & Douglass, M. J. (2007). Broaching the subjects of race, ethnicity, and culture during the counseling process. *Journal of Counseling & Development, 85*(4), 401–409. https://doi.org/10.1002/jcad.12069

DeRicco, J. N., & Sciarra, D. T. (2005). The immersion experience in multicultural counselor training: Confronting covert racism. *Journal of Multicultural Counseling and Development, 33*(1), 2–16. https://doi.org/10.1002/j.2161-1912.2005. tb00001.x

Devine, P. G. (1989). Stereotypes and prejudice: Their automatic and controlled components. *Journal of Personality and Social Psychology*, *56*(1), 5–18. https://doi.org/10.1037/0022-3514.56.1.5

Devine, P. G., Forscher, P. S., Austin, A. J., & Cox, W. T. L. (2012). Long-term reduction in implicit bias: A prejudice habit-breaking intervention. *Journal of Experimental Social Psychology*, *48*(6), 1267–1278. https://doi.org/10.1016/j.jesp.2012.06.003

Fazio, R. H. (1990). Multiple processes by which attitudes guide behavior: The MODE model as an integrative framework. *Advances in Experimental Social Psychology*, *23*, 75–109.

Fazio, R. H., Jackson, J. R., Dunton, B. C., & Williams, C. J. (1995). Variability in automatic activation as an unobtrusive measure of racial attitudes: A bona fide pipeline? *Journal of Personality and Social Psychology*, *69*(6), 1013–1027. https://doi.org/10.1037/0022-3514.69.6.1013

Fuller, P., Murphy, M., & Chow, A. (2020). *The leader's guide to unconscious bias: How to reframe bias, cultivate connection, and create high performing teams*. Simon & Schuster.

Gushue, G. V. (2004). Race, color-blind racial attitudes, and judgments about mental health: A shifting standards perspective. *Journal of Counseling Psychology*, *51*(4), 398–407. https://doi.org/10.1037/0022-0167.51.4.398

Gushue, G. V., & Constantine, M. G. (2007). Color-blind racial attitudes and white racial identity attitudes in psychology trainees. *Professional Psychology: Research and Practice*, *38*(3), 321–328. https://doi.org/10.1037/0735-7028.38.3.321

Hall, W. J., Chapman, M. V., Lee, K. M., et al. (2015). Implicit racial/ethnic bias among health care professionals and its influence on health care outcomes: A systematic review. *American Journal of Public Health*, *105*(12), e60–e76. https://doi.org/10.2105/AJPH.2015.302903

Harris, R. (2019). *ACT made simple* (2nd ed.). New Harbinger.

Helms, J. E. (1995). An update of Helm's White and people of color racial identity models. In J. G. Ponterotto, J. M. Casas, L. A. Suzuki, & C. M. Alexander (Eds.), *Handbook of multicultural counseling* (pp. 181–198). Sage Publications, Inc.

Helms, J. E. (2014). A review of White racial identity theory: The sociopolitical implications of studying White racial identity in psychology. In S. Cooper & K. Ratele (Eds.), *Psychology serving humanity: Proceedings of the 30th International Congress of Psychology, Vol. 2. Western psychology* (pp. 12–27). Psychology Press.

Hook, J. N., Davis, D., Owen, J., & DeBlaere, C. (2017). *Cultural humility: Engaging diverse identities in therapy*. American Psychological Association. https://doi.org/10.1037/0000037-000

Jadaszewski, S. (2017). Ethically problematic value change as an outcome of psychotherapeutic interventions. *Ethics & Behavior*, *27*(4), 297–312. https://doi.org/10.1080/10508422.2016.1195739

Johnson, A., & Jackson Williams, D. (2015). White racial identity, color-blind racial attitudes, and multicultural counseling competence. *Cultural Diversity and Ethnic Minority Psychology*, *21*(3), 440–449. https://doi.org/10.1037/a0037533

Johnson, M., & Melton, M. L. (2021). *Addressing race-based stress in therapy with Black clients*. Routledge.

Kluckhohn, C. (1951). Values and value orientations in the theory of action: An exploration in definition and classification. In T. Parsons & E. A. Shils (Eds.), *Toward a general theory of action* (pp. 388–433). Harper & Row.

Malott, K. M., Paone, T. R., Schaefle, S., Cates, J., & Haizlip, B. (2015). Expanding White racial identity theory: A qualitative investigation of Whites engaged in antiracist action. *Journal of Counseling & Development, 93*(3), 333–343. https://doi.org/10.1002/jcad.12031

Matthews, J. J., Barden, S. M., & Sherrell, R. S. (2018). Examining the relationships between multicultural counseling competence, multicultural self-efficacy, and ethnic identity development of practicing counselors. *Journal of Mental Health Counseling, 40*(2), 129–141. https://doi.org/10.17744/mehc.40.2.03

Middleton, R. A., Erguner-Tekinalp, B., Williams, N. F., Stadler, H. A., & Dow, J. E. (2011). Racial identity development and multicultural counseling competencies of White mental health practitioners. *International Journal of Psychology and Psychological Therapy, 11*(2), 201–218.

Middleton, R. A., Stadler, H. A., Simpson, C., Guo, Y.-J., Brown, M. J., Crow, G., Schuck, K., Alemu, Y., & Lazarte, A. A. (2005). Mental health practitioners: The relationship between White racial identity attitudes and self-reported multicultural counseling competencies. *Journal of Counseling & Development, 83*(4), 444–456. https://doi.org/10.1002/j.1556-6678.2005.tb00366.x

Ottavi, T. M., Pope-Davis, D. B., & Dings, J. G. (1994). Relationship between White racial identity attitudes and self-reported multicultural counseling competencies. *Journal of Counseling Psychology, 41*(2), 149–154. https://doi.org/10.1037/0022-0167.41.2.149

Owen, J., Imel, Z., Tao, K. W., Wampold, B., Smith, A., & Rodolfa, E. (2011). Cultural ruptures in short-term therapy: Working alliance as a mediator between clients' perceptions of microaggressions and therapy outcomes. *Counselling & Psychotherapy Research, 11*, 204–212. https://doi.org/10.1080/14733145.2010.491551

Payne, J. S. (2014). Social determinants affecting major depressive disorder: Diagnostic accuracy for African American men. *Best Practices in Mental Health, 10*(2), 78–95.

Phinney, J. S., & Ong, A. D. (2007). Conceptualization and measurement of ethnic identity: Current status and future directions. *Journal of Counseling Psychology, 54*(3), 271–281. https://doi.org/10.1037/0022-0167.54.3.271

Phipps, A. (2021). White tears, White rage: Victimhood and (as) violence in mainstream feminism. *European Journal of Cultural Studies, 24*(1) 81–93. https://doi.org/10.1177/1367549420985852

Pope-Davis, D. B., Breaux, C., & Liu, W. M. (1997). A multicultural immersion experience: Filling a void in multicultural training. In D. B. Pope Davis & H. L. K. Coleman (Eds.), *Multicultural counseling competencies: Assessment, education and training, and supervision* (pp. 227–241). Sage.

Rivers, A. M., Sherman, J. W., Rees, H. R., Reichardt, R., & Klauer, K. C. (2020). On the roles of stereotype activation and application in diminishing implicit bias. *Personality and Social Psychology Bulletin, 46*(3), 349–364. https://doi.org/10.1177/0146167219853842

Shannonhouse, L. R., Myers, J. E., & Barrio Minton, C. A. (2018). Cultural immersion in counselor education: Trends, prevalence, and common components. *Journal of Multicultural Counseling and Development, 46*(4), 283–296. https://doi.org/10.1002/jmcd.12115

Shipp, P. L. (1983). Counseling Blacks: A group approach. *The Personnel and Guidance Journal, 62*, 108–111.

Sue, D. W., Sue, D., Neville, H. A., & Smith, L. (2019). *Counseling the culturally diverse: Theory and practice* (8th ed.). John Wiley & Sons, Inc.

Tjeltveit, A. C. (2015). Appropriately addressing psychological scientists' inescapable cognitive and moral values. *Journal of Theoretical and Philosophical Psychology*, *35*(1), 35–52. https://doi.org/10.1037/a0037909

Vandiver, B. J., Fhagen-Smith, P. E., Cokley, K. O., Cross, W. E., Jr., & Worrell, F. C. (2001). Cross's Nigrescence model: From theory to scale to theory. *Journal of Multicultural Counseling and Development*, *29*(3), 174–200. https://doi.org/10.1002/j.2161-1912.2001.tb00516.x

Vinson, T. S., & Neimeyer, G. J. (2003). The relationship between racial identity development and multicultural counseling competency: A second look. *Journal of Multicultural Counseling and Development*, *31*(4), 262–277. https://doi.org/10.1002/j.2161-1912.2003.tb00354.x

Watkins, D. C., & Neighbors, H. W. (2013). Social determinants of depression and the Black male experience. In H. M. Treadwell, C. Xanthos, & K. B. Holden (Eds.), *Social determinants of health among African-American men* (pp. 39–62). Jossey-Bass/Wiley.

Chapter 5

Facilitating Culturally Responsive Therapeutic Relationships

Among novice therapists, there is often a misperception that CBT focuses on client cognitions and behaviors to the exclusion of other concerns such as the therapeutic relationship. True CBT therapists, however, know that the therapeutic relationship has long been considered a critical aspect of the therapeutic process in CBT (Matu, 2018). In fact, from its inception, the originators of first and second wave CBT theories have emphasized the role of the therapeutic relationship in the reduction of client symptoms and in overall treatment outcomes. Wolpe (1958), for example, noted that clients who seemed to like him showed signs of improvement earlier in therapy when compared to those who did not. Similarly, A. T. Beck and his colleagues (1979) described good CBT therapists as those who demonstrate counselor dispositions traditionally emphasized in psychodynamic theories, such as warmth, empathy, genuineness, and acceptance (Matu, 2018). Accordingly, Beck dedicated a significant amount of his writing to emphasizing the importance of these characteristics, as well as other critical aspects of the therapeutic relationship, such as trust, rapport, and collaboration (Dobson, 2022).

In similar fashion, decades of research conducted since CBT was initially developed confirms the link between the quality of the therapeutic relationship and positive therapeutic outcomes (Zilcha-Mano et al., 2020). One recent meta-analytic review, for example, found a positive correlation between the therapeutic alliance and treatment outcomes in CBT for depression across both early and later stages of therapy (Cameron et al., 2018). Another meta-analysis of research also found a statistically significant relationship between the therapeutic alliance and treatment outcomes across several forms of therapy, including CBT (Flückiger et al., 2012). Meta-analytical studies moreover confirm the relationship between the therapeutic alliance and treatment outcomes for children and adolescents, in couples and family settings, and in group therapy (Flückiger, 2022).

Despite the vast literature base emphasizing the importance of the therapeutic relationship in CBT, perceptions of the theory as cold and mechanized

DOI: 10.4324/9781003196303-5

continue to prevail within the broader mental health community (J. S. Beck, 2020). Castonguay et al. (2018) identified two primary reasons for this prevailing notion. First, the therapeutic relationship in CBT is different than in some other approaches to therapy in terms of its structured and highly directive qualities. Second, CBT traditionally emphasizes interventions and techniques as the source of therapeutic change, while other theories place a more direct emphasis on the therapeutic relationship. In furthering their discussion on this matter, however, Castonguay et al. (2018) also note that given the totality of how CBT has been described over time, belief that its directive and structured nature indicates neglect of the therapeutic relationship represents an unsophisticated and incomplete understanding of CBT's core foundation. Instead, the therapeutic relationship in CBT can more accurately be conceptualized as a critical (albeit insufficient) aspect of change in the therapeutic process, particularly in terms of collaboration and guided discovery (Dobson, 2022).

When working with African American clients on issues such as race and racism, the therapist's ability to build strong therapeutic relationships is even more critical to the process of change given the sensitive nature of race and racism and the amount of vulnerability required to discuss these topics. This chapter addresses the importance of culturally responsive therapeutic relationships and describes key considerations in facilitating these relationships. Accordingly, research describing the role of the therapeutic relationship with African American clients is briefly reviewed and specific aspects of the therapeutic alliance are discussed. Steps to managing cultural ruptures that may occur in the therapeutic relationship are then explored, and the chapter is concluded with a case illustration of these steps.

Therapeutic Alliance and Treatment Outcomes with African American Clients

Across theories, the therapeutic relationship, or more specifically, the *therapeutic alliance* is broadly defined as "the working relationship that exists between the therapist and the client" (Waltman et al., 2021, p. 30). Conceptually, the therapeutic alliance is understood to consist of three interrelated components, which include: (1) client and therapist agreement on treatment goals, (2) client and therapist agreement on the tasks that will be used to achieve those goals, and (3) a bond between the client and therapist that is experienced as secure, warm, and friendly (Bordin, 1979; Boswell & Constantino, 2022, pp. 113–114). According to the common factors literature, 30 percent of the outcome variance in therapy is said to be attributable to this alliance, while only 15 percent of outcome variance is said to occur as a result of specific theory and treatment techniques (Norcross & Lambert, 2011 as cited in Wenzel et al., 2016). This means that while the theory-specific interventions and techniques implemented during therapy do have a significant impact on therapeutic outcomes, a larger percentage of these outcomes can be ascribed to the quality of the working relationship between the therapist and the client.

Therapeutic outcomes are the changes that occur within an individual as a result of their experiences with therapy. In clinical settings, these changes typically refer to a reduction of symptoms, improvements in one's interpersonal relationships, or satisfaction with one's social roles. Although relatively few studies have been published on the topic, much of the extant research suggests that the quality of the therapeutic alliance has a unique impact on treatment outcomes with African American clients. A study of the relationship between the working alliance and treatment outcomes among partner-violent men, for example, found that the interaction between client race/ethnicity and working alliance was a significant predictor of treatment outcome at six-month follow-up (Walling et al., 2012). Specifically, racial/ethnic minority participants (95.8% African American) who reported significant growth in the working alliance over the course of treatment benefited from treatment to the same degree as Caucasian participants; however, minority participants who did not report significant growth in working alliance reported fewer benefits from treatment at the six-month follow-up assessment when compared to their White counterparts. Similarly, a study of urban adolescents also found a significant effect between the therapeutic alliance and treatment outcomes in that a positive therapeutic alliance predicted reductions in delinquent behavior and did so to an even greater extent among youth who were higher in callous–unemotional traits (Mattos et al., 2017). Thus, while additional research is needed, existing studies suggest that the therapeutic alliance appears to be an important factor in facilitating change in African American clients, even among populations that are difficult to engage (Mattos et al., 2017; Walling et al., 2012). Moreover, these studies further suggest that when considering the impact of the therapeutic alliance on various treatment outcomes, therapists should also be mindful of the need to promote growth in the alliance across the different stages of therapy (Walling et al., 2012).

Therapeutic Alliance in CBT

Broadly, African Americans tend to score lower on measures of the therapeutic alliance when compared to their White counterparts (Eliacin et al., 2018). Often, these differences can be attributed to perceived or actual cultural biases within the therapy dyad (Walling et al., 2012). A study of racial microaggressions against African American clients in cross-racial therapy dyads, for example, found that greater perceived racial microaggressions by African American clients were predictive of a weaker therapeutic alliance with White therapists (Constantine, 2007). Likewise, other cultural factors such as trustworthiness, cultural knowledge, and willingness to connect have also been found to affect the therapeutic relationship. As such, racial and cultural factors may be understood as significant mediators between the therapeutic alliance and change experienced as a result of therapy, warranting deliberate consideration within the interpersonal dynamics of the therapy context.

Establishing a Bond

So, with the above research findings in mind, how do therapists facilitate a strong therapeutic alliance with African American clients during CBT? At a minimum, therapists must be able to integrate the use of basic counseling techniques throughout therapy in order to develop a bond between client and therapist that is perceived as secure, warm, and friendly. This includes use of encouragers such as head nods and facial gestures, as well as skills such as empathy, probes, reflection of feeling, and open-ended questions. Consider the differences in two brief opening exchanges with Lisa, a 17-year-old adolescent seeking counseling due to generalized and social anxiety. At intake, Lisa presented as quiet and reserved in her responses to the therapist's probes regarding the nature of her difficulties with anxiety. In the first exchange, the therapist rigidly attends to the task of gathering data needed to form a diagnostic impression and formulate broad therapy goals, while in the second exchange, the therapist attends to these tasks while also implementing basic skills to establish a rapport with Lisa.

Exchange 1

Therapist: Hello, Lisa. Because today is our initial evaluation session, I'm going to focus on getting information needed to determine your diagnosis and set treatment goals.
Lisa: Ok.
Therapist: Tell me, how would you describe the issues bringing you to therapy today?

Exchange 2

Therapist: Hello, Lisa. It's nice to meet you today. Because this is our first session together, we'll focus mostly on getting an understanding of what's bringing you to therapy. If at the end the session you decide you want to continue therapy with me, we'll start working on the problems you tell me about today the next time we meet. Does that sound ok?
Lisa: Ok.
Therapist: Good. So, tell me, what brings you to therapy today?

In these two brief exchanges, we see vastly different attention to the therapeutic relationship. In Exchange 1, the therapist started the session by greeting Lisa, which is generally welcoming provided that the therapist greets the client with warmth and authenticity. Unfortunately, little was done to establish rapport with Lisa in Exchange 1 beyond welcoming her to therapy. Instead, the therapist focused solely on the primary task of an evaluation session, which is to obtain data necessary to make a diagnosis and formulate treatment goals. Conversely, the therapist in Exchange 2 focused on obtaining information needed to make an evaluation, while also integrating several basic counseling skills to communicate care and collaboration in the exchange. First, the therapist used language that was accessible to the client given her age and stage of development. Specifically, while the therapist in Exchange 1 used jargon such as "diagnosis" and "treatment goals" to describe the purpose of the session, the therapist in Exchange 2 used friendlier language, describing the purpose of the session as "getting an understanding of what's bringing you to therapy." Second, the therapist in Exchange 2 also began to establish norms around collaboration by seeking to share power and involve Lisa in decision making during therapy. This was accomplished by highlighting Lisa's choice to continue therapy or not. Collaboration was additionally illustrated in the session through the simple use of the check-out question, "Does that sound ok?" This type of collaborative stance is known as *collaborative empiricism* and is considered a hallmark feature of CBT (Beck, 2020). Further development of collaborative empiricism in the relationship would involve skillfully guiding Lisa in the discovery of the automatic thoughts contributing to her current distress and their underlying cognitions, while working together to identify tasks to address these cognitions (Wong, 2013).

In addition to broad efforts to establish rapport and develop collaborative relationships, therapists working with African American clients on issues such as race and racism should also be intentional in their use of the counseling technique known as validation. *Validation* refers to the therapist's ability to communicate that they understand the client's reactions and that these reactions make sense given their current life context or situation (Linehan, 1997). According to Linehan (1997), there are six basic ways therapists may communicate validation to their clients: (1) active listening and observing, (2) accurate reflection of the client's thoughts and feelings, (3) articulation of unverbalized emotions and meanings, (4) expressing that behavior is understandable given prior events, (5) expressing that behavior is understandable given current events, and (6) believing and responding to the client as if they are capable of achieving change and their long-term goals, something Linehan (1997) calls "radical genuineness" (p. 377). Other basic validation skills include being tolerant and maintaining a non-judgmental stance during therapy.

Because of its insidious nature, clients' experiences with racism are not always validated during therapy. Factors such as colorblind racial attitudes, racial microaggressions, or poor knowledge of the effects of racism on one's well-being, for example, may lead to reactions that actually invalidate a person's experience with racism (Burris, 2012). Some of these reactions include: (a) minimization of impact (e.g., "You're strong. Don't let them ruin your day"), (b) disbelief that it was racism (e.g., "Do you really think this was about race?"), (c) highlighting innocent intentions (e.g., "I don't think they meant to be racist"), (d) rush to problem-solving (e.g., "You should report this immediately!"), (e) defending the status quo (e.g., "The older generation had a different way of thinking about things"), (f) personal defensiveness and the need to not be seen as racist (e.g., "I just want to understand both sides of the story" and "You know I'm not racist, right?"), and (g) empathic failure (i.e., ignoring emotions that occur as a result of experiences with racism) (Mai & Whitlock, 2022; Pierson et al., 2022). Consider the following dialogue with Zena, a 42-year-old African American woman who has expressed distress over recently publicized police brutality in her community. Notice how although meant well, the therapist's response to Zena's story invalidates some of the emotion and meanings Zena appears to associate with the events happening in her community. Additionally, as you read the dialogue, try to identify specific types of reactions from the list above that characterize these invalidating responses.

Examples of Invalidating Statements by the Therapist

Zena: I've been so upset by the news lately. I just don't know how many more stories of unarmed Black men being killed I can take.

Therapist: I'm so sorry to hear that, Zena. Please, tell me more about what you've been experiencing.

Zena: Well, for days now they've been showing footage of the murder on social media. Then, every night when I get home from work, there's more about it on the news. On one network there are constant interviews with family members who are obviously devastated by what's happened. On the other network the political pundits are debating over the rights of police to "protect" themselves. It's like there's no escape. Either I'm dealing with the heartache of generations of trauma in my community or the anger of knowing that Black lives literally mean nothing to some people simply because of the color of our skin. Like I said, I just don't know how much more of this I can take.

Therapist: Zena, I can understand how you would be upset by what you're seeing on social media and the news. Let's talk about ways you can minimize your exposure to these images so that they have less of an effect on how you're feeling right now.

In reviewing the dialogue between Zena and her therapist, several areas for growth are noted in the therapist's ability to validate Zena's current experience with racism. First, while the therapist did demonstrate some empathic responses to the emotion and content shared in Zena's story (i.e., "I'm so sorry to hear that" and "I can understand how you would be upset"), empathic failure is nevertheless observed in the therapist's ability to respond specifically to the context of race and racism in Zena's life. For example, the therapist's decision to acknowledge Zena's distress without also acknowledging the source of that distress could easily be perceived as a way to avoid discussing racism, which in turn could be interpreted as fear, discomfort, or even disagreement with Zena's conclusions on the nature of race and racism in today's society. This potentiality is problematic given research findings which suggest that failure to broach racial concerns during therapy may be viewed as a microaggressive act (Day-Vines et al., 2021), negatively impacting perceived counselor competence (Constantine, 2007), psychological wellbeing (Owen et al., 2011, 2014), satisfaction with counseling (Constantine, 2007), and future help seeking (Crawford, 2011).

A second area of concern in the therapist's response to Zena's story is the therapist's rush to problem-solving evidenced by a focus on strategies to direct Zena's attention away from distressing stimuli. While this approach may be appropriate within the context of broader goal setting and treatment planning objectives, failing to first acknowledge and validate race in Zena's story could limit future disclosures of racial content, restricting the therapist's ability to obtain information necessary to conceptualize racially salient cognitions contributing to her current difficulties with mood or interpersonal relationships. Moreover, by focusing on limiting Zena's exposure to social media and the news, the therapist may communicate the message that Zena's distress is a result of her own behavior rather than the realities of racism. This message, in turn, could be interpreted as belittling or even offensive, as no therapeutic intervention can erase the difficulties of being Black in a racialized society.

In contrast to the approach illustrated in the therapist dialogue with Zena, validating a client's experience with racism requires the therapist to express care and compassion for the wounds that occur as a result of these experiences. Mai and Whitlock (2022), for example, suggested that the three elements of self-compassion; that is, mindfulness, common humanity, and kindness, may be a useful framework for fostering compassionate responses to racism. In this framework, *mindfulness* refers to the therapist's ability to be aware of and manage their own defensiveness when the topic of racism is discussed within the therapy dyad, while *common humanity* refers to the act of letting clients know that they are not alone, and that the therapist is there to support them as they deal with the hurt caused by racism. *Kindness*, on the other hand, refers to the therapist's ability to show a sincere desire to help. This may be achieved by offering words of encouragement and affirmation, or by helping the client to develop a plan of action to address racism. Examples of validating statements you may use with clients based on the three elements of compassion and Linehan's (1997) six levels of validation include the following:

- "The situation you describe sounds like racism"
- "The things that are happening to you are wrong"
- "I may not know what it is like to be mistreated because of the color of my skin but I want you to know that I believe that what you're saying is real and it hurts"
- "Thank you for trusting me enough to share something so painful"
- "I am sorry this happened to you"
- "It makes sense that you would experience anger [guilt, shame, frustration, humiliation, etc.] as a result of this situation"
- "Please let me know how I can support any actions you may take"

With these examples in mind, let's return to our case illustration, Zena. The dialogue that follows demonstrates how her therapist could use the three elements of compassion (Mai & Whitlock, 2022) and Linehan's (1997) techniques to communicate validation in the session with Zena. This time, as you read the dialogue, see if you are able to identify the specific elements of compassion and levels of validation evidenced in the therapist's reaction to Zena's story.

Examples of Validating Statements by the Therapist

Zena: I've been so upset by the news lately. I just don't know how many more stories of unarmed Black men being killed I can take.

Therapist: I'm so sorry to hear that, Zena. I've seen these stories on the news as well. While I may not know what it's like to be discriminated against because of the color of my skin, I understand that this is deeply painful. I want you to know that I am here to support you. Please, tell me more about what you've been experiencing.

Zena: Well, for days now they've been showing footage of the murder on social media. Then, every night when I get home from work, there's more about it on the news. On one network there are constant interviews with family members who are obviously devastated by what's happened. On the other network the political pundits are debating over the rights of police to "protect" themselves. It's like there's no escape. Either I'm dealing with the heartache of generations of trauma in my community or the anger of knowing that Black lives literally mean nothing to some people simply because of the color of our skin. Like I said, I just don't know how much more of this I can take.

Therapist: Zena, it makes sense that you would feel like there is no escape from the pain of racism. It seems as though just as one story of injustice ends another one begins. Could we take some time to explore the impact this is having on you in greater detail?

As described by Linehan (1997), validation communicates to clients that their reactions make sense given their past or current life experiences. For African American clients dealing with racism, acts of validation are critical to the development of the therapeutic alliance, as they convey caring and contribute to the sense of safety experienced in the therapeutic dyad (Day-Vines et al., 2021). In the therapist dialogue with Zena, validating communications were evidenced in each of the therapist statements made in response to Zena's story. In particular, both statements demonstrated each of the elements of compassion described by Mai and Whitlock (2022). The therapist's willingness to acknowledge the aspects of racism evident in Zena's story, for example, illustrated mindfulness on the part of the therapist in terms of their ability to bracket any fears or discomfort they might have been experiencing due to differences in racial group membership between Zena and the therapist. Common humanity, on the other hand, was demonstrated through the statement "I want you to know that I am here to support you," which let Zena know that she was not alone in her struggle. The other aspect of compassion, kindness, was demonstrated through statements such as "I'm sorry to hear that," which expressed sympathy, and "I understand that this is deeply painful," which reflected the emotion within Zena's story and communicated empathy.

Acknowledgment of the pain conveyed in Zena's story also demonstrated Linehan's (1997) third level of validation, accurate reflection of the client's thoughts and feelings. Levels of validation which communicate to the client that their reactions make sense given past and current events were moreover demonstrated through the therapist's statement, "It makes sense that you would feel like there is no escape from the pain of racism. It seems as though just as one story of injustice dies down another one begins." Contrary to the approach taken in the initial dialogue, these responses opened opportunities to explore Zena's reactions to the events happening in her community, which according to research, may have been experienced as cathartic and provided the therapist with additional data in the formulation of a working hypothesis and treatment goals (Day-Vines et al., 2007, 2020; Steele & Newton, 2022).

Activity 5.1: Validating Statements

Imagine that you are the therapist working with Zena. Read the continuation of the dialogue between Zena and the therapist below, and then develop your own validating response to her thoughts concerning the impact of racism on her mental health and well-being.

Therapist: Zena, it makes sense that you would feel like there is no escape from the pain of racism. It seems as though just as one story of injustice ends another one begins. Could we take some time to explore the impact this is having on you in greater detail?

Zena: Yes. It's actually pretty hard for me to describe. It's kind of like a burden that's constantly weighing me down. I feel so angry. And hopeless too. It's like I want to do something but there's nothing I can do.

Your response:

Reflection Questions

- Which elements of compassion or levels of validation did you use in your response?
- How might your response affect the alliance between Zena and the therapist?
- What other ways could you offer validation to Zena at this point in the session?

Agreeing on Treatment Goals

Recall that the therapeutic alliance consists of: (a) client and therapist agreement on treatment goals, (2) client and therapist agreement on the tasks that will be used to achieve those goals, and (3) a bond between the client and therapist (Bordin, 1979). The previous section explored factors that help to establish a strong bond with clients, including the use of basic counseling techniques to communicate friendliness and safety, collaborative empiricism, and validation. In this section, I discuss the process of developing treatment goals with clients, emphasizing identification of problems and operationalization of goals.

Most scholars define the therapeutic alliance according to the conceptualization of the construct developed by Edward Bordin in 1979, which was provided above. While other theorists such as Carl Rogers (1951) had previously defined the concept primarily within the context of qualities such as empathy, congruence, and unconditional positive regard, Bordin (1979) expanded notions of the therapeutic alliance to include other factors that promote mutuality within the therapeutic relationship; namely, agreement on goals and tasks. Elaborating on this idea, Bordin (1979) explained that beyond the bond developed between the therapist and the client, mutual agreement on goals and the tasks used to achieve identified goals increases confidence in the therapeutic process, thus enabling the client to accept, follow, and believe in the treatment (Ardito & Rabellino, 2011). Accordingly, agreement on treatment goals and the tasks used to achieve them are widely accepted as factors critical to the development of the therapeutic alliance.

Consistent with the premise described by Bordin (1979), as well as the principle of collaborative empiricism, goal setting in CBT should be based on a shared understanding of the client's motivation for therapy and approached mutually (Beck, 2020). To begin this process, therapists should first spend time identifying the problems the client is experiencing. Generally, *problems* refer to the situations that contribute to the client's psychological distress, interpersonal difficulties, or social role impairments. They may be identified both at intake and during weekly sessions as the therapist and client work together to develop a session agenda.

Regardless of when problems are identified, specific problem characteristics that therapists should be intentional in paying attention to include dysfunction (i.e., symptoms, instability in relationships, or skill deficits), urgency (i.e., severity or intensity), impairment (i.e., disruptions in the client's ability to fulfill daily roles or tasks), and risk (i.e., chance of harm to self or others) (Schwitzer & Rubin, 2012). Examples of questions to consider as the therapist and the client discuss problems are provided in the list below. A session excerpt illustrating how to gather data about the problem follows the list.

- How does the client describe the problem?
- In which situations does the problem arise?
- What symptoms (cognitive, affective, behavioral, or physiological) are associated with the problem?
- To what extent does the client feel upset or behave dysfunctionally as a result of the problem?
- In what ways does the problem affect the client's ability to function at home or in school, work, or social settings?

Therapist: Let's talk about the problems you would like to discuss during our time together.

Client: Well, I've been worried about my children. My wife and I live in a tough neighborhood and our eldest son has gotten into a lot of trouble at school lately. It seems like the teachers have it out for him and I'm concerned about how this is going to affect him in the long-run.

Therapist: I can understand why this would be upsetting. How specifically has this affected you?

Client: Like I said, I've been pretty upset, and my wife and I are arguing more. She thinks I'm worrying too much and being too hard on our son. I think she's ignoring all of the statistics that say Black students are disproportionately represented in special education and receive harsher punishments than other students. I'm afraid my son is going to be labeled and experience a negative impact on his success way into the future.

Therapist: Okay. I hear that you're upset and worried, and that you and your wife are arguing more often. What other thoughts and feelings do you have as a result of this situation?

Client: I'm just frustrated and a little bit afraid too. Poor Black children already have two strikes against them. I can't protect him if he's going to keep acting up.

Therapist: It sounds like you're feeling kind of helpless.

Client: Pretty much.

Therapist: Well, you know, when people feel upset and worried like you're feeling, they often experience physical complaints as well, things like headaches or stomachaches. Have you had any physical complaints as a result of the stress you're under right now?

Client: Sometimes, especially when my wife and I are arguing, I feel a sharp pain in my chest.

Therapist: Wow, I can see this is very serious. What impact has all of this had on your ability to take care of things at home or at work?

Client: I'm able to keep up, but I'll admit I have an attitude when I'm at home. If I'm not helping the kids with their homework or chores, I basically keep to myself.

Therapist: Thank you for sharing all of this with me. If I've heard you correctly, the problem you're experiencing right now is upset and worry about your son who is having some difficulties at school right now. These difficulties are especially worrisome for you because of the inequities Black children face in school. In addition to worry, you and your wife are arguing more and you're staying somewhat isolated when you're at home. Is this right?

Client: Yes.

Therapist: Is there anything I left out?

Client: Well, I thought the part about me feeling kind of helpless was important too.

Therapist: Yes, thank you. Is there anything else I left out or anything you want to tell me?

Client: No, I think that pretty much sums it up.

After helping clients clarify their problems, therapists are then in a position to begin goal setting. In therapy, goals are operational statements that describe expected treatment outcomes (Schwitzer & Rubin, 2012). Typically, these goals focus on the client's thoughts, feelings, behaviors, or physiology. They are operationalized by stating how therapy will increase wellness habits, decrease negative symptoms, or eliminate problematic behaviors. Examples of operationalized counseling goals include:

- Decreased symptoms of depression, including sadness, tearfulness, and feelings of hopelessness
- Decreased negative thinking, including self-blame, perfectionism, and over-responsibility
- Increased use of anger management skills that reduce irritability, anger, and aggressive behavior
- Reduced frequency and intensity of anger outbursts
- Increased ability to display a full range of emotions without experiencing loss of control

Good treatment goals are explicitly agreed upon by both client and therapist. However, depending on the therapist, agency, or setting, the detail of the goal may vary. For example, the goals on the list provided earlier were very broad and focused generally on increasing, reducing, or eliminating certain behaviors and symptoms. Other therapists approach goals in a more elaborate manner, focusing not only on reducing symptoms and increasing desired behaviors, but also on making the goals emotionally compelling to the patient, realistic, measurable, and specific about when they have been met (Persons, 2008). Wenzel (2019), for example, described a SMART goal approach to goal setting, wherein goals are operationalized to be specific, measurable, achievable, realistic, and time-limited. Using this approach, the goal "Reduced frequency of anxious thoughts" might be restated as "Reduce the frequency of anxious thoughts to no more than five times per day" or "Reduced intensity of anxiety symptoms as measured by the Beck Anxiety Inventory at the 2-week follow-up assessment." As illustrated in both SMART goal statements, a specific targeted change is identified (i.e., reduced anxiety) in a manner that is measurable (i.e., number of times per day/BAI scores), achievable, realistic, and limited to the period of time during which the client will be in therapy.

Whether a simple or elaborate approach to goal setting is taken, once developed, goals should be listed in priority order (Persons, 2008). In many cases, goals are a direct reflection of the items on the problem list; however, it may be unrealistic to address all of the issues listed, resulting in a list of treatment goals that is shorter than the problem list. For example, clients may identify problems that cannot be addressed within therapy (e.g., medical problems like a broken leg or environmental issues like problems with housing), or if discussing acute issues, problems that cannot be addressed within the timeframe of an individual session (Persons, 2008). When this occurs, therapists may nevertheless elect to include these problems on the problem list but then encourage clients to prioritize goals that can be addressed during therapy. Community resources can be provided to assist with medical or environmental concerns.

The session excerpt that follows continues the previous client/therapist dialogue, illustrating how the therapist may approach goal setting once problems have been identified. Notice the collaborative approach taken by the therapist as they work together to turn the problems the client has identified into operationalized goals to be achieved during therapy.

Therapist: Alright, let's focus on turning the problems you've identified into goals we can work on together during therapy. Based on what we've talked about today, it sounds like you have two major problems. The first problem is that you're feeling pretty upset, worried, and helpless about the difficulties your son is having at school. The second problem is arguing between you and your wife. Is that correct?

Client: Yes.

Therapist: Okay. As we're developing goals to address these problems, we should keep track of what we come up with. Would you like to write the goals down, or should I?

Client: I can write them down.

Therapist: Great. Now, the first problem you mentioned was worry and helplessness about your son's difficulties at school. It can be helpful to think about goals as the flipside of the problem. So, for this problem, we might think of the goal as reduced feelings of worry and helplessness. Does this sound like a good place to start?

Client: Yes.

Therapist: Good. If you were feeling less worried and helpless, what would be different?

Client: Well, I guess I would be calmer and more relaxed. I would also be more proactive in talking to my son and his teachers to get a better understanding of what's going on.

Therapist: Okay. So then, it sounds like your first goal would be to decrease worry and feelings of helplessness by being calmer, more relaxed, and more proactive. Did I say that right? Is there anything else you'd like to add?

Client: No, I think that sounds about right.

Therapist: Good. Then why don't you write that down.

Client: Okay.

Therapist: Great. Now, let's move on to your second problem, which is the frequency of arguments between you and your wife. What would you like to be different there?

Client: Well, I'd like for us to come to some sort of agreement on how we're going to handle the problem. I guess neither one of us has done much compromising.

Therapist: Okay. So, how would you state this as a goal?

Client: I'd say I'd like to strengthen my use of communication and conflict resolution skills in my relationship with my wife.

Therapist: That's great, I'm impressed! Don't forget to write that down.

Client: Okay.

Therapist: Alright. As we're winding down our goal setting, let's summarize what we've come up with today. You have two primary goals that you'd like to work on. The first goal is decreasing your worry and feelings of helplessness by being calmer, more relaxed, and more proactive. The second goal is strengthening your use of communication and conflict resolution skills in your relationship with your wife. Is that correct?

Client: Yes.

Therapist: Okay. Between these two goals, which would you like to address first?

Client: I'd like to talk about my worry and feelings of helplessness first. I think if I can do better with that, it might actually help the problems I have with my wife.

As illustrated in the preceding dialogue, the therapist and the client worked together to identify treatment goals to focus therapy. In their discussion of the first goal, the therapist provided information on how to set goals (i.e., "It can be helpful to think about goals as the flipside of the problem") and then modeled application of this information ("So, for this problem, we might think of the goal as reduced feelings of worry and helplessness"). The therapist then worked with the client to operationalize each goal by asking the client what would be different if they achieved the goal. This encouraged the client to identify specific changes in cognition or behavior, which ultimately provides an indication of the tasks needed to achieve their goals.

Agreeing on Tasks

Once goals have been identified, the therapist and client should work together to make decisions regarding how to go about treating the problems they face. As mentioned in Chapter 1, in CBT, this process not only involves consideration of the client's goals but their overall cognitive conceptualization as well (J. S. Beck, 2020). Recall that a cognitive conceptualization refers to the summary of data describing (a) the client's relevant childhood experiences and societal influences, (b) their central beliefs about themselves, (c) attitudes and rules they use to navigate the world in light of their beliefs, (d) cognitive, affective, and behavioral strategies they use to adhere to their rules, and (e) examples of how such data are translated into negative automatic thoughts and reactions in daily situations (J. S. Beck, 2020; Steele, 2020). From a CBT perspective, this data is critical to the selection of tasks, which are otherwise referred to as interventions, as it informs the formulation of the therapist's working hypothesis. This working hypothesis (i.e., the understanding of the basic beliefs and behavioral patterns influencing the nature of the client's presenting concerns and their subsequent goals for therapy), in turn, directs the therapist's attention to the interventions that are likely to be most efficacious in addressing the client's chief complaints (J. S. Beck, 2020). For example, clients with goals concerned with decreasing severely depressed mood may initially focus on behavioral activation tasks, while clients with phobias may initially focus treatment on the development of emotional regulation skills and graduated exposure exercises.

According to Matu (2018), the skillful selection and implementation of tasks fosters a good therapeutic alliance in several ways. First, careful selection and implementation of tasks demonstrates the therapist's competence, which builds trust between the client and the therapist. Second, effective intervention implementation also helps clients experience a decline in distressing symptoms, which reduces the burden of their psychological problems and helps them to function more effectively in daily life. This builds further trust in the therapeutic relationship and generates positive feelings toward the therapist. Finally, when tasks are decided upon and agreed to mutually, there are additional opportunities to foster collaboration in the relationship.

Cultural Ruptures

While it is important to know how to build a strong therapeutic alliance with clients, it is equally important to understand what may cause potential ruptures to the therapeutic alliance and how to respond to them. According to Zlotnick et al. (2020), "a rupture in the therapeutic alliance may be defined as tension or a breakdown in the collaborative relationship between patient and therapist" in any of the interrelated components of the alliance—bond, goals, or tasks (p. 860). *Cultural ruptures* may be more specifically defined as intentional and unintentional statements that portray insensitivity, disrespect, and/or negligent attention to some salient aspect of the client's cultural heritage (Hook et al., 2017). Broadly, the impact of cultural rup-tures include: (a) limitations to client disclosure level, (b) early termination of the therapy session, (c) increased self-doubt and decreased self-esteem, (d) feelings of embarrassment, worthlessness, shame, and anger in the client, and (e) reinforcement of the client's presenting problems (Miles et al., 2021). Let's look at a brief clinical example wherein the therapist commits the microaggressive act of overidentification to illustrate how cultural ruptures may occur during therapy.

Case Illustration: Hasan

Hasan is 20-year-old African American student athlete on the football team of a small mid-western college. He's seeking therapy due to ongoing difficul-ties with his teammates. Hasan explained that his teammates often use racial slurs to describe people of color on other teams, which makes Hasan won-der what they say about him when he's not in the room. Hasan also reported that although he played quarterback in high school, he was never even con-sidered for the position on his current team. Hasan believes that this is due to old stereotypes that say African Americans don't have enough intelligence and leadership qualities for the role. Attempting to empathize and establish a connection with Hasan, the therapist replied, "You know, as a gay person, I know what it's like to be discriminated against." Instead of building a con-nection, however, Hasan feels annoyed and frustrated by his therapist's response, and decides not to return to therapy.

As illustrated in the case example, cultural ruptures often occur due to discernible cultural insensitivities. However, Zlotnick and his colleagues (2020) noted that although therapeutic ruptures are typically viewed as major, acute incidents, ruptures may also occur due to subtle fluctuations in alliance. In other words, therapeutic ruptures vary in frequency, severity, intensity, and duration across treatment and across therapist-client dyads (Aspland et al., 2008).

When ruptures occur, it is important to openly acknowledge and seek to repair them. An *alliance repair* is defined as "a situation where, following a rupture, the patient and therapist resume collaboration on the work of therapy at the level of collaboration that they had before or at a greater level" (Zlotnick et al., 2020, p. 860). These repairs are significant, as rup-tures with no repairs are associated with poor outcomes, while repaired ruptures are associated with better outcomes (Zlotnick et al., 2020, p. 860). According to Matu (2018), two common sources of ruptures to the thera-peutic alliance include unrealistic beliefs about the therapist and fears on the client's part that the therapist may become upset when the therapist learns about their negative automatic thoughts and find out that the client really is defective and worthless. Similarly, based on their review of related research, Aspland et al. (2008) suggested that ruptures may occur when clients: (a) do not feel safe to explore their emotional experience with their therapist, (b) question the purpose and value of therapy, (c) have different expectations of the therapist's role in treatment, and (d) find that the therapist applies the CBT framework in a rigid, inflexible manner, particularly when therapists persist in the use of techniques despite client concern.

Research into specific cultural factors that lead to therapeutic ruptures shows that missed opportunities to broach race during therapy with clients from diverse racial/ethnic backgrounds, as well as microaggressions committed by the therapist in the course of therapy may additionally weaken the therapeutic alliance (Day-Vines et al., 2018; Fuertes et al., 2006; Owen et al., 2011). In particular, microaggressions that occur during therapy reinforce historic distrust of the mental health system among individuals from marginalized groups and have been found to result in early termination, low treatment utilization, negative treatment outcomes, and feelings of anger, shame, and being misunderstood (Miles et al., 2021). Moreover, microaggressions have also been found to create psychological harm for some clients including a worsening of mood. Therefore, beyond the common sources of therapeutic ruptures identified above, therapists should also be alert to the unique potential for cultural ruptures to influence the therapeutic alliance and engage in regular assessment of the level of cultural humility exhibited in the relationship. Let's look at another clinical example to illustrate this point.

Case Illustration: Charles

Charles was a 40-year-old man who self-referred to therapy after a volatile argument with his 15-year-old daughter. Charles reported that while the argument did not escalate to physical violence, Charles was frightened by his level of anger. Charles explained that he had been feeling overwhelmed due to frequent disagreements between himself and his daughter, and what Charles perceived as disrespect. Frustrated, Charles stated to the therapist, "I get enough disrespect from the outside world as a Black man. I don't want that in my home," to which his therapist replied, "You know, I don't see you as Black, I just see you as a regular person. Tell me more about that."

Can you identify the microaggression in this statement? While the therapist was appropriate in his attempt to probe and learn more about Charles's experience as a Black man, the therapist's assertion that he did not see Charles as Black but as a regular person was actually a subtle put down. First, denying Charles's identity as a Black man negates his experience with racism and a large part of his identity. Second, the idea that the therapist sees Charles not as Black but as "regular" implies that Black people somehow aren't regular. These put downs were felt by Charles in the session who responded by shutting down and saying very little for the remainder of the session.

As illustrated in the case of Charles, these ruptures may have a significant impact on the therapeutic alliance and treatment outcomes among African Americans (Miles et al., 2021). Accordingly, cultural ruptures and their repair are discussed in greater detail in the following section.

Repairing Cultural Ruptures

Clients are often reluctant to bring up concerns about the therapeutic relationship with their therapists, as illustrated in the case of Charles. Therefore, therapists should take responsibility for repairing therapeutic ruptures. A first task in this process is recognizing the signs of therapeutic ruptures. According to Safran and Muran (2000), clients engage in certain types of behaviors once a therapeutic rupture has occurred. These behaviors can be categorized into two types: (1) withdrawal markers and (2) confrontation markers. Withdrawal ruptures are when the client disengages from therapy through behaviors such as denial, minimal response, intellectualization, and disengagement (Gaztambide, 2012). These ruptures typically lead to poor treatment outcomes (Okamoto & Kazantzis, 2021). Confrontation ruptures on the other hand, are evidenced by directly expressed dissatisfaction with the therapist or aspects of therapy, for example, criticisms of therapist or therapy and skepticism about progress in therapy (Gaztambide, 2012). These ruptures typically result in premature termination, preceded by increased confrontation and withdrawal before dropout from CBT (Okamoto & Kazantzis, 2021).

A second task in addressing ruptures involves changing behavior and encouraging clients to engage by becoming more helpful and collaborative in interpersonal interactions with clients (Aspland et al., 2008). Okamoto and Kazantzis (2021) identified eight specific steps to accomplish this task. These steps include: (1) identifying and acknowledging the rupture, (2) validating the client's experience, (3) exploring the circumstances that led to the rupture in collaboration with the client, (4) sharing decision making on how to proceed with the resolution process, (5) incorporating the client's direct experience in the rupture resolution process and evaluating its effectiveness, (6) using Socratic questions to explore the situation, (7) inviting feedback from the client and responding to it, and (8) engaging in self-reflection, self-practice, and mindfulness. When ruptures to the therapeutic alliance are cultural in nature, responding from a multicultural orientation (i.e., cultural humility, cultural opportunities, and cultural comfort) as described in Chapter 4 can also be beneficial. Chang et al. (2021) described another similar six stage process to assist with this task, which includes: (1) attending to the rupture marker, (2) analyzing the rupture, (3) exploring the meaning of the rupture, (4) exploring the avoidance, (5) affirming the relationship, and (6) repairing the rupture. Because clients from marginalized backgrounds often perceive the therapist as an authority figure, this process also includes paying special attention to issues of power, privilege, and identity (Chang et al., 2021).

Let's return to our case example, Charles to take a closer look at the steps in repairing cultural ruptures. Recall that Charles was a 40-year-old man who self-referred to therapy after a volatile argument with his 15-year-old daughter. During a session with his therapist, Charles expressed frustration with the amount of disrespect he receives due to his identity as a Black man, to which his therapist replied, "You know, I don't see you as Black, I just see you as a regular person. Tell me more about that." Although meant well, this statement negated a significant aspect of Charles's identity and his experience with racism. In discussing the situation with his supervisor, the therapist realized the potential impact of his statement and decided to address it with Charles at their next session. The following session excerpt details the therapist's attempt to repair the rupture.

Therapist: Charles, as we're getting started today, I would like to discuss something with you.

Charles: Okay.

Therapist: Last week, I noticed that you became kind of silent and withdrawn toward the end of our session. I discussed the issue with my supervisor who pointed out that when I said that I see you as a regular person and not as a Black person, I may have unintentionally been communicating messages that suggest I don't understand the importance of your identity as a Black man, and that Black people aren't "regular." Charles, I want to sincerely apologize for this. I understand now how what I said may have been deeply hurtful. Could we spend some time talking about how you felt?

Charles: Okay.

Therapist: Thank you. How did you feel about what I said?

Charles: Well, to tell you the truth, I was offended. I know you didn't mean anything by it, but that just goes to show how much you don't get what it's like to be a Black person. That's why I just stopped talking.

Therapist: Charles, I understand why you felt that way. And you're right. I will never really know what it's to experience racism the way that you do. Nevertheless, I should have been able to empathize with what you were saying and instead I minimized it.

Charles: Yes! It was just more of what I experience on an everyday basis.

Therapist: I see. Charles, I think I am beginning to understand even more about how you felt last week. You were trying to tell me what it's like to be disrespected as a Black man, and then I disrespected you. I feel terrible about this. I really want to thank you for sharing your feelings with me this week. I realize that what you were saying was extremely important. Would you like to talk about it today?

Charles: Okay...

In the above dialogue, the therapist took several steps to repair the cultural rupture in the therapeutic relationship with Charles (Chang et al., 2021; Okamoto & Kazantzis, 2021). As recommended by Chang et al. (2021), the therapist attended to the rupture marker by acknowledging that Charles had become silent and withdrawn toward the end of their session together. The therapist then discussed the situation in supervision, which provided opportunities for critical self-reflection and analysis of the rupture. Through this process, the therapist was able to recognize the microaggression in their response to Charles and the need to apologize and repair the rupture. Upon meeting with Charles at their next session, the therapist took the opportunity to be accountable for the rupture and acknowledged the hurt it might have caused. The therapist then elicited feedback from Charles and sought to repair the rupture by providing space to explore his initial concerns.

In conclusion, the therapeutic relationship is a significant aspect of the therapeutic process, affecting factors such as treatment outcomes (Walling et al., 2021), perceived counselor competence (Constantine, 2007), psychological wellbeing (Owen et al., 2011, 2014), satisfaction with counseling (Constantine, 2007), and future help seeking (Crawford, 2011). To strengthen the therapeutic relationship, therapists should work to establish bonds with their clients and promote mutuality through collaboration in the development of treatment goals and selection of interventions to achieve those goals. When cultural ruptures occur, therapists should be intentional in repairing these ruptures by taking steps to acknowledge the rupture, elicit feedback, apologize, and move forward in the relationship.

References

Ardito, R. B., & Rabellino, D. (2011). Therapeutic alliance and outcome of psychotherapy: Historical excursus, measurements, and prospects for research. *Frontiers in Psychology, 2*, 270. https://doi.org/10.3389/fpsyg.2011.00270

Aspland, H., Llewelyn, S., Hardy, G. E., Barkham, M., & Stiles, W. (2008). Alliance ruptures and rupture resolution in cognitive-behavior therapy. *Psychotherapy Research, 18*(6), 699–710. https://doi.org/10.1080/10503300802291463

Beck, A. T., Rush, A. J., Shaw, B. F., & Emery, G. (1979). *Cognitive therapy of depression*. Guilford Press.

Beck, J. S. (2020). *Cognitive behavior therapy: Basics and beyond* (3rd ed.). Guilford Press.

Bordin, E. S. (1979). The generalizability of the psychoanalytic concept of the working alliance. *Psychotherapy: Theory, Research & Practice, 16*(3), 252–260. https://doi.org/10.1037/h0085885

Boswell, J. F., & Constantino, M. J. (2022). *Deliberate practice in cognitive behavioral therapy*. American Psychological Association.

Burris, J. L. (2012). On enhancing competent work with African American clients: Challenging persistent racial disparity trends by examining the role of the working alliance. *Journal of Applied Rehabilitation Counseling, 43*(3), 3–12. https://doi.org/10.1891/0047-2220.43.3.3

Cameron, S. K., Rodgers, J., & Dagnan, D. (2018). The relationship between the therapeutic alliance and clinical outcomes in cognitive behaviour therapy for adults with depression: A meta-analytic review. *Clinical Psychology & Psychotherapy, 25*(3), 446–456. https://doi.org/10.1002/cpp.2180

Castonguay, L. G., Youn, S. J., Xiao, H., & McAleavey, A. A. (2018). The therapeutic relationship: A warm, important, and potentially mutative factor in cognitive-behavioral therapy. In O. Tishby & H. Wiseman (Eds.), *Developing the therapeutic relationship: Integrating case studies, research, and practice* (pp. 157–179). American Psychological Association. https://doi.org/10.1037/0000093-008

Chang, D. F., Dunn, J. J., & Omidi, M. (2021). A critical-cultural-relational approach to rupture resolution: A case illustration with a cross-racial dyad. *Journal of Clinical Psychology, 77*(2), 369–383. https://doi.org/10.1002/jclp.23080

Constantine, M. G. (2007). Racial microaggressions against African American clients in cross-racial counseling relationships. *Journal of Counseling Psychology, 54*(1), 1–16. https://doi.org/10.1037/0022-0167.54.1.1

Crawford, E. P. (2011). Stigma, racial microaggressions, and acculturation strategies as predictors of likelihood to seek counseling among Black college students [Doctoral dissertation, Oklahoma State University]. ProQuest Information & Learning.

Day-Vines, N. L., Ammah, B. B., Steen, S., & Arnold, K. M. (2018). Getting comfortable with discomfort: Preparing counselor trainees to broach racial, ethnic, and cultural factors with clients during counseling. *International Journal for the Advancement of Counselling, 40*(2), 89–104. https://doi.org/10.1002/jcad.12304

Day-Vines, N. L., Cluxton-Keller, F., Agorsor, C., & Gubara, S. (2021). Strategies for broaching the subjects of race, ethnicity, and culture. *Journal of Counseling & Development, 99*(3), 348–357. https://doi.org/10.1002/jcad.12380

Day-Vines, N. L., Cluxton-Keller, F., Agorsor, C., Gubara, S., & Otabil, N. A. A. (2020). The multidimensional model or broaching behavior. *Journal of Counseling & Development, 98*(1), 107–118. https://doi.org/10.1002/jcad.12304

Day-Vines, N.L., Wood, S. M., Grothaus, T., Craigen, L., Holman, A., Dotson-Blake, K., & Douglass, M. J. (2007). Broaching the subjects of race, ethnicity, and culture during the counseling process. *Journal of Counseling & Development, 85*(4), 401–409. https://doi.org/10.1002/jcad.12069

Dobson, K. S. (2022). The therapeutic relationship. *Cognitive and Behavioral Practice, 29*(3), 541–544. https://doi.org/10.1016/j.cbpra.2022.02.006

Eliacin, J., Coffing, J. M., Matthias, M. S., Burgess, D. J., Bair, M. J., & Rollins, A. L. (2018). The relationship between race, patient activation, and working alliance: Implications for patient engagement in mental health care. *Administration and Policy in Mental Health, 45*(1), 186–192. https://doi.org/10.1007/s10488-016-0779-5

Flückiger, C. (2022). Alliance. *Cognitive and Behavioral Practice, 29*(3), 549–553. https://doi.org/10.1016/j.cbpra.2022.02.013

Flückiger, C., Del Re, A. C., Wampold, B. E., Symonds, D., & Horvath, A. O. (2012). How central is the alliance in psychotherapy? A multilevel longitudinal meta-analysis. *Journal of Counseling Psychology, 59*(1), 10–17. https://doi.org/10.1037/a0025749

Fuertes, J. N., Stracuzzi, T. I., Bennett, J., Scheinholtz, J., Mislowack, A., Hersh, M., & Cheng, D. (2006). Therapist multicultural competency: A study of therapy dyads. *Psychotherapy: Theory, Research, Practice, Training, 43*(4), 480–490. https://doi.org/10.1037/0033-3204.43.4.480

Gaztambide, D. J. (2012). Addressing cultural impasses with rupture resolution strategies: A proposal and recommendations. *Professional Psychology: Research and Practice, 43*(3), 183–189. https://doi.org/10.1037/a0026911

Hook, J. N., Davis, D., Owen, J., & DeBlaere, C. (2017). *Cultural humility: Engaging diverse identities in therapy*. American Psychological Association. https://doi.org/10.1037/0000037-000

Linehan, M. M. (1997). Validation and psychotherapy. In A. C. Bohart & L. S. Greenberg (Eds.), *Empathy reconsidered: New directions in psychotherapy* (pp. 353–392). American Psychological Association.

Mai, T., & Whitlock, J. (2022, November 28). *How to respond with compassion when someone is hurt by racism*. https://accelerate.uofuhealth.utah.edu/equity/how-to-respond-with-compassion-when-someone-is-hurt-by-racism

Mattos, L. A., Schmidt, A. T., Henderson, C. E., & Hogue, A. (2017). Therapeutic alliance and treatment outcome in the outpatient treatment of urban adolescents: The role of callous–unemotional traits. *Psychotherapy, 54*(2), 136–147. https://doi.org/10.1037/pst0000093

Matu, S. A. (2018). Cognitive therapy. In A. Vernon and K. A. Doyle (Eds.), *Cognitive behavior therapies: A guidebook for practitioners* (pp. 75–108). American Counseling Association.

Miles, J. R., Anders, C., Kivlighan, D. M. III, & Belcher Platt, A. A. (2021). Cultural ruptures: Addressing microaggressions in group therapy. *Group Dynamics: Theory, Research, and Practice, 25*(1), 74–88. https://doi.org/10.1037/gdn0000149

Okamoto, A., & Kazantzis, N. (2021). Alliance ruptures in cognitive-behavioral therapy: A cognitive conceptualization. *Journal of Clinical Psychology, 77*(2), 384–397. https://doi.org/10.1002/jclp.23116

Owen, J., Imel, Z., Tao, K. W., Wampold, B., Smith, A., & Rodolfa, E. (2011). Cultural ruptures in short-term therapy: Working alliance as a mediator between clients' perceptions of microaggressions and therapy outcomes. *Counselling & Psychotherapy Research, 11*, 204–212. https://doi.org/10.1080/14733145.2010.491551

Owen, J., Tao, K. W., Imel, Z. E., Wampold, B. E., & Rodolfa, E. (2014). Addressing racial and ethnic microaggressions in therapy. *Professional Psychology: Research and Practice, 45*(4), 283–290. https://doi.org/10.1037/a0037420

Persons, J. B. (2008). *The case formulation approach to cognitive-behavior therapy.* Guilford Press.

Pierson, A. M., Arunagiri, V., & Bond, D. M. (2022). "You didn't cause racism, and you have to solve it anyways:" Antiracist adaptations to dialectical behavior therapy for White therapists. *Cognitive and Behavioral Practice, 29*(4), 796–815. https://doi.org/10.1016/j.cbpra.2021.11.001

Rogers, C. R. (1951). *Client-centered therapy.* Houghton Mifflin.

Safran, J. D., & Muran, J. C. (2000). Resolving therapeutic alliance ruptures: Diversity and integration. *Journal of Clinical Psychology, 56*(2), 233–243. https://doi.org/10.1002/(SICI)1097-4679(200002)56:2<233::AID-JCLP9>3.0.CO;2-3

Schwitzer, A. M., & Rubin, L. C. (2012). *Diagnosis and treatment planning skills for mental health professionals: A popular culture casebook approach.* Sage Publications, Inc.

Steele, J. M. (2020). A CBT approach to internalized racism among African Americans. *International Journal for the Advancement of Counselling, 42*(3), 217–233. https://doi.org/10.1007/s10447-020-09402-0

Steele, J. M., & Newton, C. S. (2022). Culturally adapted cognitive behavior therapy as a model to address internalized racism among African American clients. *Journal of Mental Health Counseling, 44*(2), 98–116. https://doi.org/10.17744/mehc.44.2.01

Walling, S. M., Suvak, M. K., Howard, J. M., Taft, C. T., & Murphy, C. M. (2012). Race/ethnicity as a predictor of change in working alliance during cognitive behavioral therapy for intimate partner violence perpetrators. *Psychotherapy, 49*(2), 180–189. https://doi.org/10.1037/a0025751

Waltman, S., Codd, R., III, McFarr, L., & Moore, B. (2021). *Socratic questioning for therapists and counselors: Learn how to think and intervene like a cognitive behavior therapist.* Routledge. https://doi.org/10.4324/9780429320392

Wenzel, A. (2019). *Cognitive behavioral therapy for beginners.* Routledge.

Wenzel, A., Dobson, K. S., & Hays, P. A. (2016). Culturally responsive cognitive behavioral therapy. In A. Wenzel, K. S. Dobson, & P. A. Hays, *Cognitive behavioral therapy techniques and strategies* (pp. 145–160). American Psychological Association. https://doi.org/10.1037/14936-008

Wolpe, J. (1958). *Psychotherapy by reciprocal inhibition.* Stanford University Press.

Wong, C. W. (2013). Collaborative empiricism in culturally sensitive cognitive behavior therapy. *Cognitive and Behavioral Practice, 20*(4), 390–398. https://doi.org/10.1016/j.cbpra.2012.08.005

Zilcha-Mano, S., Eubanks, C. F., Bloch-Elkouby, S., & Muran, J. C. (2020). Can we agree we just had a rupture? Patient-therapist congruence on ruptures and its effects on outcome in brief relational therapy versus cognitive-behavioral therapy. *Journal of Counseling Psychology, 67*(3), 315–325. https://doi.org/10.1037/cou0000400

Zlotnick, E., Strauss, A. Y., Ellis, P., Abargil, M., Tishby, O., & Huppert, J. D. (2020). Reevaluating ruptures and repairs in alliance: Between- and within-session processes in cognitive–behavioral therapy and short-term psychodynamic psychotherapy. *Journal of Consulting and Clinical Psychology, 88*(9), 859–869. https://doi.org/10.1037/ccp0000598

Chapter 6

Assessment, Cognitive Conceptualization, and Treatment Planning

Individuals seek help for their psychological problems from a variety of sources. As discussed in Chapter 3, some informal sources of help within the African American community include family, friends, trusted elders, community organizations, and religious groups. With recent efforts to reduce stigma around mental health services in this population, professional counselors, psychologists, and social workers are slowly becoming another source of help many African Americans also look to. While both informal and formal sources of help provide wellness benefits to those who seek them, mental health professionals are differentiated from lay helpers through their specialized knowledge and training. In particular, mental health professionals have education in mental health and human development principles that provide them with unique insight into the development and maintenance of psychological problems. Moreover, through assessment, case conceptualization, and treatment planning, mental health professionals are able to apply their knowledge of these principles in order to empower clients to achieve their mental health and wellness goals.

This chapter explores assessment, cognitive conceptualization, and treatment planning with African American clients, focusing on how these aspects of clinical practice may be used to address psychological distress resulting from experiences with racism. Accordingly, the chapter begins with a discussion of culturally sensitive assessment practices, highlighting assessment during both intake and the working phase of therapy. Specific assessment of the impacts of racism through both quantitative and qualitative approaches is then explored. Next, cognitive conceptualization based on information obtained throughout the course of therapy is discussed. The chapter concludes with a discussion of treatment planning according to the cognitive conceptualization.

DOI: 10.4324/9781003196303-6

Culturally Sensitive Assessment

In CBT, assessment begins in the first session and continues throughout the remainder of therapy as the therapist gathers data needed to develop a diagnosis and then refine their conceptualization of the client's presenting concerns (Matu, 2018). Typically, during the initial session, this data includes information about the nature of the client's presenting problems, symptoms, and their duration, severity, and impact on client functioning. Relevant histories necessary for a biopsychosocial formulation should also be taken at this time. Specific biopsychosocial information of interest includes: (a) the client's psychiatric, medical, developmental, educational, vocational, family, and substance use histories, (b) their expectations for therapy, and (c) any strengths, adaptive coping strategies, and protective factors that may assist with the treatment process. Once this initial data has been obtained, assessment continues as the therapist gathers information to determine precipitants to the client's current illness as well as cross-sectional and longitudinal views of the client's maladaptive cognitions (J. S. Beck, 2020).

Traditionally, assessment data in CBT is obtained through two primary sources: (1) the clinical interview and (2) quantitative measures of client symptomatology. In Chapter 1, I highlighted some of the quantitative strategies commonly used to (a) gauge clients' baseline report of symptoms at intake and (b) monitor progress over the course of therapy. These strategies include tools such as the weekly client mood check and assessments such as the Beck depression and anxiety inventories (A. T. Beck, 1990; A. T. Beck et al., 1996). As mentioned in Chapter 1, *mood checks* are quick assessments of symptoms the client has experienced in the time since the last session. Therapists may conduct mood checks by asking clients a question such as, "Over the past week, how would you rate your depression on a scale from 1 to 10?" or by having the client point to a number or image on a visual representation of the intensity of their symptomatology. Measures such as the Beck depression and anxiety inventories, on the other hand, are more formalized assessments of specific disorders. These assessments have undergone psychometric development to ensure the accuracy and consistency of their results. Consequently, use of these assessments has the added benefit of reducing bias in the interpretation of a simple mood check and increasing confidence that information the therapist has obtained actually represents how clients are feeling (Creed, 2019).

Other more global assessments of client symptomatology are also helpful in obtaining baseline scores and examining treatment outcomes across the course of therapy. The Outcome Questionnaire 45.2 (OQ-45.2; Lambert & Burlingame, 1996), for example, measures client progress in three areas: (1) Symptom Distress (i.e., depression and anxiety), (2) Interpersonal Relationships (i.e., loneliness, conflict with others, and marriage and family difficulties), and (3) Social Role (i.e., difficulties in the workplace, school, or home duties). When compared to disorder-specific assessments, these measures have the added benefits of alerting the therapist to other clinically significant symptomatology that might not otherwise be captured. For example, the OQ-45.2 includes a risk assessment of suicidality, substance abuse, and potential violence that provides the therapist with information they may not have otherwise been alerted to without direct examination of these topics.

In terms of the clinical interview, open-ended questions designed to elicit information about the client's presenting concerns provide the therapist with data needed to corroborate and gain a fuller understanding of scores obtained on any quantitative measures utilized during the assessment process. The clinical interview also allows the therapist to gain a fuller picture of coping strategies, strengths, sources of support, and cultural factors that should be considered in the cognitive conceptualization and treatment planning process (Matu, 2018).

While some therapists take an informal approach to the clinical interview, others utilize more structured formats. The Cultural Formulation Interview (CFI) is an example of a structured approach that examines the impact of culture on key aspects of a client's clinical presentation and care (American Psychiatric Association, 2013). This tool, located in the Emerging Measures and Models section of the *DSM-5* (American Psychiatric Association, 2013) emphasizes four areas of assessment: (1) Cultural Definition of the Problem; (2) Cultural Perceptions of Cause, Context, and Support; (3) Cultural Factors Affecting Self-Coping and Past Help Seeking; and (4) Cultural Factors Affecting Current Help Seeking. In this interview protocol, the Cultural Definition of the Problem section guides the therapist in assessing the client's cultural perspective on the development of their problem as well as the impact of this problem on their functioning. The next section, Cultural Perceptions of Cause, Context, and Support, further assesses the client's cultural explanations for the development of their problems, as well as psychosocial stressors, supports, and aspects of the client's identity that make a difference to their problems. The third section, Cultural Factors Affecting Self-Coping and Past Help Seeking, explores cultural factors influencing coping, help-seeking, and barriers to help-seeking. The final section, Cultural Factors Affecting Current Help Seeking, explores cultural preferences in treatment and the clinician-patient relationship.

Whether approached using the CFI or through less structured formats, culturally sensitive assessment requires the therapist to be intentional in broaching race and culture in the client's presenting concerns and in the therapeutic relationship itself. Chapter 4, Activity 4.7: Introducing Race Into the Therapeutic Process, guided you in developing a broad approach to exploration of racial and cultural factors in the therapeutic process; however, more direct exploration of the psychological impacts of racism requires therapists to also obtain specific information about the client's history of racial experiences. According to Carter and Pieterse (2020), examples of questions that may be used to obtain this history include:

1. When did the client become aware of race and racial issues?
2. How did these issues get discussed, if at all, in the family and community?
3. How did the client come to think of themselves as a racial being?
4. Did they encounter racial incidents, and, if so, how were they handled?
5. Were race and racial issues discussed in school? If so, how; if not, how was that understood?

(p. 162)

When exploring a specific incidence of racial trauma, the clinical interview should also address the following:

1. The characteristics of the actors involved (race/ethnicity, extent of power, and influence over the claimant)
2. The number, nature, and duration of the events
3. The client's perception of the negativity, controllability, and suddenness of the event
4. The extent to which the event constituted a threat or caused feelings of fear and helplessness
5. How the client tried to adapt or respond to the incident

(Carter & Pieterse, 2020, p. 194)

Reviewing these questions with clients provides the therapist with insight into the client's racial worldview. It also provides the therapist with information necessary to determine if experiences with racism have resulted in trauma; that is, the extent to which race-based incidents were experienced as sudden, negative, and out of one's control, leading to symptoms that include avoidance, arousal, and intrusion (Carter, 2007). Table 6.1 provides an example of the write-up for an initial evaluation that integrates information from traditional and cultural formulation approaches to assessment for Jessica Johnson, a 45-year-old African American woman who experienced an unlawful arrest two months prior to intake.

Activity 6.1: Exploring One's Racial History

Carter and Pieterse (2020) suggest that documentation of the client's racial history and background is a critical feature of culturally sensitive assessment. Yet, as stated elsewhere throughout this text, research also suggests that many therapists are uncomfortable exploring race and racism with their clients (Knox et al., 2003). Practice outside of the therapy dyad can help

Table 6.1 Example Assessment Report

Identifying Information: Jessica Johnson is a 45-year-old cisgender African American woman who identifies as heterosexual. When questioned about religious or spiritual beliefs, Jessica reported being raised in the Christian faith but discontinuing regular church attendance once reaching adulthood.

Chief Complaint: Ms. Johnson is referred to the current clinician by her primary care physician for an assessment of posttraumatic stress disorder. At the time of the assessment, Ms. Johnson reported the following symptoms: decreased appetite, trouble concentrating, distressing memories, difficulty sleeping, nightmares, hypervigilance, low motivation, isolation from others, fatigue/low energy, depressed mood, anxiety, and worry about the future. Additional assessment of the client's current symptomatology was made through administration of the General Anxiety Disorder-7 (GAD-7), the Patient Health Questionnaire-9 (PHQ-9), and the Posttraumatic Stress Disorder Checklist (PCL). Findings are reported in the Assessment Results section below.

History of Current Complaint: Ms. Johnson reports being referred to therapy by her primary care physician after sustaining injuries in an unlawful arrest two months prior to intake. Ms. Johnson explains that on the date of the arrest, she was driving home from a friend's house when she was pulled over by police officers. During the traffic stop, Ms. Johnson was instructed to exit her vehicle at which time the vehicle was searched. When Ms. Johnson objected, officers attempted to restrain Ms. Johnson and a struggle ensued. Ms. Johnson was charged with resisting and obstructing as a result of the incident; however, upon review of body camera footage, the charges were later dropped. Ms. Johnson reports that since her charges were dropped, she continues to experience distressing flashbacks of the event, as well as frequent nightmares. Ms. Johnson believes that she was unfairly profiled because she was an African American woman driving a nice car. She, therefore, additionally reports avoiding travel away from her home unless going to work or to provide care for her children due to fear of being profiled and assaulted again.

Psychiatric History: Ms. Johnson denies past or present thoughts, plan, or intent to commit suicide. She further denies previous hospitalization for psychiatric reasons or use of psychopharmacological medications. Ms. Johnson reports that she was seen in individual counseling for approximately six months after her divorce was finalized two years ago. Treatment was terminated once Ms. Johnson met her treatment goals. Ms. Johnson denies thoughts or urges to hurt others. She further denies history of substance use disorder.

(Continued)

Table 6.1 (Continued)

Personal and Social History: Ms. Johnson is currently divorced and unpartnered. She is the mother of two children who are eight and ten years old. At the time of the assessment, Ms. Johnson was employed as a cosmetologist at a local hair salon. She graduated from high school and earned an associate degree in business administration before enrolling in cosmetology school and becoming a cosmetologist. Ms. Johnson denies prior legal history outside of the current situation, other than receiving some traffic and parking tickets. In terms of her family of origin, Ms. Johnson reports that her parents are still married, and she has three biological siblings. Ms. Johnson reports being the eldest child in her family, and states that she has good relationships with both her parents and her siblings.

History of Racial Experiences: Ms. Johnson reports she first became aware of herself as a racial being during elementary school, describing this awareness as "being different." According to Ms. Johnson, as a toddler, all of her family members and family friends were African American; however, once entering Kindergarten, Ms. Johnson was exposed to a more racially diverse group of peers. Ms. Johnson, who was one of only two Black students in her Kindergarten class, recalls being questioned about her skin color and hair by some of her White peers, causing Ms. Johnson to feel shame and embarrassment. Ms. Johnson noted that these feelings of shame and embarrassment followed her throughout grade school, as most of the African American history she was taught in school focused on slavery. When positive African American exemplars were discussed, they were typically persons from the Civil Rights Movement, which for Ms. Johnson, continued to root the African American experience in pain, trauma, and shame.

Ms. Johnson reports that in her family home, positive African American history was not frequently discussed. Most conversations on race and racism focused on the dangers faced in life due to racism and the importance of disconfirming stereotypes. Upon entering adulthood, she began to learn more about Black history through her own reading and some of the college courses she took. Ms. Johnson described this process as an "awakening," characterized by greater knowledge and appreciation for African American culture and traditions. In terms of the Black community, Ms. Johnson notes that as a result of this education, she believes that African Americans have a wealth of inner resources and should focus on "pulling themselves up by their own bootstraps" in order to improve the community.

Behavioral Observations: Ms. Johnson completed one assessment session by the time of this report. During the session, Ms. Johnson was fully oriented to person, place, and time, with a generally euthymic mood. She presented appropriately groomed and attired, and displayed no articulation problems, using a normal rate and volume of speech. Ms. Johnson displayed a normal activity level throughout the session and had an alert level of consciousness. Ms. Johnson does not have any identified impairments in intelligence and did not display problems with impulse control or judgment during the session. Her spontaneous speech was unremarkable, and her perceptual processes appear to be within normal limits.

Assessment Results

Generalized Anxiety Disorder-7 (GAD-7): The GAD-7 is a 7-item scale that was designed primarily as a screening and severity measure for generalized anxiety disorder in adults. Total scores from 5 to 9 indicate mild anxiety; scores from 10 to 14 indicate moderate anxiety; and scores from 15 to 21 indicate severe anxiety.

GAD-7 test score summary: Ms. Johnson's total score on the GAD-7 was 11, which indicates a moderate level of anxiety. The GAD-7 also includes a functional health assessment. This asks the patient how emotional difficulties or problems impact work, things at home, or relationships with other people. Patient responses can be one of four: *not difficult at all, somewhat difficult, very difficult,* or *extremely difficult.* Ms. Johnson endorsed somewhat difficult, which suggests her functionality is somewhat impaired due to her anxiety.

Patient Health Questionnaire-9 (PHQ-9): The PHQ-9 is a 9-item scale that was designed primarily as a screening and severity measure for depression in adults. Total scores from 5 to 9 indicate mild depression; scores from 10 to 14 indicate moderate depression; scores from 15 to 19 indicate moderately severe depression, and scores from 20 to 27 indicate severe depression.

PHQ-9 test score summary: Ms. Johnson's total score on the PHQ-9 was 19, which indicates a moderately severe level of depression. The PHQ-9 also includes a functional health assessment. This asks the patient how emotional difficulties or problems impact work, things at home, or relationships with other people. Patient responses can be one of four: *not difficult at all, somewhat difficult, very difficult,* or *extremely difficult.* Ms. Johnson endorsed somewhat difficult, which suggests her functionality is somewhat impaired due to her depression.

Posttraumatic Stress Disorder Checklist (PCL): The PCL is a 20-item self-report measure that assesses PTSD symptoms according to the *DSM-5.* Total scores range from 0 to 80. A cutoff score between 31 and 33 is indicative of probable PTSD. Cluster severity scores can be obtained by summing the scores for the items within a given cluster, i.e., Cluster B (items 1 to 5), Cluster C (items 6 and 7), Cluster D (items 8 to 14), and Cluster E (items 15 to 20). A provisional PTSD diagnosis can be made by treating each item rated as 2 = "Moderately" or higher as a symptom endorsed, then following the *DSM-5* diagnostic rule which requires at least: 1 B item (questions 1 to 5), 1 C item (questions 6 and 7), 2 D items (questions 8 to 14), and 2 E items (questions 15 to 20).

PCL test score summary: Ms. Johnson's total score on the PCL was 40, which is above clinical significance. According to her scores on the assessment, Ms. Johnson met criteria for each of the four clusters assessed on the PCL, endorsing four items on Cluster B (i.e., memories, dreams, flashbacks, and cued physical reactions), one item on Cluster C (i.e., avoiding external reminders), three items on Cluster D (i.e., loss of interest, detachment, and estrangement), and three items on Cluster E (i.e., hypervigilance, concentration, and sleep).

(Continued)

Table 6.1 (Continued)

Conclusion: Based on the results of her clinical interview and scores on the GAD-7, PHQ-9, and PCL, Ms. Johnson exhibits signs and symptoms of posttraumatic stress disorder. Ms. Johnson experienced serious injury as a result of a race-based encounter with police in her community. Ms. Johnson perceived this encounter as sudden, negative, and out of her control. As a result, Ms. Johnson reports symptoms of avoidance, arousal, and intrusion, making the event traumatic. These reports are corroborated by Ms. Johnson's scores on the assessment administered during her evaluation. Ms. Johnson had a clinically significant total score on the PCL and met all four clusters of PTSD assessed on the PCL; i.e., four items on Cluster B (i.e., memories, dreams, flashbacks, and cued physical reactions), one item on Cluster C (i.e., avoiding external reminders), three items on Cluster D (i.e., loss of interest, detachment, and estrangement), and three items on Cluster E (i.e., hypervigilance, concentration, and sleep). Ms. Johnson additionally reports current elevations in anxiety and depressive symptoms, indicated by her scores on the GAD-7 and the PHQ-9. Functional health assessments on the GAD-7 and PHQ-9 indicate her functioning is somewhat impaired. During the evaluation session, Ms. Johnson was visibly upset as she recalled details of her encounter with police. She continues to suffer and would benefit from ongoing therapy to address her psychological distress and functional impairment.

Initial Diagnostic Impression: Initial diagnostic impression is F43.10 Posttraumatic Stress Disorder increase comfort exploring these topics. It can also enhance your skill in guiding clients through this exploration. For this activity, practice exploring your own racial history using the following questions from Carter and Pieterse's (2020) guidelines on conducting the clinical interview: When did you become aware of race and racial issues? How did these issues get discussed, if at all, in your family and community? How did you come to think of yourself as a racial being? Did you encounter racial incidents, and, if so, how were they handled? Were race and racial issues discussed in school? If so, how; if not, how was that understood? (p. 162). Once you have answered these questions for yourself, practice engaging this dialogue with a colleague or a supervisor—someone who's able to give you direct feedback on your interview skills. After completing the activity, consider the following reflection questions.

Reflection Questions

- Were some of the questions easier or more difficult to answer than others? Why might this be?
- What did you learn about how you view yourself as a racial being?
- How might this view affect your work with clients?
- What did you notice about how your body reacts when having conversations about race and racism with others?
- What steps do you need to take to increase your comfort discussing race and racism?

Assessing the Impact of Racism

The clinical interview offers therapists insight into the cultural lens through which clients view, explain, and cope with their problems (American Psychiatric Association, 2013). When considering the impacts of racism, however, therapists must also be intentional in their exploration of symptoms associated with race-based traumatic stress in their clients. As evidenced in the case of Jessica Johnson, diagnostically, the impacts of racism often result in trauma disorders such as PTSD. Yet, there may be noteworthy differences in the presentation of race-based traumatic stress symptoms and traditional trauma symptoms (Carter & Pieterse, 2020). One recent study of Black Americans, for example, found that among participants who experienced racial stress, depression, intrusion, anger, and low self-esteem primarily drove the relationship between race-based traumatic stress symptoms and trauma reactions (i.e., arousal, intrusion, avoidance); however, hypervigilance, a common trauma symptom, was not predictive of trauma reactions within this group (Roberson & Carter, 2022). These findings were contrary to the results of other studies which suggest that hypervigilance is the most common symptom of trauma for African Americans and warrants further exploration (Smith & Patton, 2016); nevertheless, based on these findings, the study's authors suggest that when assessing and treatment planning for race-based traumatic stress, caution should be taken, as hypervigilance may not be as prevalent. Low self-esteem may need to be emphasized instead. Moreover, arousal may be an adaptive coping strategy used to navigate racially charged situations and increase safety. As such, therapists may need to take caution in how they attempt to help clients eliminate avoidant behaviors, especially within the context of the current sociopolitical environment.

While research suggests there are similarities between racial trauma and PTSD, it is important to note that individuals who experience racial trauma may or may not meet criteria for a diagnosis of PTSD. To meet *DSM-5* criteria for PTSD, an individual must experience or witness an event that leads to actual or threatened death, serious injury, or sexual violence (American Psychiatric Association, 2013). In some cases, the traumatic events leading to racial trauma meet this criterion. Williams et al. (2018a), for example, identified several race-based events that meet *DSM-5* criteria for PTSD, including overt racially motivated threats of violence, physical assaults or threats from law enforcement, racially motivated threats of violence in the workplace, community violence, medical mistreatment, physical or sexual assault while in prison, and deportation. Other types of race-related experiences such as repeated microaggressions, being denied access or services, being stereotyped, being ignored, verbal assaults, or being profiled, however, do not qualify as traumatic events as defined by the *DSM-5*. Nevertheless, these events when varied, chronic, pervasive, uncontrollable, and stressful in nature frequently lead to the full clinical syndrome of PTSD symptoms (Abdullah et al., 2021; Kirkinis et al., 2021). Accordingly, therapists should be careful to conduct a full assessment of trauma symptoms, even when the client has not experienced or witnessed an event that leads to actual or threatened death, serious injury, or sexual violence. Table 6.2 provides a list of assessments that explore trauma symptoms specifically within the context of racism, as well as a description of the specific constructs measured on each assessment.

Of the assessments listed in Table 6.2, one of the more well-researched and empirically validated assessments of race-based traumatic stress is a measure titled the Race-Based Traumatic Stress Symptom Scale (RBTSSS, Carter et al., 2013). On this scale, race-based traumatic stress is conceptualized and assessed along seven clusters of symptoms that occur after a race-based event: (1) depression, (2) intrusion, (3) anger, (4), hypervigilance, (5) physical reactions, (6) low self-esteem, and (7) avoidance. The assessment begins by asking clients to describe three of the most memorable events of racism they have experienced in their lives, and then from these three events,

Table 6.2 Quantitative Measures of Race-Based Stress

Assessment	Description
Race-Based Traumatic Stress Symptom Scale (RBTSSS; Carter et al., 2013)	A 52-item measure of race-based traumatic stress that assesses symptoms across seven scales: (1) Depression, (2) Anger, (3) Physical Reactions, (4) Avoidance, (5) Intrusion, (6) Hypervigilance/Arousal, and (7) Low Self-Esteem.
Racial Trauma Scale (RTS; Williams et al., 2022)	A 30-item measure of racial trauma that assesses symptoms across three subscales: (1) Lack of Safety, (2) Negative Cognitions, and (3) Difficulty Coping.
The Trauma Symptoms of Discrimination Scale (TSDS; Williams et al., 2018b)	A 21-item measure that focuses on anxiety-related trauma symptoms surrounding the experience of discrimination across four domains: (1) Uncontrollable Hyperarousal, (2) Feelings of Alienation, (3) Worries About Future Negative Events, and (4) Perceiving Others as Dangerous.
Index of Race-Related Stress–Brief Version (IRRS-B; Utsey, 1999)	A 22-item measure of race-related stress among African Americans that assesses symptoms across three subscales: (1) Cultural Racism, (2) Institutional Racism, and (3) Individual Racism.
The Racial Microaggressions Scale–Modified (RMAS; Torres-Harding et al., 2012)	A 35-item assessment that measures the frequency and distress caused by experiences with six types of racial microaggressions: (1) Invisibility, (2) Criminality, (3) Low-Achieving/Undesirable Culture, (4) Sexualization, (5) Foreigner/Not Belonging, and (6) Environmental Invalidations.
Schedule of Racist Events (SRE; Klonoff & Landrine, 1999)	An 18-item assessment that measures the frequency of racial discrimination across three subscales: (1) Recent Racist Events, (2) Lifetime Racist Events, and (3) Appraised Racist Events.
Perceived Racism Scale (PRS; McNeilly et al., 1996)	A 51-item measure that assesses perceptions of the frequency of racism in five domains: (1) Workplace Setting, (2) Academic Setting, (3) Public Setting Overtly, (4) Public Setting Covertly, and (5) Racist Statements in the past year.

to select the most memorable. After identifying the most memorable event, clients are then asked if the event was experienced as (1) negative (i.e., emotionally painful), (2) beyond their control, and (3) sudden in its occurrence. Recalling that these factors define racialized trauma, the client's response gives the clinician one point of data to assess if the event was experienced as traumatic. Next, the client is presented with the items of the scale and the following prompt: "Below is a list of reactions or feelings that people sometimes have after an upsetting event. Read each reaction carefully and circle the number that best describes your reactions or feelings *right after the event* (within one month)" (Carter et al., 2013, p. 4). The intensity of the client's reactions is rated on a 5-point Likert-type scale that ranges from 0 (does not describe my reaction) to 4 (this reaction would not go away). Summed scores are then converted to *t*-scores to allow comparisons across subscales. The full version of the assessment also asks clients to rate these reactions More Recently or Now, and if anyone has noticed a change in the client's behavior or personality with respect to the reaction, with a yes or no response to each item (Carter & Sant-Barket, 2015).

To illustrate how specific measures of race-based trauma such as the RBTSSS may enhance the assessment process, let's return to the case of Jessica Johnson. Jessica is a 45-year-old African American woman seeking an evaluation of trauma due to an unlawful arrest. During her intake interview, Jessica's therapist explored her symptoms to a greater extent using the RBTSSS. Jessica described three incidents of racism she has experienced in the past and then selected the most memorable, the encounter with police, to base her responses to the scale's items. In exploring this incident, Jessica endorsed reactions from each of the seven symptoms clusters, having *t*-scores of 72 for Depression, 61 for Intrusion, 80 for Anger, 65 for Hypervigilance, 50 for Physical Reactions, 64 for Low Self-Esteem, and 68 for Avoidance. In discussing her difficulties with Depression and Anger, her two highest scores, Jessica explained that while racism is something she has experienced throughout her life, she believed that things would become more equal and fairer once she obtained a certain level of education and success. The fact that she experienced an unprovoked assault left Jessica feeling hopeless and angry about her powerlessness to change her situation. At times, Jessica also wonders if there is something she is doing wrong, or some standard she is not living up to. She was visibly distraught while discussing these issues during the session, crying and holding her chest. Although not reported during the initial clinical interview, Jessica admitted that she often experiences panic symptoms when discussing the situation, including chest pain and shortness of breath.

During the interpretation of her assessment, Jessica and her therapist discussed the nature of racial trauma in further depth, with her therapist explaining that racial trauma is a response to race-based events that are perceived as sudden, out of one's control, and highly negative or emotionally painful. This helped to normalize Jessica's experience, which she had previously been interpreting as weakness on her part. With this new understanding of racial trauma in mind, Jessica and her therapist agreed to develop goals focused on managing the physical, emotional, and cognitive symptoms of her experience. The next section discusses cognitive conceptualization, which would further inform Jessica's therapy goals.

Cognitive Conceptualization

Cognitive conceptualization is the map that depicts the relationship between the client's core beliefs, conditional assumptions, and automatic thoughts (J. S. Beck, 2020). As stated in Chapter 1, this map consists of data describing: (a) the client's relevant childhood experiences, (b) the client's central beliefs about themselves, (c) attitudes and rules they use to navigate the world in light of their beliefs, (d) cognitive, affective, and behavioral strategies they use to adhere to their rules, and (e) examples of how such data are translated into negative automatic thoughts and reactions in daily situations. CBT therapists who take a Beckian approach to therapy often utilize a tool called the cognitive conceptualization diagram to assist in their development of the client's cognitive conceptualization (J. S. Beck, 2020). Figure 6.1 illustrates this diagram completed for the case of Jessica Johnson, which I will return to at the end of this section. On the diagram, the lower portion illustrates

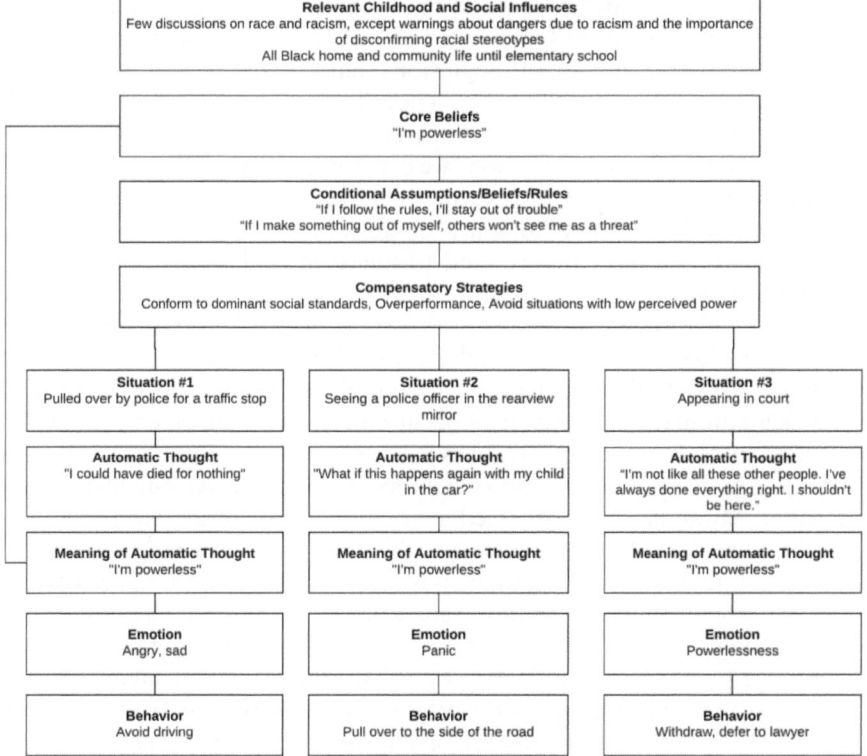

Figure 6.1 Jessica's Cognitive Conceptualization Diagram. Adapted from Beck, J. S. (2020). *Cognitive behavior therapy: Basics and beyond* (3rd ed.). Guilford Press.

specific examples of the generic cognitive model; that is, client perceptions that lead to their emotional, behavioral, and physiological reactions. The upper portion of the diagram depicts the childhood experiences, underlying cognitions, and compensatory strategies that influence these perceptions.

In the paragraphs that follow, I discuss each aspect of cognitive conceptualization and provide new case examples. I begin with a discussion of the generic cognitive model, focusing on automatic thoughts. I then discuss the underlying cognitions that influence automatic thoughts and various compensatory strategies, highlighting core beliefs, schemas, and compensatory strategies specific to the experience of racism. I conclude the section with a discussion of a complete cognitive conceptualization diagram for the previous case example, Jessica Johnson.

The Cognitive Model

The cognitive model, one of CBT's primary tenets, states that our reactions, that is, our feelings, behaviors, and physiological responses, are not caused by what happens to us, but by how we think about what happens to us (J. S. Beck, 2020). In this model, the cognitions that lead to our various responses are known as automatic thoughts. These thoughts, which may be fleeting and unintentional, in turn, lead to the emotions we have, the behaviors we exhibit, and the physical sensations we experience in our bodies. While automatic thoughts may be positive or negative, it is typically the negative thoughts that lead to psychological distress. Negative automatic thoughts, therefore, are the thoughts we tend to focus on challenging and replacing during therapy.

Automatic thoughts often take the form of words and phrases; however, they may also consist of mental pictures or memories (Greenberger & Padesky, 2015). Let's look at a clinical example to illustrate the various forms in which automatic thoughts may occur and the ways in which they lead to psychological distress. Miranda was a 17-year-old adolescent seeking treatment for both generalized and social anxiety disorder. At our fifth session together, Miranda and I discussed a situation she recorded on her thought record homework. Miranda described the situation as receiving a phone call from her father who wanted to encourage her to be careful on her drive to school that morning, as the roads were more icy than usual. Her initial automatic thoughts were, "I might get into an accident," "I might slide," and "I might die or get paralyzed." However, Miranda also remembered hitting someone else's car a couple of weeks prior when the roads were icy and imagined herself getting into an even worse accident. These thoughts resulted in Miranda feeling anxious and scared, and caused her to seek permission to stay home from school that day. Figure 6.2 shows the connection between Miranda's automatic thoughts and her reactions.

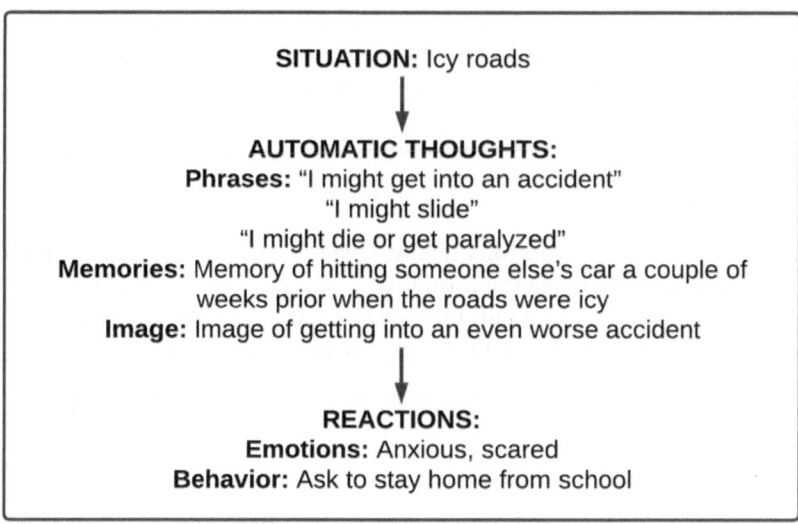

Figure 6.2 Cognitive Model in the Case of Miranda.

As shown in this example, clients often have more than one automatic thought in any given situation. In fact, most clients experience a stream of thoughts that vary in terms of their rationality and the extent to which they are psychologically or emotionally distressing (J. S. Beck, 2020). During therapy, the primary goal is to identify the thoughts that are the most dysfunctional and emotionally charged. Noted CBT experts Dennis Greenberger and Christine Padesky (2015) call these thoughts "hot thoughts." Returning to the case example, Miranda, it is noted that she was able to identify several automatic thoughts as she reflected on the phone call from her father; however, each of these thoughts varied in the extent to which they were emotionally charged and connected to her feelings of anxiety and fear. For example, during the session, Miranda revealed that the thoughts "I might get into an accident" and "I might slide" contributed very little to the distressing emotions she experienced. The thought, "I might die or get paralyzed," her memory of the car accident she was in a couple of weeks prior, and the mental picture of her getting into an even worse accident, however, elicited a very intense emotional response from Miranda and therefore could be described as the hot thoughts.

Activity 6.2: Identifying Automatic Thoughts

Let's test your ability to identify automatic thoughts. Below, you will find two hypothetical situations. After reading each situation, write down the automatic thoughts you might have in each situation. Remember, emotions provide clues to negative automatic thoughts, so in addition to writing down your automatic thoughts, also write down the feelings you might experience in the situation.

Let's Practice!

Read the hypothetical situations below. Imagine yourself in each situation and write down your automatic thoughts. Then, write down the feelings you would have in each situation and rate the intensity at which you would experience each feeling from 0 to 100% using the following scale:

0%	25%	50%	75%	100%
Less Intense				More Intense

Example: You receive an unexpected bill in the mail.
Thought(s): If it's not one thing, it's another. I'll never get ahead.
Emotion(s): Frustrated (70%); Hopeless (60%)

Situation 1: A friend invites you to a party where it's likely you will not know any of the other guests.
Thought(s):
Emotion(s):

Situation 2: While driving to work, you realize you've forgotten an important file and going back home to get the file will make you ten minutes late for the morning staff meeting.
Thought(s):
Emotion(s):

When you're finished, examine your level of awareness during this exercise. Did you actually identify thoughts where you were supposed to identify thoughts and feelings where you were supposed to identify feelings? How well do the thoughts and feelings you identified match up with each other? Is it likely that the thoughts you identified would produce the feelings you listed?

Core Beliefs

Much of the initial work in CBT focuses on teaching clients to identify, challenge, and replace their negative automatic thoughts. Over time, thematic patterns may emerge in the client's automatic thoughts that reveal their core beliefs. *Core beliefs* refer to central ideas about oneself, others, and the world (J. S. Beck, 2020). They may be negative or positive, and typically develop in response to early childhood experiences and societal messages about one's various social group identities (Steele, 2020). Core beliefs are significant because they serve as the underlying cognitions that lead to negative automatic thoughts and errors in thinking in daily situations. For this reason, a line is drawn on the cognitive conceptualization diagram connecting core beliefs to automatic thoughts (J. S. Beck, 2020). Let's look at another clinical example to illustrate the connection between core beliefs and automatic thoughts.

Sierra was a 32-year-old woman who came to therapy due to the recent breakup of her romantic relationship and worsening problems with anxiety. Sierra, who was still living with her ex-girlfriend, was now facing the challenge of finding a new apartment to live in on her own. During therapy, Sierra and I explored her thoughts and feelings about the situation, using the cognitive model as an organizing framework. Together, we came up with the conceptualization shown in Figure 6.3. As depicted in the diagram, when reflecting on the process of moving out of the apartment, Sierra had the automatic thought "I'm 32 years old and I should have figured this out by now." Her emotional reaction was to become sad, and her behavioral response was to stay at a friend's house and avoid packing. To explore the core belief behind this thought, I used the downward arrow technique, asking Sierra about the meaning the automatic thought would have to the client's life if it were true. As Sierra responded to the technique, it became clear

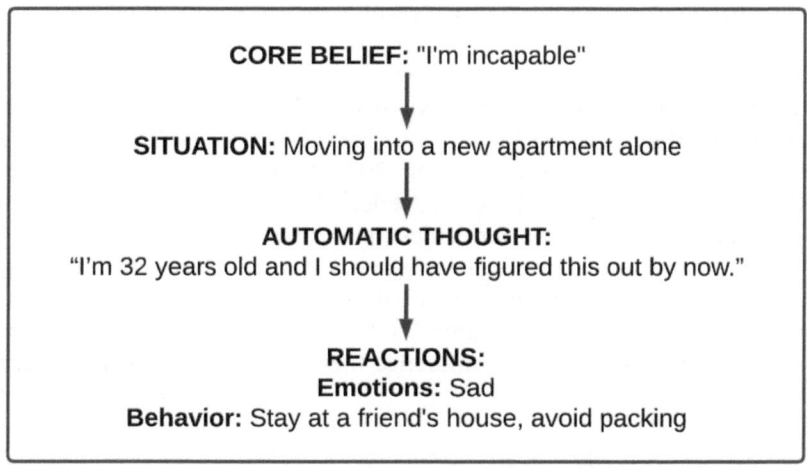

Figure 6.3 Extended Cognitive Model in the Case of Sierra.

that the automatic thoughts she was having in response to this situation originated from the core belief "I'm incapable," which we were eventually able to see evidenced in her thoughts about other situations as well. A goal for our work together, then, became the modification of this belief, as modification of core beliefs can decrease the likelihood clients will process situations in a maladaptive way in the future (J. S. Beck, 2020).

During therapy, the core beliefs that are of most interest to therapists are those that are negative in nature, as these beliefs shape how clients process the information they receive from the environment and the negative automatic thoughts they develop. According to J. S. Beck (2020), negative core beliefs generally fall into three categories: (1) helplessness, (2) unlovability, and (3) worthlessness. Helplessness core beliefs reflect ideas about personal incompetence, vulnerability, and inferiority (Schaffner, 2021). Examples of these core beliefs include "I am incompetent" and "I am a victim." Clients with unlovability core beliefs, on the other hand, perceive themselves as unlikable and incapable of intimacy. Examples of beliefs in this category include "I am unattractive" and "I am bound to be rejected." Last, clients with worthlessness core beliefs perceive themselves as inherently bad and/or a burden to others. Examples of these beliefs include "I am worthless" and "I don't deserve to live."

Core beliefs are often self-focused, as illustrated in the examples of helplessness, unlovability, and worthlessness provided above. However, as mentioned previously, core beliefs may also focus on others or the world. Examples of core beliefs about others include cognitions such as "People can't be trusted" and "Everyone is out for themselves." Core beliefs about the world, on the other hand, are typically even more broad, as exemplified in core beliefs such as "Things never work out for me," "The universe is against me," and "The world is a dangerous place."

Elsewhere, I have delineated several core beliefs commonly associated with internalized racism, which may be considered one psychological manifestation of racism (Steele & Newton, 2022; Banks et al., 2021). These core beliefs, which are listed in Table 6.3, reflect themes around inferiority, inadequacy, personal blame, powerlessness, and belief in a just world. They not only suggest the source of clients' negative automatic thoughts but also provide insight into the avoidance or numbing compensatory strategies clients enact to manage their racial trauma. Let's look at another clinical example to illustrate how these beliefs influence the ways in which clients interpret various situations.

Case Illustration: Rashida

Rashida is a 43-year-old African American woman who grew up in a lower-middle-class neighborhood in the Bay Area of California. She and her

Table 6.3 Core Beliefs, Schemas, and Compensatory Strategies Associated with Internalized Racism

Core Beliefs/Schemas

Inferiority	Believing, either consciously or unconsciously, in the supremacy of White culture (Bailey et al., 2014). "Being Black is at times embarrassing or shameful."
Inadequacy	Ascribing to personal inferiority beliefs surrounding being Black (Bailey et al., 2014). "I'm not good enough. I can't be successful unless I adopt certain interests, communication styles, and standards of beauty."
Personal blame	Taking complete responsibility for failures or difficulties even when prejudice and discrimination are factors (Prilleltensky & Gonick, 1996). "All of my difficulties in life are my own fault."
Powerlessness	Perceiving the inability to initiate change to be greater than the actual limitations of one's social context (Prilleltensky & Gonick, 1996). "Things will always stay the same. Nothing I do matters."
Belief in a just world	Believing there must be just reasons for the inequalities among racial groups, such as low morals or inferior intellectual abilities (Prilleltensky & Gonick, 1996). "Everyone gets what they deserve."

Compensatory Strategies

Avoidance	Attempting to cope with feelings of shame, embarrassment, and alienation by distancing oneself from aspects of one's racial group membership, for example, concealing the neighborhood one is from or isolating oneself from individuals and social settings perceived to confirm negative stereotypes (Watts-Jones, 2002).
Conformity	Adjusting one's speech, appearance, and behavior to be more similar to the dominant culture, ranging on a continuum from code-switching to overt stigmatization of one's own cultural norms (Bailey et al., 2014).
Overperformance	Overperforming in occupational, academic, or social settings to meet real or perceived expectations greater than those held for members of the dominant racial group (Palmer & Walker, 2020).
Learned helplessness	Doing nothing when challenged by racism in response to the belief that one has no control over what happens (Bivens, 2005; Prilleltensky & Gonick, 1996).

Source: Steele, J. M., & Newton, C. S. (2022). Culturally adapted cognitive behavior therapy as a model to address internalized racism among African American clients. *Journal of Mental Health Counseling, 44*(2), 98–116. https://doi.org/10.17744/mehc.44.2.01

younger sister were raised by their paternal grandmother until returning to live with their mother in high school. Although the community Rashida grew up in was racially diverse, socioeconomic status was clearly stratified according to race. Additionally, the elementary and middle schools Rashida attended had larger percentages of White students than other schools in her town and the majority of the teaching staff at the schools were White or Asian American as well. Although Rashida was naturally a shy child, she made friends with both the Black children in her neighborhood and the White students at her school. In spite of this, Rashida never felt as though she truly fit in with either group of children. At times, the Black children in her neighborhood teased her for "sounding White," while the White children occasionally teased Rashida for having a "Black" sounding name, wearing braided hairstyles, and the neighborhood in which she lived. During one session, Rashida recalled being invited to a friend's house for a sleepover in middle school. The friend's father agreed to pick Rashida up for the sleepover, as Rashida's grandmother did not drive outside of their neighborhood. Upon being invited to their home, Rashida's friend blurted out, "This is where you live?" Rashida, who felt embarrassed and ashamed, hung her head in silence in response to the friend's comment. The friend's father, mortified, scolded his daughter and took the girls away for their visit.

Rashida's childhood experiences with race had a significant impact on the goals she later developed for herself as an adult. In particular, Rashida became determined to prove she was just as good as anyone, and that she has what it takes to be successful. Accordingly, Rashida did well throughout grade school, became a first-generation college student, and went on to pursue a law degree from an Ivy League school. During her education, she was always careful to wear "the right" clothes and hairstyles, and to speak using vernacular that would be acceptable to mainstream America. Recently, Rashida passed the California bar exam and was hired as a junior associate at a prestigious corporate law firm. In spite of her credentials and experience, Rashida finds that her contributions are often ignored, and she is often tasked with paperwork while her White colleagues are mentored and given opportunities to assist directly on cases.

Rashida initiated counseling after being passed over for an opportunity to assist on yet another one of her firm's larger cases. Rashida reports feeling frustrated with the poor institutional support, exclusion from informal networks, and challenges to her credibility she receives. She additionally finds herself feeling disconnected from her job and avoids socializing with coworkers because she feels unheard and devalued. As she reflects on her situation, Rashida finds herself thinking "I just can't win" and is considering quitting the law profession. She reports feeling like a failure and has now entered therapy to address the increasing severity of her symptoms of anxiety and depression.

As mentioned previously, therapists are often alerted to their clients' core beliefs through the themes reflected in the client's automatic thoughts over time. Therapists can also help clients identify these beliefs by working with them to confirm, disconfirm, or modify hypothesized core beliefs as the client presents data (J. S. Beck, 2020). In the case of Rashida, several of her responses to childhood experiences with race suggest core beliefs of inferiority and inadequacy. In particular, these beliefs were evidenced in the shame and embarrassment she felt in response to her friend's disdain of Rashida's home environment, as well as in Rashida's belief that she had to adopt Eurocentric styles of communication and dress in order to be successful. Core beliefs reflecting powerlessness (i.e., "I just can't win") and personal blame (i.e., "I'm a failure") are also reflected in the content of Rashida's story. However, because internalized racism is largely an unconscious process, the therapist would need to be intentional in working with Rashida to articulate these beliefs and their impact on her cognitive appraisals. Once doing so, the therapist and Rashida would then be in position to identify the specific rules and maladaptive coping strategies she implements to circumvent these beliefs.

Intermediate Beliefs

When core beliefs are negative, it can be helpful to know how these beliefs are mediated by an intermediate level of cognition called intermediate beliefs. *Intermediate beliefs* are the attitudes, rules, and conditional assumptions clients develop in response to their negative core beliefs (J. S. Beck, 2020). In other words, intermediate beliefs describe the mindsets, guidelines, and "if-then" conditions clients develop to prevent their core beliefs from being true.

Let's first continue with the previous example of Sierra to illustrate what these attitudes, rules, and conditional assumptions might look like. Recall that Sierra was a 32-year-old woman who came to therapy due to the recent breakup of her romantic relationship and worsening problems with anxiety. At the beginning of therapy, Sierra was still living with her ex-girlfriend and was in the process of finding and moving into a new apartment on her own. Sierra had several negative automatic thoughts about this situation, including the thought, "I'm 32 years old and I should have figured this out by now." Using the downward arrow technique, Sierra and I discovered that the underlying core belief in this situation was "I'm incapable." In examining this core belief, Sierra and I also discovered the attitude "It's embarrassing to make a mistake," the rule "Don't try if it's too hard," and the conditional assumption, "If I get information and the opinions of others before I form my thoughts and make a decision, I'll be ok." You can review Sierra's hierarchy of beliefs and automatic thoughts in Figure 6.4.

Intermediate beliefs can also be identified in the case of Rashida. Recall that Rashida is a 43-year-old African American woman who initiated

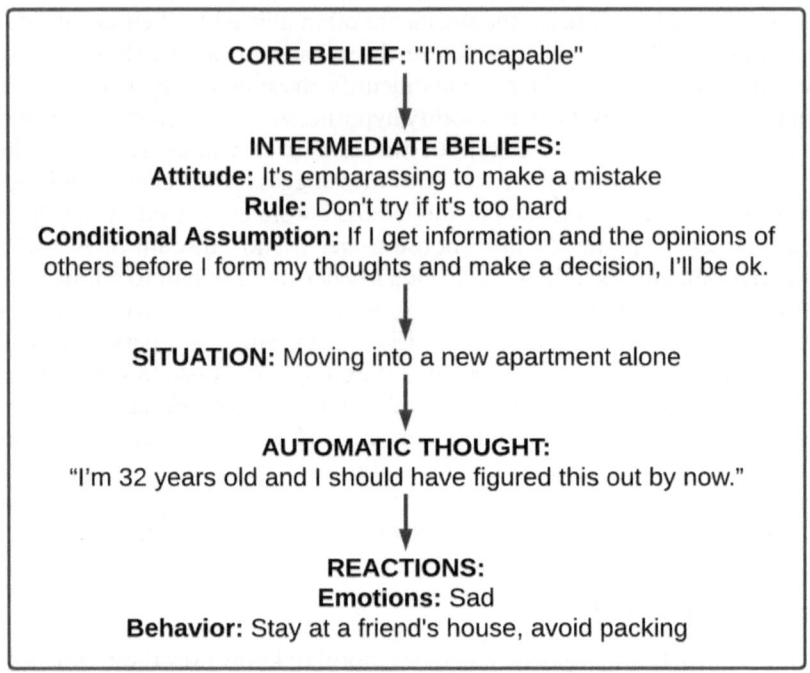

Figure 6.4 Sierra's Hierarchy of Beliefs and Automatic Thoughts.

therapy due to problems in her employment as a corporate lawyer at a prestigious law firm. In discussing her presenting concerns and childhood experiences, the therapist suspected that core beliefs associated with internalized racism (i.e., beliefs reflecting inferiority, inadequacy, powerlessness, and personal blame) had been activated by the situation with Rashida's employer. Rashida confirmed her therapist's hypothesis, which then allowed for further discussion of the intermediate beliefs she had developed to cope with her painful core beliefs. Specifically, through a process of guided discovery, Rashida realized she had developed the attitude "It's terrible to be different," the rule "Conform whenever possible," and the conditional assumption, "If I work hard and fit in, I will succeed." As previously mentioned, Rashida also developed behavioral strategies to enable her intermediate beliefs to cope with her feelings of inferiority, inadequacy, powerlessness, and personal blame.

Compensatory Strategies

Compensatory strategies refer to the methods clients use to cope with, compensate for, or protect themselves from their negative core beliefs

(Beck Institute, n.d.). While many individuals think about strategies that are overtly destructive when they hear this term, most compensatory strategies actually represent normal behaviors that are overused at the expense of more functional strategies (J. S. Beck, 2020). For instance, examples of compensatory strategies that could in some ways be viewed by clients as positive include perfectionism, people pleasing, being overly controlling, seeking recognition, avoiding confrontation, and their opposites (i.e., purposely appearing incompetent, distancing oneself from others, and abdicating control to others) (J. S. Beck, 2020). Other compensatory strategies, however, do have obviously negative impacts on clients and their relationships. Among individuals with personality disorders, for example, overdeveloped compensatory strategies tend to include lying, manipulating or taking advantage of others, threatening or attacking others, resisting control from others, and acting impulsively. Underdeveloped strategies, on the other hand, include cooperating with others, following societal rules, and thinking about consequences (Beck Institute, n.d.).

Returning one final time to the case of Sierra, strategies developed to cope with her core belief "I'm incapable" included relying on others, avoiding responsibility, trying to please others, and avoiding confrontation. Sierra believed that enacting these strategies would save her from failure and the embarrassment of making a mistake. As such, Sierra's initial response to her housing difficulties was to retreat to a friend's home and avoid dealing with the situation. Rashida's compensatory strategies, however, were more specific to the compensatory strategies associated with internalized racism described in Table 6.3, particularly conformity and overperformance. Conformity was evidenced in Rashida's efforts to adhere to Eurocentric styles of dress and communication, which she believed would allow her to "fit in" and avoid the feelings of shame and embarrassment she experienced as a child. Likewise, Rashida also believed she would be able to avoid feelings of shame and inferiority by meeting the Eurocentric standards of success dictated to her by society.

Jessica's Cognitive Conceptualization

Thus far, I have discussed various aspects of cognitive conceptualization and provided examples of the information used to inform the conceptualization. I now return to the earlier case of Jessica Johnson to illustrate what a complete cognitive conceptualization might look like, using the cognitive conceptualization diagram as a tool to further clarify the relationship between Jessica's underlying cognitions and automatic thoughts in daily situations (see Figure 6.1).

Jessica is a 45-year-old African American woman referred to therapy by her primary care physician for an assessment of posttraumatic stress disorder.

During the assessment, Jessica reported that she sustained physical injuries in an unlawful arrest two months prior to intake. Explaining the situation further, Jessica reported that during a traffic stop, she was instructed to exit her vehicle at which time the vehicle was searched. When she objected, officers attempted to restrain Jessica and a struggle ensued. Jessica was charged with resisting and obstructing as a result of the incident; however, upon review of body camera footage, the charges were later dropped. Since her charges were dropped, Jessica continues to experience distressing flashbacks of the event, as well as frequent nightmares. She believes that she was unfairly profiled because she was an African American woman driving a nice car. Jessica, therefore, additionally reports avoiding travel away from her home unless going to work or to provide care for her children due to fear of being profiled and assaulted again.

At the time of the assessment, Jessica endorsed the following symptoms: decreased appetite, trouble concentrating, distressing memories, difficulty sleeping, nightmares, hypervigilance, low motivation, isolation from others, fatigue/low energy, depressed mood, anxiety, and worry about the future. Results of quantitative assessments revealed elevated scores on measures of PTSD, anxiety, depression, and racial trauma, as well. Specifically, Jessica's scores revealed that she met criteria for each area of PTSD and had a moderate level of anxiety, a moderately severe level of depression, and elevated scores on all seven areas of racial trauma assessed during the evaluation session. Based on these results, the therapist's initial diagnostic impression was F43.10 Posttraumatic Stress Disorder. Given this diagnosis, Jessica decided to continue therapy to decrease her current psychological distress and learn new coping strategies.

As indicated in the case of Jessica, precipitating events leading to her current symptomatology were the incidents of her arrest and subsequent legal charges. The individual situations described on her cognitive conceptualization diagram provide insight into the cross-sectional view of Jessica's cognitions and behaviors subsequent to these precipitating events. During one session, Jessica reported that she often considers what could have gone wrong during the traffic stop, thinking, "I could have died for nothing." This thought caused Jessica to feel angry and sad, and to avoid driving except to go to work or care for her children. In another situation, Jessica described seeing a police officer in her rearview mirror while driving her youngest child home from soccer practice one afternoon. In this situation, Jessica's thought was "What if this happens again with my child in the car?" In response, Jessica had a panic attack, causing her to pull over on the side of the road until her symptoms subsided and she could no longer see the police unit. In the last situation illustrated on the diagram, Jessica recalled the final court appearance addressing her resisting and obstruction charges. During this situation, she thought, "I'm not like all these other people. I've always done everything right. I shouldn't be here." The emotion she felt was powerlessness, and her behavioral response was to withdraw within herself and defer to her lawyer.

When considering the impact of race and racism in Jessica's cognitive conceptualization, it is noted that the automatic thoughts in her cross-sectional view of cognitions and behaviors exemplify characteristics of both racial trauma and internalized racism, as discussed throughout this text. In particular, recall that racial trauma according to the race-based traumatic stress injury model refers to mental and emotional injury caused by encounters with racial harassment, racial discrimination, or discriminatory harassment (Carter, 2007). While Jessica's symptoms are consistent with traumatic stress due to violence, they are further impacted by the perceived role of race in her interactions with police. Accordingly, it is essential that her therapist acknowledge the impact of race in Jessica's presenting concerns in order to broach any relevant race-related beliefs or negative self-appraisals she may have developed as a result of the situation. As mentioned, elements of internalized racism are also evidenced in Jessica's cross-sectional view of cognitions and behaviors in that Jessica's thought "I'm not like all these other people. I've always done everything right. I shouldn't be here" appears to reflect a mentality that places the blame for oppression solely on its victims without considering the role of societal structures that also influence the marginalization of various communities (Prilleltensky & Gonick, 1996). As such, Jessica appears to be experiencing elements of shame and self-criticism that additionally warrant exploration during therapy.

The racial themes evident in Jessica's cross-sectional view of cognitions and behaviors also have a direct impact on the longitudinal view of her cognitions and behaviors, as described in the top half of Figure 6.1. Jessica was the product of a two-parent home where race and racism were rarely discussed, except within the context of the need to be aware of the dangers faced in life due to racism and the importance of disconfirming racial stereotypes. According to Jessica, her parents felt less compelled to discuss race during her early years given the racial homogeneity of their homelife and neighborhood environment. Upon entering the more racially diverse environment of her elementary school, however, Jessica's parents became more intentional in warning Jessica about the chance of unjust treatment by authority figures because of her race and the need to be mindful of how others perceived her. This warning, known colloquially in the African American community as "the talk," is a common discussion many African American parents have with their children in order to prepare them for the realities of living in a racially oppressed society (Solis, 2021). While scholars note that the content of this talk varies to some extent across generations, it generally consists of admonitions against trusting members of other races and conversations about the importance of being cautious when in public, respectful to people in authority, and careful not to dress, walk, or talk in ways that make members of other races uncomfortable.

As Jessica listened to these warnings throughout her life, she interpreted them to mean that Black people are vulnerable to the whims of more dominant racial groups, making the world a dangerous place she was incapable of changing. As Jessica internalized this idea, she developed the core belief "I'm powerless." In order to cope with this belief, she developed the conditional assumption "If I follow the rules, I'll stay out of trouble" and "If I make something out of myself, others won't see me as a threat." The compensatory strategies she enacted in response to her core and intermediate beliefs included conformity, overperformance, and avoidance.

To summarize, cognitive conceptualization is a critical aspect of CBT, as it not only provides the framework for understanding the client's problems but also directs the interventions used during treatment (Matu, 2018). While cognitive conceptualization begins during the first session, it continues throughout therapy as more is discovered about the client's automatic thoughts and the deeper-level cognitions underlying these thoughts (J. S. Beck, 2020). Given the ongoing nature of cognitive conceptualization, any interpretations or hypotheses formed during the conceptualization process should be viewed as tentative and therapists should regularly check-in with clients to determine the accuracy of the conceptualization, modifying it as necessary.

Activity 6.3: Developing a Cognitive Conceptualization

In Activity 6.1: Exploring One's Racial History, you practiced investigating an individual's history of racial experiences using your own self-reflection as well as data obtained from a colleague or supervisor. In this exercise, use the information acquired either from your self-reflection or from your colleague to complete a blank cognitive conceptualization diagram. If necessary, continue your self-reflection or return to your colleague to gather any missing data needed to complete the diagram. Then, work to identify any racial themes apparent in the relevant experiences and underlying cognitions identified on the diagram. If you are a White therapist with difficulty identifying specific aspects of White culture influencing your racial worldview, consider reading Judith Katz's (1985) seminal article, "The Sociopolitical Nature of Counseling."

Reflection Questions

• What did the cognitive conceptualization diagram teach you about the relationship between a client's underlying cognitions and automatic thoughts?
• How might this information be useful in your work with clients?
• To what extent were you able to identify racial themes in the underlying cognitions identified by you or your colleague?
• What additional cultural knowledge do you need to adequately identify racial content in a client's underlying cognitions?
• What can you do to obtain this knowledge?

Treatment Planning

Broadly, therapists use treatment plans as a way to identify clients' problems, set goals, and choose interventions. Because client/therapist agreement on the approach taken to treatment is a mediator of the therapeutic alliance (Bordin, 1979), basic aspects of identifying client problems, goal setting, and intervention selection were discussed in Chapter 5. In this section, greater attention is given to these three aspects of treatment planning, with additional considerations for mental health impacts due to racism. The section concludes with an example treatment plan for the case of Jessica Johnson.

Identifying the Problem

Recall that problems refer to the situations that contribute to the client's psychological distress, interpersonal difficulties, or social role impairments. When identifying problems, specific characteristics therapists should be intentional in paying attention to include dysfunction (i.e., symptoms, instability in relationships, or skill deficits), urgency (i.e., severity or intensity), impairment (i.e., disruptions in the client's ability to fulfill daily roles or tasks), and risk (i.e., chance of harm to self or others) (Schwitzer & Rubin, 2012). Symptom dysfunction can be separated into four broad categories: emotional symptoms, cognitive symptoms, behavioral symptoms, and physiological symptoms. Emotional symptoms refer to internal reactions to various stimuli in the environment (Brady, 2020). Examples of these symptoms include anger, anxiety, disgust, and sadness. Typically, emotional symptoms experienced during a specific situation are called *affect*, while *mood* refers to the client's emotional state over the course of time and fits into one of six categories: euthymic (i.e., normal), dysphoric (e.g., sad, down, upset, frustrated, worthless, hopeless), euphoric (i.e., manic), angry (e.g., irritable), anxious (e.g., fearful, worried, tense), and apathetic (e.g., dull, bland, flat)

(Polanski & Hinkle, 2000, p. 359). According to the conceptualization of racial trauma provided by Carter et al. (2013), emotional symptoms that tend to characterize clients' response to negative race-based encounters include depression and anger. Other scholars also describe irritability, humiliation, shame, guilt, fear, anxiety, grief, worthlessness, and hopelessness as common emotions experienced in response to racism as well (Williams et al., 2018b).

In contrast to emotional symptoms, cognitive symptoms refer to difficulties processing information or errors in thinking. Examples of cognitive symptoms include problems with concentration, poor decision making, or perfectionism. Cognitive symptoms often associated with racial trauma include hypervigilance, flashbacks, distressing memories, dissociation, low self-esteem, self-alienation, self-blame, pessimism, and cultural mistrust (Carter et al., 2013; Polanco-Roman et al., 2016; Williams et al., 2018b). Behavioral symptoms, on the other hand, refer to persistent or repetitive behaviors that are unusual, disruptive, or inappropriate. General examples of these symptoms include aggression, arguing, self-harm, crying, and social withdrawal. Behavioral symptoms that may occur due to encounters with racism include avoidance, substance use, smoking, and nonparticipation in behaviors that promote good health such as cancer screening, diabetes management, and condom use (Carter et al., 2013; Pascoe & Smart Richman, 2009). Finally, physiological symptoms refer to the physical sensations clients experience in their bodies. Examples of these symptoms include rapid heart rate, difficulty breathing, sweating, trembling, fainting, blushing, or having a shaky voice, any of which may occur due to racism.

Having a good understanding of the different types of symptoms clients may have in response to experiences with racism allows the therapist to ask questions that result in greater specificity in the list of problems identified. This is especially important given that racism is not always recognized as a stressor that leads to such a breadth of symptoms. Moreover, some African Americans are socialized to refrain from expressing helplessness and vulnerability, which further necessitates direct exploration of symptoms in the identification of problems (Payne, 2014). The assessments mentioned earlier can provide insight into which symptoms clients may endorse. Questions therapists may also pose directly to clients to help identify problems due to racism include:

• What are your most memorable experiences with racism?
• Have you ever been in a situation where you suspected that someone's attitude or behavior toward you was due to racism, but you could not prove it? [Provide examples of microaggressions or colorblind racial attitudes if necessary]

- Do you have any strong emotions as a result of these experiences? If so, what are they?
- Do you have any negative thoughts or feelings about yourself or others as a result of these experiences? If so, what are they?
- Do you experience any physical sensations in your body when you recall your experiences?
- Do you find yourself reliving what happened, either through your thoughts, dreams, memories, or flashbacks?
- Do you avoid things that remind you of the event?
- Did you experience changes in your relationships with others after these experiences?
- Do any of your reactions to these experiences make it difficult to manage your life?

Below is an example of a problem list created in response to Jessica's self-report on the RBTSS and her answers to some of these questions.

Jessica's Problem List

1. Depression, especially social withdrawal, fatigue, and poor concentration
2. Anger, especially irritability, humiliation, and resentment toward others
3. Reliving the trauma, including flashbacks and distressing memories
4. Difficulty leaving the house
5. Panic, including chest pain and shortness of breath

Developing Treatment Goals

So far, you've learned that experiences with racism result in a variety of outcomes that are physical, emotional, and psychological in nature. Therefore, when developing treatment goals to mitigate the impacts of racism, it is important to identify goals that address symptoms the client is experiencing in each of these areas. During this process, therapists should focus on providing clients with a safe space to: (a) verbalize their experience with racism, (b) explore and modify negative emotions and views of self that develop as a result of racism, and (c) identify actions that can be taken to increase the client's sense of empowerment. Based on a review of the literature, other areas of focus for treatment goals include self-regulation, insight, processing strong emotions, and resilience (Bryant-Davis & Ocampo, 2006; Bryant-Davis et al., 2021; Chioneso et al., 2020; Comas-Díaz, 2016).

Self-regulation is often discussed within the context of helping children manage their emotions and behaviors; however, the ability to self-regulate is an important skill for both children and adults. This is especially true when dealing with the reactive nature of trauma response and the effects of racism on mental health. *Self-regulation* refers to

> the ability to manage your emotions and behavior in accordance with the demands of the situation. It includes being able to resist highly emotional reactions to upsetting stimuli, to calm yourself down when you get upset, to adjust to a change in expectations, and to handle frustration.
>
> (Child Mind Institute, 2022)

African Americans often feel upset or frustrated in response to racism, and rightly so. However, research shows that negative coping strategies such as rumination, confrontation, and avoidance are often employed when dealing with these emotions (Hoggard et al., 2012). While these strategies may provide temporary relief of symptoms, they ultimately worsen the experience of racial trauma by increasing distress associated with the seven symptom clusters of race-based stress. Therefore, treatment goals around the development of more positive self-regulation strategies such as mindfulness, self-compassion, and cognitive reframing are often essential to offsetting the emotional and psychological harm of racism (Sawyer, 2019; Steele & Newton, 2023).

Another way to help clients offset the emotional and psychological weight of racism is through insight. *Insight* refers to increased understanding of oneself and the origin of one's problems. Given the varied, chronic, and pervasive nature of racism, individuals who have experienced racial trauma may not always be aware of the source of their trauma or its impact. Helping clients develop insight into the relationship between racism and their problems, therefore, can be therapeutic by reducing guilt, self-blame, and feelings of worthlessness. Treatment goals that may produce insight include increasing awareness of (a) societal influences leading to racial trauma and other related psychological phenomena and (b) the ways in which racial trauma manifests in the lives of people of color. For example, during therapy with my clients who are dealing with racial trauma, I often discuss the ways in which dominant culture influences how people of color are perceived by others and how they perceive themselves, and how negative self-perceptions reflect aspects of internalized racism such as a sense of inferiority, powerlessness, and learned helplessness. These discussions typically begin with me as the therapist providing the client with information on these topics and then using basic counseling and theory specific techniques such as Socratic questioning to explore how these issues present in the client's own life. I also highlight the symptoms of their race-based stress as they are illustrated in the content of their stories.

As mentioned, avoiding the painful emotions of race-based stress is a coping strategy employed by many individuals who experience racial trauma;

however, this strategy often has the opposite intended effect, instead deepening and worsening the pain. Teaching clients how to process strong emotions can reduce reliance on avoidance as a coping strategy and help provide clients the catharsis they need. *Emotions* refer to internal reactions to various stimuli in our environment (Brady, 2020). As previously discussed, individuals with racial trauma experience emotions such as sadness, anger, hopelessness, fear, guilt, shame, and humiliation. Brady (2020) identified three basic steps to processing emotions that may be beneficial in helping African American clients manage these feelings. These steps include: (1) identifying and labeling one's feelings, (2) giving oneself the time and space needed to experience feelings without judgment, and (3) deciding how to handle feelings, either through problem-solving if one has control over the issue or through coping if not.

The next area of focus for treatment goals when working with the impacts of racism is resilience. *Resilience* refers to the ability to maintain or regain mental health despite experiencing adversity (Wald et al., 2006). Racial trauma not only results from direct race-based incidents, but also occurs as a result of disparate social and developmental outcomes including poverty, violent neighborhoods, and higher mortality rates due to disease, necessitating a need for strategies that facilitate an ability to overcome difficulties (Brown, 2008). Examples of such strategies include developing an ability to sit with difficult emotions, adapting to change, and empowering oneself through recognition of one's value and worth. It is important to note, however, that promotion of resilience without equal consideration of the need for change in racist and discriminatory policies and practices has the effect of perpetuating the status quo and various systems of oppression. Accordingly, therapists should make an effort to contextualize the discussion of resilience to reflect the importance of drawing on personal strengths without sacrificing one's mental health, and while also holding those in positions of power accountable.

Finally, *psychological empowerment* refers to an awareness of factors that impinge upon one's ability to structure their life and committed action to initiate change (Curtis-Tweed, 2003; Zimmerman, 1995). One important aspect of psychological empowerment is critical consciousness. *Critical consciousness* is "the capacity of oppressed or marginalized people to critically analyze their social and political conditions, endorsement of societal equality, and action to change perceived inequities" (Diemer et al., 2017, p. 461). I'll discuss this in greater depth in Chapter 8. As it relates to goal setting, Zimmerman (1995) identified the following goals associated with psychological empowerment: being more informed, being more skilled, being healthier, and being more involved in decision making. When dealing with racial trauma, this may include learning more about racism or engaging in activism.

Let's return to our case example, Jessica, to illustrate what therapy goals based on these characteristics might look like. Recall that Jessica had elevated scores on all seven subscales of the RBTSSS and identified five specific problems she would like to address throughout the course of therapy: (1) depression (i.e., social withdrawal, fatigue, and poor concentration), (2) anger (i.e., irritability, humiliation, and resentment toward others), (3) reliving the trauma (i.e., flashbacks and distressing memories), (4) difficulty leaving the house, and (5) panic (i.e., chest pain and shortness of breath). To address these problems in a way consistent with recommended approaches to the treatment discussed above, Jessica's initial goals for therapy were to:

1. Reduce the amount of emotional and mental distress experienced when thinking about or discussing the trauma (modify the negative self-appraisals in response to the event)
2. Reduce the occurrence of intrusive thoughts, arousal, and avoidance associated with the trauma
3. Increase the use of self-regulation skills and other positive coping strategies such as diaphragmatic breathing, mindfulness, self-compassion, prayer, positive racial identity development, and connections with social supports
4. Increase her sense of power in addressing the legal aspects of her unlawful arrest

Selecting Interventions

Throughout this text, the similarities between racial trauma and other trauma disorders such as PTSD have been emphasized. Given these similarities, it can be helpful to think about interventions as they are traditionally conceptualized in the trauma literature when developing treatment plans to address the psychological effects of racism; that is, in terms of top-down and bottom-up approaches (van der Kolk, 2014). Top-down approaches refer to strategies designed to help clients identify and challenge unhelpful thinking and behavioral patterns, solve problems more effectively, and develop a sense of empowerment. These approaches include cognitive restructuring, as well as strategies such as role-plays, consciousness-raising, and psycho-education on microintervention strategies for confronting, disarming, or counteracting the effects of microaggressions in one's environment. Other strategies with even greater emphasis on empowerment such as collective healing, community participation, and responding to White fragility; that is, the need to sooth White people when they feel unsafe or uncomfortable are also beneficial in addressing cognitive aspects of racial trauma (Menakem, 2017). More is said about top-down cognitive restructuring strategies and empowerment interventions in Chapters 7 and 8. For the purpose of intervention selection, it can be helpful to understand cognitive interventions as those designed to address the maladaptive cognitions and behavioral responses that develop in response to experiences with racism.

Bottom-up approaches describe body-centric techniques focused on helping clients cope with their raw emotions and physiological reactions. These techniques consist of strategies such as breathing, mindfulness, and relaxation exercises (Menakem, 2017). Use of these body-centric strategies to address the mental health impacts of racism among African Americans is discussed in great detail in a book I co-authored with Dr. Charmeka Newton, titled, *Black Lives are Beautiful: 50 Tools to Heal from Trauma and Promote Positive Racial Identity*. I refer readers to this text for specific scripts and worksheets clients can use to learn various breathing, mindfulness, and relaxation strategies.

Because racial trauma in many ways represents the body's protective response to race-based events, racial trauma experts such as Resmaa Menakem (2017) recommend beginning treatment with psychoeducation that highlights the physiological aspects of trauma and emphasizes the importance of healing through the body. A second step is to teach clients exercises to increase awareness of their body's trauma responses, when and where they activate, the emotions they give rise to, and how to settle these emotions and physiological responses (Menakem, 2017). Broadly, Menakem (2017) conceptualized this process as a five-part model that consists of: (1) soothing yourself to quiet your mind, calm your heart, and settle your body, (2) noticing the sensations and emotions in your body, (3) accepting any discomfort you are experiencing rather than attempting to flee from it, (4) staying present in your body as your pain unfolds and responding to it from the best parts of yourself, and (5) safely discharging any remaining energy (p. 168). From a CBT perspective, this may involve teaching mindfulness-integrated CBT or acceptance and commitment therapy techniques in culturally responsive ways that incorporate cultural values, culturally-familiar terminology, and cultural resources (Watson-Singleton et al., 2019).

Once clients have developed the ability to experience their pain without fleeing from it, they can then begin using top-down strategies to reconceptualize their understanding of themselves and their abilities to cope, as well as reduce unhelpful thinking patterns that contribute to their symptoms. For example, using the CBT technique Socratic questioning, clients can explore the ways in which they expect catastrophic outcomes or think negatively about themselves, and then begin to develop more balanced and effective thinking patterns and core beliefs. A final treatment plan inclusive of both the top-down and bottom-up interventions selected to address Jessica's treatment goals is presented in Table 6.4.

Table 6.4 Jessica's Final Treatment Plan

Problem List

1. Depression, especially social withdrawal, fatigue, and poor concentration
2. Anger, especially irritability, humiliation, and resentment toward others
3. Reliving the trauma, including flashbacks and distressing memories
4. Difficulty leaving the house
5. Panic, including chest pain and shortness of breath

Treatment Goals

1. Reduce the amount of emotional and mental distress experienced when thinking about or discussing the trauma (modify the negative self-appraisals in response to the event)
2. Reduce the occurrence of intrusive thoughts, arousal, and avoidance associated with the trauma
3. Increase the use of self-regulation skills and other positive coping strategies such as diaphragmatic breathing, mindfulness, self-compassion, prayer, positive racial identity development, and connections with social supports
4. Increase her sense of power in addressing the legal aspects of her unlawful arrest

Interventions

1. Psychoeducation focused on consciousness-raising and the nature of racial trauma
2. Relaxation and mindfulness training including the use of breathing exercises and loving-kindness meditations
3. Cognitive restructuring including the use of Socratic questioning, thought records, and review and modification of core beliefs
4. Participation in community support groups

References

Abdullah, T., Graham-LoPresti, J. R., Tahirkheli, N. N., Hughley, S. M., & Watson, L. T. J. (2021). Microaggressions and posttraumatic stress disorder symptom scores among Black Americans: Exploring the link. *Traumatology, 27*(3), 244–253. https://doi.org/10.1037/trm0000259

American Psychiatric Association. (2013). *Diagnostic and statistical manual of mental disorders* (5th ed.). American Psychiatric Association. https://doi.org/10.1176/appi.books.9780890425596

Bailey, T.-K. M., Williams, W. S., & Favors, B. (2014). Internalized racial oppression in the African American community. In E. J. R. David (Ed.), *Internalized oppression: The psychology of marginalized groups* (pp. 137–162). Springer Publishing Company, Inc.

Banks, K. H., Goswami, S., Goodwin, D., Petty, J., Bell, V., & Musa, I. (2021). Interrupting internalized racial oppression: A community based ACT intervention. *Journal of Contextual Behavioral Science, 20*, 89–93. https://doi.org/10.1016/j.jcbs.2021.02.006

Beck, A. T. (1990). *Manual for the Beck Anxiety Inventory*. Pearson.

Beck, A. T., Steer, R. A., & Brown, G. K. (1996). *Manual for the Beck Depression Inventory-II*. Pearson.

Beck, J. S. (2020). *Cognitive behavior therapy: Basics and beyond* (3rd ed.). Guilford Press.

Beck Institute. (n.d.). Basics of CBT: Essentials I: Online course. https://beckinstitute.org/training/online-training

Bivens, D. K. (2005). What is internalized racism? *Flipping the Script: White Privilege and Community Building, 1*, 43–51.

Bordin, E. S. (1979). The generalizability of the psychoanalytic concept of the working alliance. *Psychotherapy: Theory, Research & Practice, 16*(3), 252–260. https://doi.org/10.1037/h0085885

Brady, K. (2020, May 20). *What does processing your feelings even mean? Experts offer strategies to help you sit with, and learn from, uncomfortable emotions*. https://www.shondaland.com/live/body/a32601217/what-does-processing-your-feelings-even-mean/

Brown, D. L. (2008). African American resiliency: Examining racial socialization and social support as protective factors. *Journal of Black Psychology, 34*(1), 32–48. https://doi.org/10.1177/0095798407310538

Bryant-Davis, T., Fasalojo, B., Arounian, A., Jackson, K. L., & Leithman, E. (2021). Resist and rise: A trauma-informed womanist model for group therapy. *Women & Therapy*. Advance online publication. https://doi.org/10.1080/02703149.2021.1943114

Bryant-Davis, T., & Ocampo, C. (2006). A therapeutic approach to the treatment of racist-incident-based trauma. *Journal of Emotional Abuse, 6*(4), 1–22. https://doi.org/10.1300/J135v06n04_01

Carter, R. T. (2007). Racism and psychological and emotional injury: Recognizing and assessing race-based traumatic stress. *The Counseling Psychologist, 35*(1), 13–105. https://doi.org/10.1177/0011000006292033

Carter, R. T., Mazzula, S., Victoria, R., Vazquez, R., Hall, S., Smith, S., Sant-Barket, S., Forsyth, J., Bazelais, K., & Williams, B. (2013). Initial development of the Race-Based Traumatic Stress Symptom Scale: Assessing the emotional impact of racism. *Psychological Trauma: Theory, Research, Practice, and Policy, 5*(1), 1–9. https://doi.org/10.1037/a0025911

Carter, R. T., & Pieterse, A. L. (2020). *Measuring the effects of racism: Guidelines for the assessment and treatment of race-based traumatic stress injury*. Columbia University Press. https://doi.org/10.7312/cart19306

Carter, R. T., & Sant-Barket, S. M. (2015). Assessment of the impact of racial discrimination and racism: How to use the Race-Based Traumatic Stress Symptom Scale in practice. *Traumatology, 21*(1), 32–39. https://doi.org/10.1037/trm0000018

Child Mind Institute. (2022). How can we help kids with self-regulation? https://childmind.org/article/can-help-kids-self-regulation/

Chioneso, N. A., Hunter, C. D., Gobin, R. L., McNeil Smith, S., Mendenhall, R., & Neville, H. A. (2020). Community healing and resistance through storytelling: A framework to address racial trauma in Africana communities. *Journal of Black Psychology, 46*(2–3), 95–121. https://doi.org/10.1177/0095798420929468

Comas-Díaz, L. (2016). Racial trauma recovery: A race-informed therapeutic approach to racial wounds. In A. N. Alvarez, C. T. H. Liang, & H. A. Neville (Eds), *The cost of racism for people of color: Contextualizing experiences of discrimination* (pp. 249–272). American Psychological Association. https://doi.org/10.1037/14852-000

Creed, T. A. (2019). *Clinical measures in CBT: A hassle or a help?* https://beckinstitute. org/blog/clinical-measures-in-cbt-a-hassle-or-a-help/

Curtis-Tweed, P. (2003). Experiences of African American empowerment: A Jamesian perspective on agency. *Journal of Moral Education, 32*(4), 397–409. https://doi. org/10.1080/0305724032000161295

Diemer, M. A., Rapa, L. J., Park, C. J., & Perry, J. C. (2017). Development and validation of the Critical Consciousness Scale. *Youth & Society, 49*(4), 461–483. https://doi.org/10.1177/0044118X14538289

Greenberger, D., & Padesky, C. A. (2015). *Mind over mood: Change how you feel by changing the way you think* (2nd ed.). Guilford Press

Hoggard, L. S., Byrd, C. M., & Sellers, R. M. (2012). Comparison of African American college students' coping with racially and nonracially stressful events. *Cultural Diversity and Ethnic Minority Psychology, 18*(4), 329–339. https://doi.org/10.1037/a0029437

Katz, J. H. (1985). The sociopolitical nature of counseling. *The Counseling Psychologist, 13*(4), 615–624. https://doi.org/10.1177/0011000085134005

Kirkinis, K., Pieterse, A. L., Martin, C., Agiliga, A., & Brownell, A. (2021). Racism, racial discrimination, and trauma: A systematic review of the social science literature. *Ethnicity & Health, 26*(3), 392–412. https://doi.org/10.1080/13557858.2018. 1514453

Klonoff, E. A., & Landrine, H. (1999). Cross-validation of the Schedule of Racist Events. *Journal of Black Psychology, 25*(2), 231–254. https://doi.org/10.1177/00957 98499025002006

Knox, S., Burkard, A. W., Johnson, A. J., Suzuki, L. A., & Ponterotto, J. G. (2003). African American and European American therapists' experiences of addressing race in cross-racial psychotherapy dyads. *Journal of Counseling Psychology, 50*(4), 466–481. https://doi.org/10.1037/0022-0167.50.4.466

Lambert, M. J., & Burlingame, G. M. (1996). *Outcome Questionnaire 45.2 (OQ-45.2)*. OQ Measures LLC.

Matu, S. A. (2018). Cognitive therapy. In A. Vernon and K. A. Doyle (Eds.), *Cognitive behavior therapies: A guidebook for practitioners* (pp. 75–108). American Counseling Association.

McNeilly, M. D., Anderson, N. B., Armstead, C. A., Clark, R., Corbett, M., Robinson, E. L., Pieper, C. F., & Lepisto, E. M. (1996). The Perceived Racism Scale: A multidimensional assessment of the experience of White racism among African Americans. *Ethnicity & Disease, 6*(1–2), 154–166.

Menakem, R. (2017). *My grandmother's hands: Racialized trauma and the pathway to mending our hearts and bodies*. Central Recovery Press.

Palmer, R. T., & Walker, L. J. (2020, July 6). Proposing a concept of the Black tax to understand the experiences of Blacks in America. *Diverse Issues in Higher Education*. https://diverseeducation.com/article/182837/

Pascoe, E. A., & Smart Richman, L. (2009). Perceived discrimination and health: A meta-analytic review. *Psychological Bulletin, 135*(4), 531–554. https://doi.org/10. 1037/a0016059

Payne, J. S. (2014). Social determinants affecting major depressive disorder: Diagnostic accuracy for African American men. *Best Practices in Mental Health, 10*(2), 78–95.

Polanco-Roman, L., Danies, A., & Anglin, D. M. (2016). Racial discrimination as race-based trauma, coping strategies, and dissociative symptoms among emerging adults. *Psychological Trauma: Theory, Research, Practice, and Policy, 8*(5), 609–617. https://doi.org/10.1037/tra0000125

Polanski, P. J., & Hinkle, J. S. (2000). The mental status examination: Its use by professional counselors. *Journal of Counseling & Development, 78*(3), 357–364. https://doi.org/10.1002/j.1556-6676.2000.tb01918.x

Prilleltensky, I., & Gonick, L. (1996). Polities change, oppression remains: On the psychology and politics of oppression. *Political Psychology, 17*(1), 127–148. https://doi.org/10.2307/3791946

Roberson, K., & Carter, R. T. (2022). The relationship between race-based traumatic stress and the Trauma Symptom Checklist: Does racial trauma differ in symptom presentation? *Traumatology, 28*(1), 120–128. https://doi.org/10.1037/trm0000306

Sawyer, B. A. (2019). *Emotion regulation and the experience of racial microaggressions* [Doctoral dissertation, University of Louisville]. https://ir.library.louisville.edu/etd/3189/

Schaffner, A. K., (2021, June 6). Identifying and challenging core beliefs: 12 helpful worksheets. *Positive, Psychology,* https://positivepsychology.com/core-beliefs-worksheets/

Schwitzer, A. M., & Rubin, L. C. (2012). *Diagnosis and treatment planning skills for mental health professionals: A popular culture casebook approach.* Sage Publications, Inc.

Smith, J. R., & Patton, D. U. (2016). Posttraumatic stress symptoms in context: Examining trauma responses to violent exposures and homicide death among Black males in urban neighborhoods. *American Journal of Orthopsychiatry, 86*(2), 212–223. https://doi.org/10.1037/ort0000101

Solis, G. (2021, March 10). For Black parents, 'the talk' binds generations and reflects changes in America. *USC Today.* https://today.usc.edu/the-talk-usc-black-parents-children-racism-america/

Steele, J. M. (2020). A CBT approach to internalized racism among African Americans. *International Journal for the Advancement of Counselling, 42*(3), 217–233. https://doi.org/10.1007/s10447-020-09402-0

Steele, J. M., & Newton, C. S. (2023). *Black lives are beautiful: 50 tools to heal from trauma and promote positive racial identity.* Routledge.

Steele, J. M., & Newton, C. S. (2022). Culturally adapted cognitive behavior therapy as a model to address internalized racism among African American clients. *Journal of Mental Health Counseling, 44*(2), 98–116. https://doi.org/10.17744/mehc.44.2.01

Torres-Harding, S. R., Andrade, A. L., Jr., & Romero Diaz, C. E. (2012). The Racial Microaggressions Scale (RMAS): A new scale to measure experiences of racial microaggressions in people of color. *Cultural Diversity and Ethnic Minority Psychology, 18*(2), 153–164. https://doi.org/10.1037/a0027658

Utsey, S. O. (1999). Development and validation of a short form of the Index of Race-Related Stress (IRRS)–Brief Version. *Measurement and Evaluation in Counseling and Development, 32*(3), 149–167.

van der Kolk, B. A. (2014). *The body keeps the score: Brain, mind, and body in the healing of trauma*. Penguin Random House.

Wald, J., Taylor, S., Asmundson, G. J., Jang, K. L., & Stapleton, J. (2006). *Literature review of concepts: Psychological resiliency* (No. DRDC-CR-2006-073). British Columbia University.

Watson-Singleton, N. N., Black, A. R., & Spivey, B. N. (2019). Recommendations for a culturally-responsive mindfulness-based intervention for African Americans. *Complementary Therapy in Clinical Practice, 34*, 132–138. https://doi.org/10.1016/j.ctcp.2018.11.013

Watts-Jones, D. (2002). Healing internalized racism: The role of a within-group sanctuary among people of African descent. *Family Process, 41*(4), 591–601. https://doi.org/10.1111/j.1545-5300.2002.00591.x

Williams, M. T., Osman, M., Gallo, J., Pereira, D. P., Gran-Ruaz, S., Strauss, D., Lester, L., George, J. R., Edelman, J., & Litman, L. (2022). A clinical scale for the assessment of racial trauma. *Practice Innovations, 7*(3), 223–240. https://doi.org/10.1037/pri0000178

Williams, M. T., Printz, D., Ching, T., & Wetterneck, C. T. (2018a). Assessing PTSD in ethnic and racial minorities: Trauma and racial trauma. *Directions in Psychiatry, 38*(3), 179–196. https://www.monnicawilliams.com/articles/Williams_RacialTrauma PTSD_2018.pdf

Williams, M. T., Printz, D. M. B., & DeLapp, R. C. T. (2018b). Assessing racial trauma with the Trauma Symptoms of Discrimination Scale. *Psychology of Violence, 8*(6), 735–747. https://doi.org/10.1037/vio0000212

Zimmerman, M. A. (1995). Psychological empowerment: Issues and illustrations. *American Journal of Community Psychology, 23*(5), 581–599. https://doi.org/10.1007/BF02506983

Chapter 7

Working with Automatic Thoughts and Underlying Cognitions

Interventions focused on helping clients identify, evaluate, and modify negative thoughts, beliefs, and behaviors are the primary means through which CBT therapists facilitate change and assist clients in achieving their goals (Wenzel, 2019). In CBT, there are three main types of thoughts therapists typically focus on: automatic thoughts, core beliefs, and intermediate beliefs (Greenberger & Padesky, 2015). According to Padesky (2020), different interventions are more ideally suited for working with each type of thought. In Chapter 1, I gave an overview of key CBT interventions. The current chapter illustrates how these interventions may be used to restructure each of the three types of thoughts typically focused on in CBT. First, the case example of Vanessa, a woman experiencing covert discrimination at her place of employment, is presented. Following the presentation of the case of Vanessa, the remainder of the chapter demonstrates how her therapist utilized different CBT interventions to address maladaptive thoughts across the various levels of cognition.

As you read through this chapter, notice how the therapist integrates several of the cultural considerations discussed thus far in this text. In particular, observe the therapist's attempt to adapt the cognitive restructuring process to be responsive to Vanessa's lived experience as a racial being. Recall from Chapter 1 that culturally adapted cognitive restructuring focuses on: (a) validating the painful emotions that arise in the face of these experiences, (b) acknowledging that we live in a society where these painful experiences occur, and (c) challenging negative thoughts about self that occur in response to these experiences rather than the experiences themselves (Graham et al., 2013, p. 104). Additionally, note the therapist's inclusion of strengths and coping practices indigenous to the African American community as she works with Vanessa to develop more adaptive thoughts and behaviors. As discussed in Chapter 3, some of these strengths and sources of coping include the African-centered worldview, positive racial socialization, religion and spirituality, and cultural healing practices. You may use Activity

DOI: 10.4324/9781003196303-7

7.1 to assist you with noting how the therapist in the case of Vanessa integrates culture into the cognitive restructuring process.

Activity 7.1: Working with Vanessa's Automatic Thoughts and Underlying Cognitions

So far, this text has emphasized the importance of several considerations when attempting to help empower African American clients heal from racism. Above, I identified culturally adapted cognitive restructuring and the inclusion of strengths and indigenous coping practices as significant considerations when working with automatic thoughts and underlying cognitions. Other important considerations include intentional broaching of race, ethnicity, and culture (Day-Vines et al., 2007), knowledge of psychological phenomena specific to the African American experience (Steele & Newton, 2022), and culturally sensitive case conceptualization (Steele, 2020). As you read this chapter, notice the therapist's attempts to address each of these considerations throughout her exploration of the case example's presenting concerns. It may be helpful to highlight these portions of the text. As you do, also consider the following questions:

- How did the therapist address culture during therapy with Vanessa?
- What opportunities to explore culture did the therapist miss?
- What other interventions may have been applicable to the case of Vanessa?
- When and how would you implement these interventions?

Case Illustration: Vanessa

Vanessa is a 35-year-old human resource worker at a large warehouse. In her role, Vanessa is often required to take on leadership responsibilities including attending to employee needs, recruiting, staffing, and covering for the human resource manager in the manager's absence. Vanessa describes herself as the person everyone goes to at the warehouse. She is knowledgeable, fair, and relatable. Due to these qualities and her exemplary work record, Vanessa was led to believe she would be promoted to an interim human resource manager during the current manager's maternity leave. Two months prior to intake, Vanessa was scheduled to train for the position but unfortunately, that training never occurred. Instead, and without notification, a temporary human resource employee was brought into the company. Since the new employee's arrival, more time has been devoted to acclimating that employee to the company's human resource procedures than has been given to preparing Vanessa for her promised promotion. Vanessa, who is the only African American in an administrative role at the warehouse, feels angry and frustrated that the time and training opportunities she has continuously requested were made immediately available to the new employee. She believes that overall, the situation at her job is an "uphill battle" and states that she is "tired of putting in double the work for half the reward."

Working with Automatic Thoughts

In Chapter 1, you learned about the cognitive model and its various components. As a reminder, the cognitive model refers to the idea that our reactions—that is, our feelings, behaviors, and physiological responses—are not caused by what happens to us, but by how we think about what happens to us (J. S. Beck, 2020). In the cognitive model, *situations* refer to the contexts that precipitate automatic thoughts. *Automatic thoughts* are the fleeting, unintentional thoughts that occur in any given situation, and *reactions* refer to the emotions, behavioral responses, and physical sensations that occur as a result of our automatic thoughts. An example of the cognitive model drawn from the case of Vanessa at intake is presented in Figure 7.1.

While many clients express their automatic thoughts as phrases like Vanessa's thought "This job is an uphill battle," these thoughts may also occur in the form of mental representations such as images or memories (Greenberger & Padesky, 2015). For example, when discussing her reaction to learning that another human resource employee had been hired in the current manager's absence, Vanessa reported having the memory of being skipped over for a promotion at a previous place of employment and imagined herself going to the warehouse parking lot to cry in her car as she had done at the previous

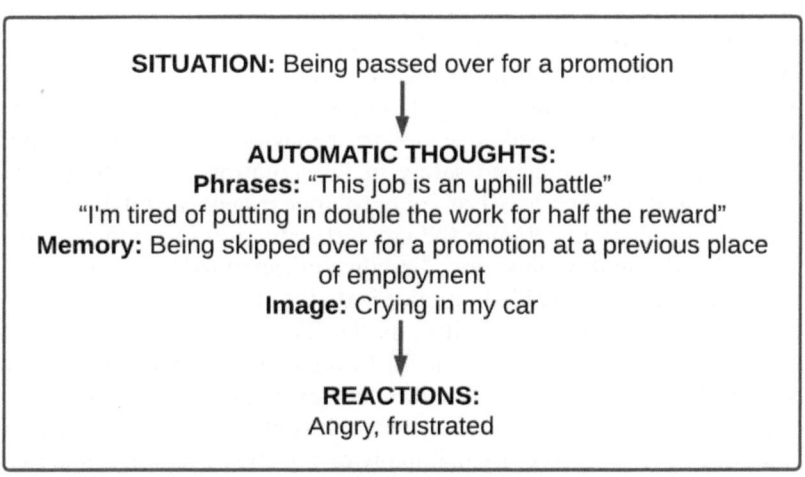

Figure 7.1 Cognitive Model in the Case of Vanessa.

job. Whether automatic thoughts occur as words, images, or memories, a primary feature of these thoughts is their fleeting nature. Automatic thoughts often occur so quickly, clients often do not realize they have even had them. Yet, according to the basic premise of the cognitive model, these thoughts are the primary source of the distressing emotions that lead clients to seek therapy. Accordingly, early sessions in CBT focus on helping clients increase their awareness of these thoughts. Questions such as "What was going through my mind just before I started to feel this way?" "What am I afraid might happen?" and "What images or memories do I have in this situation?" help to facilitate this process (Greenberger & Padesky, 2015).

Occasionally, clients have difficulty identifying their automatic thoughts even when posed with the questions presented above. In these cases, additional techniques can be helpful in eliciting automatic thoughts. According to J. S. Beck (2020), some of these techniques include requesting that the client visualize themselves in the distressing situation, role-playing the situation during therapy, and suggesting thoughts that are opposite to the automatic thoughts you suspect the client actually experienced during the situation. It can also be helpful to provide clients with guided practice before asking them to identify their own automatic thoughts. In Activity 6.2, you engaged in your own guided practice identifying automatic thoughts. I encourage you to go back and review this activity now. There are several benefits to using a similar type of guided practice with clients. First, it serves as a quick assessment of the client's ability to identify an automatic thought and provides an opportunity to offer corrective feedback if necessary. In my own clinical experience, this has been especially important, as I have observed that many clients skip over their automatic thoughts and jump right into problem-solving. For example, when completing Activity 6.2, many of my clients identify a thought such as, "I would ask someone to go with me" in response to the situation of being invited to a party where it is likely you will not know any of the other guests. However, this type of thought typically represents the beginning of a secondary behavioral response designed to address the lack of perceived safety in the situation originating from an automatic thought such as, "I'm going to appear awkward if I show up by myself." In order to experience the greatest reduction in symptoms, clients must deal with the thoughts most directly connected to their moods.

A second benefit to guided practice is that it also affords an opportunity to reeducate clients on the cognitive model. This can be achieved by posing alternative thoughts and asking clients how someone in the situation would feel were they to have those thoughts. For example, referring again to the scenario of being invited to a party where it is likely you will not know any of the other guests in Activity 6.2, many of my clients identify anxious and worried thoughts in response to this situation. To underscore the significance of the cognitive model and the importance being aware of one's automatic thoughts, I ask clients how someone would feel were they to think other thoughts such as, "This will be great, I'll have an opportunity to meet new people" or "No one is going to like me, I'm such a loser." Client responses typically include emotions such as excited and depressed, which allows me to highlight the range of emotions that may be experienced in any given situation and reemphasize the idea that it is not what happens that determines how people feel but how they think about what happens.

According to Padesky (2020), the best interventions for working with automatic thoughts are those that encourage the client to examine the evidence for or against their thoughts. However, as previously stated throughout this text, questioning clients' experiences with race-related concerns can be invalidating and may exacerbate their symptoms. Therefore, when working to address the automatic thoughts of clients who are experiencing racism, therapists should be careful to examine the negative self-appraisals and beliefs about the future that develop in response to these situations rather than the situations themselves. In the sections that follow, I illustrate this process in the case of Vanessa using two interventions commonly implemented to work with automatic thoughts—thought records and Socratic questioning.

Thought Records

A *thought record* is a specific type of journaling activity, typically in chart format, with sections for recording situations, feelings, negative automatic thoughts, and new, more functional thoughts. Use of a thought record helps clients increase insight into the automatic thoughts contributing to their mood and be more active in challenging and replacing these thoughts. During this process, a primary goal is to identify the thoughts that are the most dysfunctional and emotionally charged. Greenberger and Padesky (2015) call these thoughts *hot thoughts*.

One strategy for identifying hot thoughts when using a thought record is by rating the emotion elicited with each thought. Table 7.1 shows a simple thought record completed by Vanessa during one of her early sessions. Upon further discussion of her current work situation, Vanessa identified additional negative automatic thoughts including "Things are never going to change," "If I say something, things will get worse or I may lose my job," "It's always something," and "I have problems wherever I go." Emotions she experienced included hopelessness (80 percent), fearfulness (70 percent), sadness (60 percent), and worthlessness (65 percent). To identify her hot thoughts, the therapist asked Vanessa to provide an emotion and rating for each thought individually. As shown, the most distressing thoughts seem to be based on negative predictions about the future. This is useful information for both the therapist and the client, as it provides an indication of the types

Table 7.1 Vanessa's Thought Record

Situation	Automatic Thoughts	Emotions
Being passed over for a promotion in favor of a less qualified and less experienced temporary employee	"Things are never going to change"	Hopelessness (80%)
	"If I say something, things will get worse or I may lose my job"	Fearfulness (70%)
	"It's always something"	Sadness (60%)
	"I have problems wherever I go"	Worthlessness (65%)

of thoughts that would benefit from additional examination in future sessions. The session excerpt below illustrates how Vanessa's therapist introduced the thought record as a tool to assist in the identification of negative automatic thoughts and hot thoughts.

Therapist: Vanessa, it sounds like you're experiencing racism at your job. Does that sound accurate?

Vanessa: Yes, that's exactly what's going on.

Therapist: And I hear that the racism you've experienced at work has been deeply distressing.

Vanessa: That's right.

Therapist: In previous sessions, we talked about the idea that our emotions are not caused by what happens to us, but by how we think about what happens to us. However, it's important to keep in mind that many of our feelings are reasonable given the situations we face. For example, when people experience racism, it makes sense to feel many different emotions like anger, frustration, fear, and worry. Changing your emotions in this type of situation may not be realistic. However, if your feelings are so intense that they cause you significant pain or impair your ability to go to work, take care of your hygiene, or keep up with your chores, finding alternative ways to focus your thoughts may be helpful. Does this make sense so far?

Vanessa: Yes, it does.

Therapist: A first step in this process is to increase awareness of your automatic thoughts. I'd like to introduce you to a tool designed to help you identify, evaluate, and modify your negative automatic thoughts. It's called a thought record. Would that be okay?

Vanessa: Sure.

Therapist: Great [handing a copy of a thought record to Vanessa]. Thought records are a type of journaling activity that help you to identify negative automatic thoughts and their corresponding emotional, behavioral, or physiological reactions. This, in turn, helps you to be more active in challenging and replacing these thoughts. Over time, this will allow you to feel better and be more empowered. To start, I'd like for us to explore your situation at your job, working with the first three columns of the thought record labeled, *Situation, Automatic Thoughts*, and *Emotions*.

Vanessa: Okay.

Therapist: In your own words, how would you describe the situation taking place at your job right now?

Vanessa: Well, I'd say that I am being passed over for a promotion in favor of a less qualified and less experienced temporary employee.

Therapist: Okay. Could you write that down in the column labeled *Situation*?

Vanessa: Okay [therapist waits while Vanessa writes].

Therapist: Now, let's write down the thoughts you have about this situation in the column labeled *Automatic Thoughts*. Remember, these thoughts might be phrases but they could also be pictures or memories that go through your mind.

Vanessa: I guess I have a lot of thoughts!

Therapist: That's okay, Vanessa. Go ahead and write them down. We'll spend some time deciding which thought we should explore in more depth a little later.

Vanessa: Okay [therapist waits while Vanessa writes].

Therapist: Now, in the third column labeled *Emotions*, I'd like for you to write the specific emotion you feel with each individual thought. This is important because our emotions provide clues to our thinking. Emotions you're experiencing that aren't captured by any of the thoughts you've written down so far lets us know that there are still some additional automatic thoughts connected to this situation.

Vanessa: Okay [therapist waits while Vanessa writes].

Therapist: Is anything missing?

Vanessa: Well, I guess I am embarrassed too.

Therapist: Okay. It doesn't look like any of the thoughts you've identified so far would typically result in a person feeling embarrassed. If you visualize yourself in the moment when you first realized another HR employee had been hired, what thought comes to your mind?

Vanessa: I remember thinking that I was foolish for believing that they would really give me a promotion.

Therapist: Okay, that makes sense, Vanessa. Go ahead and write that thought down too.

Vanessa: Got it [therapist waits while Vanessa writes].
Therapist: Now, as we're beginning to work with your thoughts, dealing with the ones that are the most emotionally charged can help you to experience the greatest amount of relief. The thoughts that are the most emotionally charged are called hot thoughts. One way to identify your hot thoughts is by rating the intensity of the emotion you feel with each thought on a scale from 0 percent to 100 percent. Does this make sense?
Vanessa: Yes.
Therapist: Good. Please go ahead and write down how intensely you felt each emotion you've identified.
Vanessa: Okay [therapist waits while Vanessa writes].

As shown in the initial introduction to the thought record presented above, the therapist demonstrated several of the cultural considerations identified at the beginning of this chapter. First, the therapist was intentional in broaching some of the inter-racial dynamics (Day-Vines et al., 2007) of the case by labeling Vanessa's experience at her place of employment as racism (e.g., "Vanessa, it sounds like you're experiencing racism at your job. Does that sound accurate?"). This is significant given research which suggests that therapists who do not address race and culture during therapy may come across as authoritarian, poor listeners, or untrustworthy, causing clients to feel unsafe and, therefore, weakening the therapeutic alliance (Duncan et al., 2010; Owen et al., 2018). Second, the therapist was also careful to make appropriate adaptations to the cognitive restructuring process by validating (Graham et al., 2013) the painful emotions people have in the face of their encounters with racism (e.g., "...when people experience racism, it makes sense to feel many different emotions like anger, frustration, fear, and worry"). As discussed in Chapter 5, because of the subtle and covert nature of some forms of racism, people of color are often required to prove their experiences with racial discrimination, which can worsen their distress. By validating rather than minimizing or ignoring emotions that occur as a result of experiences with racism (Mai & Whitlock, 2022; Pierson et al., 2022), the therapist in the case of Vanessa was able to convey caring and contribute to the sense of safety experienced in the therapeutic dyad (Day-Vines et al., 2021). The therapist's validation may have also been experienced as cathartic by Vanessa, providing some relief through empathic connection (Day-Vines et al., 2007, 2020; Steele & Newton, 2022).

Now that Vanessa has identified her negative automatic thoughts and their corresponding emotions, a next step would be to complete her thought record by developing more adaptive and functional thoughts to replace her current thinking. This process, however, can be complicated for a number of reasons. First, as illustrated in the case of Vanessa, clients often have more thoughts than can be reasonably addressed in a limited amount of time (Waltman et al., 2021). Second, not all of a client's thoughts are central to their distress. Spending time working with thoughts that are not related to their core difficulties may actually worsen a client's mood, diminish their hope, and decrease their satisfaction with therapy. Third, some clients may have a poor ability to disconfirm their thinking due to limited information or errors in information processing. For example, growing up within the societal context of racism may have led to the development of maladaptive assumptions that heightened Vanessa's sense of powerlessness, which could cause her to act in ways that reinforce racism and maintain the status quo (Steele & Newton, 2022). Finally, some clients may mistakenly understand the goal of cognitive restructuring as developing alternative thoughts that are purely positive rather than thoughts that are believable and authentic to clients' lived experiences (Waltman et al., 2021). This may lessen the effectiveness of the thought record and similarly decrease the client's satisfaction with therapy.

Socratic questioning is an intervention that may assist clients and therapists with the aforementioned difficulties in developing alternative thoughts. It also serves as a way to uncover the more central ideas underlying the client's automatic thoughts, thereby providing a segue into later exploration of core beliefs. The section that follows describes a recently developed Socratic questioning framework (Waltman et al., 2021) and illustrates how this framework was used to assist Vanessa and her therapist with identifying a cognitive target, evaluating assumptions, and replacing the negative thought.

Socratic Questioning

As stated in Chapter 1, *Socratic questioning* refers to the successive use of open-ended questions to help clients monitor their thoughts and emotions, evaluate their thinking, and respond to situations that occur in life in an adaptive way (Matu, 2018). Within the literature, various typologies describe the different types of open-ended questions that may be used to facilitate Socratic dialogue in the therapeutic context (e.g., Paul & Elder, 2006; Wright et al., 2006). Overholser's (1993) synthesis of the literature, for example, resulted in a taxonomy of seven question formats, which include memory, translation, interpretation, application, analysis, synthesis, and evaluation questions. These question formats ask clients to recall information, identify meaning, articulate relationships among ideas or events, apply information to problems, break problems down into smaller parts and examine evidence, synthesize disparate information into a unified whole, and make judgments according to specific standards. More recently, Resick et al. (2016) identified a simpler four-part typology of Socratic questioning, which includes questions to clarify meaning, challenge assumptions, evaluate objective evidence, and challenge underlying core beliefs. According to Resick et al. (2016), these question formats allow the therapist to inquire about content, context, or meaning; examine beliefs about self, others, or the world; deconstruct conclusions; and help clients evaluate central beliefs about themselves that may have a negative impact on their ability to develop more adaptive ways of thinking.

Somewhat differently, J. S. Beck (2020) proposed a series of Socratic questioning strategies that include examining the evidence, devising alternative explanations, decatastrophizing and problem-solving, examining the utility, and gaining distance. These strategies involve looking for evidence for and against the thought, developing alternative explanations based on the evidence, identifying the worst that could happen in the situation and what could be done then, examining the functionality of keeping the thought versus changing the thought, and gaining distance by thinking about how one might advise a friend in a similar situation. Like other aspects of CBT, these strategies were created to help clients become their own therapists, and as such, may be implemented verbally or in worksheet format using J. S. Beck's (2020) "Testing Your Thoughts" worksheet.

While the question formats and strategies identified by researchers such as Overholser (1993), Resick et al. (2016), and J. S. Beck (2020) provide therapists with guidance on the types of questions that may encourage clients to reflect on their experiences, they offer less direction on how therapists may structure their use of these questions and strategies to examine thoughts, develop new viewpoints, and solve problems. To address this issue, Padesky (1993) developed a four-step model that has become one of the most well-known frameworks of Socratic questioning. The steps of this model include: (1) asking informational questions, (2) active listening, (3) summarizing, and (4) asking synthesizing or analytical questions. An in-depth discussion of this model illustrated can be explored in the text, *Dialogues for Discovery: Improving Psychotherapy's Effectiveness* (Padesky & Kennerley, 2023). Elsewhere, Waltman et al. (2021) developed a model based on their research concerning how expert CBT therapists conduct Socratic questioning and that be summarized across the following steps: (1) focusing on key content, (2) phenomenological understanding, (3) collaborative curiosity, and (4) summary and synthesis. A brief overview of each stage of Waltman et al.'s (2021) model along with an illustration of how the model was used in the case of Vanessa is presented in the paragraphs that follow.

Focusing on Key Content

According to Waltman et al. (2021), the first step of Socratic questioning involves helping clients focus on key content. As illustrated in the case of Vanessa, clients may have a number of thoughts associated with their presenting problems. Identifying the thoughts that are most relevant to their issue, that is, their hot thoughts, allows the therapist to plan their treatment approach and improve clinical outcomes more optimally. Earlier, I described Greenberger and Padesky's (2015) strategy for identifying hot thoughts, which consists of rating the emotion elicited with each thought on a scale of 0 percent to 100 percent. Finding a hot thought with Socratic questioning can be accomplished through a similar process of asking clients clarifying questions to determine the most upsetting elements of their story, questions such as "What was the most upsetting part?" or "Which is the most upsetting thought?"

Once the client and therapist have identified a key cognition, a second task at the focusing stage is creating a shared definition of the cognitive target. This works best if the hot thought is broken down to reflect its emotional meaning as well as its connection to the client's core beliefs or conditional assumptions. In this way, this aspect of the model takes working with automatic thoughts one step further through a burgeoning exploration of deeper underlying cognitions. One way to determine these connections is by using a strategy such as the downward arrow technique (Waltman et al., 2021). After these connections are articulated, the client and therapist can then collaboratively define the negative self-appraisals within the client's cognition to have a clearer understanding of what is being evaluated. The excerpt below provides a brief example of how a therapist may use this first step of Socratic questioning to help Vanessa further clarify and articulate her target thoughts.

Therapist: So, Vanessa, I see that you've rated several of your thoughts pretty high.

Vanessa: Yes, I have so much stress with this situation!

Therapist: I get that. As you look at what you've written down, what would you say is the most distressing thought?

Vanessa: I think it's the thought, "I'm tired of putting in double the work for half the reward."

Therapist: Vanessa, I may not know what it is like to be mistreated because of the color of my skin but I want you to know that I believe that what you're saying and that it hurts. From what I understand, this idea of working twice as hard as others, particularly one's White counterparts, is a common experience for many African Americans. Is that correct?

Vanessa: Yes.

Therapist: Okay, and could you help me understand more about this experience by telling me what's the worst part of being in a situation where you must work twice as hard?

Vanessa: It's the fact that I never know if what I'm doing is good enough.

Therapist: And what does it mean if what you're doing is not good enough?
Vanessa: I guess in a way it means that I'm not good enough.
Therapist: And when you say, "I'm not good enough," what does that mean?
Vanessa: I'll never be White. It's not like I want to be White, but I'll never be acceptable in their eyes. And I know I shouldn't feel this way, but it makes me feel embarrassed sometimes because even though I know my value, I know they're looking down on me.
Therapist: Thank you for sharing that, Vanessa, I know it's not always easy to admit that kind of painful emotion.
Vanessa: Mm hmm.

In this excerpt from the focusing step of Socratic questioning (Waltman et al., 2021), the therapist was able to collaborate with Vanessa to identify her hot thought by asking the question, "As you look at what you've written down, what would you say is the most distressing thought?" In response to Vanessa's answer, "I'm tired of putting in double the work for half the reward," the therapist offered a validating statement integrated with knowledge of the psychological effects of "working twice as hard." Subsequent use of the downward arrow technique allowed the client and therapist to then gain a better understanding of the central belief influencing Vanessa's automatic thought; that is, "I'm not good enough."

Upon discovering the underlying cognition "I'm not good enough," the therapist continued with the second element of focusing on key content, which is creating a shared definition. In this situation, Vanessa defined not being good enough as not being able to meet White standards and cultural norms. This explanation is significant as it clarified that, rather than experiencing a sense of personal inadequacy, Vanessa may feel helpless to overcome or challenge racist workplace practices. This distinction would ultimately allow for more accurate cognitive conceptualization and treatment planning.

Phenomenological Understanding

After identifying the specific cognitions to target, the next step in Waltman et al.'s (2021) approach to Socratic questioning is increasing phenomenological understanding of the cognition. This includes gaining an understanding of the experiences the client's beliefs are based on, as well as the emotional processing of those beliefs. In the case of Vanessa, the therapist has some insight into experiences that may have contributed to Vanessa's belief "I'm not good enough" (i.e., "I'll never be White") through data obtained on the thought record, such as Vanessa's experience of being passed over for a promotion at her prior place of employment. Yet, there may be many other experiences that have also contributed to Vanessa's belief. For example, Vanessa may have had childhood or early life experiences that highlighted the disparities that exist in the United States due to racial discrimination, or she may have received societal messages that led to negative schemas surrounding race (Steele & Newton, 2022). Accordingly, Socratic questioning at this step should focus on questions that provide insight into the client's subjective and objective reality. Examples of these questions include, "How long have you had these thoughts?" "What experiences are these thoughts based on?" "What is it like to believe this thought?" "When do you believe this thought more or less?" and "What do you do when these thoughts come up?" (Waltman et al., 2021). Questions that explore evidence for and against the client's thoughts may also be beneficial at this step; however, the therapist should exercise caution, being careful to explore evidence concerning negative self-appraisals rather than whether the situation may be attributed to racism. For example, in the case of Vanessa, although her belief "I'm not good enough" may appear to be a negative self-appraisal, based on her definition, "I'll never be White," a question such as "What makes you think this thought is true or not completely true?" would be inappropriate as it could be interpreted as a challenge to Vanessa's interpretation of racism in her environment or a lack of cultural sensitivity on the therapist's part.

Another important element at the phenomenological understanding stage of Socratic questioning is validation. According to Waltman et al. (2021), the in-depth exploration of the client's inner world that occurs at this step of Socratic questioning creates a unique opportunity to communicate to the client that you hear them and understand what they are saying. In Chapter 5, I discussed Linehan's (1997), six techniques for communicating validation to clients, which included: (1) active listening and observing, (2) accurate reflection of the client's thoughts and feelings, (3) articulation of unverbalized emotions and meanings, (4) expressing that behavior is understandable given prior events, (5) expressing that behavior is understandable given current events, and (6) believing and responding to the client as if they are capable of achieving change and their long-term goals. By using these techniques, the therapist can affirm the client and create the sense of safety needed for disclosure of racial content and processing of its meaning. The excerpt below illustrates how the therapist approached phenomenological understanding in the case of Vanessa.

Therapist: So, what I hear you saying is that you must work twice as hard as everyone else at work, but that only gets you half as far. And this situation seems insurmountable because you'll never be White, is that correct?

Vanessa: Yes.

Therapist: Vanessa, I really want to understand what that experience is like for you. Can we spend some time looking at that?

Vanessa: Sure.

Therapist: When did you first become of aware of this?

Vanessa: I think I first noticed differences in middle school. It seemed like the White students got all the opportunities and Black students were treated like second class citizens. For example, a bunch of my friends and I tried out for the cheerleading team one year. *None* of us made it.

Therapist: Wow, Vanessa. What did that experience say to you at the time?

Vanessa: I guess it said the same thing my current work situation says— that we aren't good enough. You know, we didn't fit the image of cute little cheerleaders with long blonde ponytails and lots of enthusiasm. I think even back then we were up against the stereotype of an angry Black woman.

Therapist: So, you've been dealing with the weight of thinking about how White people perceive Black people for a long time. I imagine that over the course of your life, this has come to feel like such a burden.

Vanessa: It really has. I think exhausting is the word I would use.

Therapist: Are there any other experiences you've had that contribute to this exhaustion and pressure that comes from not being White?

Vanessa: Well, I've already told you about being passed over for a promotion at my previous job for the same reason. Really, it's kind of just an everyday thing, you know. I can't even talk like myself when I'm around White people because it might make them feel uncomfortable or I might not fit in.

Therapist: Thank you for sharing that, Vanessa. Again, I hear you've had many experiences to reinforce this idea that not being White is a hurdle you must overcome. Has anyone ever said anything like this to you directly?

Vanessa: Well, my parents were actually pretty vocal about this part of the Black experience while I was growing up and they always told me that you have to work twice as hard as White people to get ahead in life.

Therapist: I see. So, it sounds like your parents did their best to prepare you for this bias you would experience as an adult but living through it is still difficult, nonetheless.

Vanessa: That's right.

Therapist: What else can you tell me about what it has been like emotionally to face these challenges?

Vanessa: Like I said, it's just exhausting. You work and work for very little reward and there's nothing you can do about it.

In this step of Socratic questioning, Vanessa's therapist investigated aspects of the client's inner world by exploring how long the client has believed this thought ("When did you first become of aware of this?"), examining the experiences her thought is based on ("Are there any other experiences you've had that contribute to this exhaustion and pressure that comes from not being White?"), exploring direct messages she has received about this issue ("Has anyone ever said anything like this to you directly?"), and attempting to understand what it is like to believe this thought ("What else can you tell me about what it has been like emotionally to face these challenges?"). Again, the therapist is observed doing so in a manner that is culturally nuanced. First, while attempting to gain a phenomenological understanding of the client's belief, the therapist continues the practice of validation through accurate reflection of the client's thoughts and feelings (e.g., "So, what I hear you saying is that you must work twice as hard as everyone else at work, but that only gets you half as far. And this situation seems insurmountable because you'll never be White, is that correct?"), active listening and observing (e.g., "Wow, Vanessa"), and articulation of unverbalized emotions and meanings (e.g., "…this has come to feel like such a burden"). The therapist additionally continues to integrate her knowledge of psychological phenomena relevant to the Black experience into her questions, for example, framing the idea of working twice as hard as the psychological weight of thinking about how White people perceive Black people (Palmer & Walker, 2020) and acknowledging the racial socialization practice of preparing children for bias (Okeke-Adeyanju et al., 2014). Questions about direct evidence to support or refute the belief were excluded as they may have invalidated Vanessa's experience. Therapists should keep in mind, however, that in some cases exploring evidence may be crucial to developing alternative thoughts as skipping discussion of evidence the client believes is true may cause the client difficulty in believing the new thoughts (Waltman et al., 2021).

Collaborative Curiosity

The third step in Waltman et al.'s (2021) model of Socratic questioning is collaborative curiosity. Traditionally, this may be framed as the disconfirming the evidence step of Socratic dialogue; however, as previously stated throughout this chapter and text, this should be approached with caution given the potential to invalidate the client's experience by being perceived as asking the client to prove their experience with racism. A more culturally sensitive framing of this step may be to conceptualize it as an attempt to add context in order to devise more adaptive thoughts or solutions. Accordingly, questions at this step may explore what the client is missing; that is, what the client may not see or what the client may not know due to a lack of knowledge or experience. Examples of questions that may facilitate this exploration include, "What context can we add to this belief?" "What are the consequences of having this belief?" "How does believing this thought make you feel?" "What does this belief make you do?" and "Are there any skills or problem-solving strategies that challenge this belief?" There are also a number of strategies therapists may use at this stage of Socratic questioning such as the loose thread strategy and untwisting the evidence; however, exploration of these strategies is beyond the scope of this chapter. For a fuller discussion, the reader is referred to Waltman et al. (2021). In the brief excerpt that follows, the therapist demonstrates how collaborative curiosity was approached in the case of Vanessa.

Therapist: Vanessa, what I hear you saying is the significant meaning of what you've discussed so far today is that there's nothing you can do to overcome the bias you face as an African American, is that correct?

Vanessa: Basically, yes.

Therapist: And this is based on the many experiences you've had throughout your life, as well as the messages you received from your parents while growing up, is that also correct?

Vanessa: Yes.

Therapist: Vanessa, I hear how overwhelming and exhausting this has been for you. If you recall, earlier we talked about the fact that many of our thoughts and feelings are reasonable given the situations we face. In these situations, it can be helpful to challenge your thinking to be more adaptive and empowering. Could we take some time to do this?

Vanessa: Okay.

Therapist: Good. Let's spend some time looking at what you've just said about there being nothing you can do to overcome the bias you face as an African American since this is where a lot of the meaning and emotion in this situation comes from. I think it may be helpful to first look at how this thought has been functioning in your life. How do you feel when you have this thought?

Vanessa: I feel helpless.

Therapist: I see. And what do you do when you have this thought?

Vanessa: I guess I don't do anything. I just keep working and hoping that things might be fair this time, but they never are.

Therapist: Okay. So, what I hear you saying is that having the thought "there's nothing I can do about it" leads you to feel helpless and you get caught up in a cycle of working hard but not experiencing any change in the bias you encounter in your work environment, is that accurate?

Vanessa: Yes.

Therapist: I can understand how this has been overwhelming. Vanessa, you may not know how you can think about this situation differently right now, but if there was a more adaptive way of thinking, what would be the benefit of having a more functional thought to focus on?

Vanessa: Well, maybe I wouldn't feel so bad.

Therapist: And what would happen if your thoughts stayed the same?

Vanessa: I guess everything else would stay the same and I would continue to feel bad.

Therapist: Okay, so do you think it's worth continuing to look at other ways of viewing this situation?

Vanessa: Definitely.

Therapist: Great. Let's continue our exploration and look at if there's any missing information that might change your perspective on this situation. Earlier we discovered that working twice as hard was one way your parents prepared you to deal with the racial bias you might encounter throughout life. What other ways of addressing bias do you know of?

Vanessa: Besides protesting or quitting my job, I don't really know of any.

Therapist: And how do those two options sound to you?

Vanessa: Not very realistic. I mean, I've got to work to live.

Therapist: I understand that. Like most of us, you have the reality of needing a job to put food on the table and pay bills.

Vanessa: Exactly.

Therapist: So, any strategies you'd be willing to implement would have to allow you to address bias while minimizing risk to your job, but you don't know of any, is that correct?

Vanessa: Yes.

Therapist: Okay. It seems what we are discovering is that one challenge in this situation is a lack of information on how to address bias. What does this discovery mean to you?

Vanessa: It means that maybe I need to learn more about how to deal with racism!

Therapist: Along those lines, some people might more specifically describe the experience you are having at work as a microaggression. Are you familiar with this term?

Vanessa: No, I'm not.

Therapist: Well, microaggressions refer to subtle acts or messages that reflect prejudice or discrimination (Sue et al., 2019b). One obvious way microaggressions are expressed is by what people say to each other; however, another common way microaggressions are delivered is through an organization's physical environment. For example, the fact that you are the only African American in

	administration at your job and that you keep getting passed over for promotions could be considered a microaggression because it communicates the message that Black people don't belong in leadership roles.

Vanessa: That's right. It's like they're okay with us doing the work but not having the titles.

Therapist: Actually, there are strategies for confronting, disarming, or counteracting the effects of microaggressions in one's environment. These strategies are called *microinterventions*. In my work with clients, I've found that learning and trying out different types of microinterventions helps to provide a greater sense of self-determination and empowerment in these situations. What I'm noticing in your case is that we're challenging this thought that there's nothing you can do about the fact that you're not White and as a result experience racism; however, you haven't had much opportunity to test this belief out because you weren't really aware of any strategies you could use to address bias or microaggressions at work. I am wondering how does knowing this influence how strongly you believe this idea "there's nothing I can do?"

Vanessa: I guess it changes things a bit…

Although brief, the excerpt above illustrates the way in which the collaborative curiosity phase may take up the bulk of Socratic questioning. In the case of Vanessa, the therapist began by restating the client's thoughts and the reasons she believes them. This allowed the therapist to ensure she had a good understanding of the client's perceptions and the client's subjective experience of these perceptions (Waltman et al., 2021). From there, the therapist utilized questions that would allow Vanessa to examine the utility of her current thinking (e.g., "How do you feel when you have this thought?" "And what do you do when you have this thought?" "What would be the benefit of having a more functional thought to focus on?"). Realizing that she could benefit from changing her thinking may have increased her openness and motivation to do so.

After examining the utility of Vanessa's thinking, the therapist focused on obtaining missing information that may broaden Vanessa's perspective on options in her work situation. This was initiated with the question "What other ways of addressing bias do you know of?" and expounded upon through enhanced psychoeducation on microaggressions and microinterventions (Sue et al., 2019a, 2021). As discussed in Chapter 1, enhanced psychoeducation situates clients' concerns within their broader social context, normalizing clients' experiences and providing insight needed for more effective problem solving (Graham et al., 2013). The enhanced psychoeducation in Vanessa's case had several benefits, including providing a direct connection to Vanessa's experience with bias in her work environment and increasing hope that there may be alternatives.

Summary and Synthesis

Finally, the last step of Waltman et al.'s (2021) model of Socratic questioning involves summary and synthesis of the information obtained through the previous steps of the model. The primary goal here is to make new learning explicit in order to develop alternative thoughts that are more balanced. This process includes summarizing what was discussed, stating an alternative thought, indicating a level of belief in the alternative thought, and identifying appropriate behavioral change. Questions that might facilitate this process at this stage include, "How would you summarize what we've talked about today?" "How does everything fit together?" "Based on your summary, what's another way of viewing this situation?" "How much do you believe this to be true?" and "What should you do now?" (Waltman et al., 2021). In the concluding excerpt of Socratic questioning in the case of Vanessa that follows, the therapist demonstrates how summary and synthesis was utilized to assist Vanessa in developing a new thought based on the evaluation of her current belief.

Therapist: Vanessa, I hear you saying your view there's nothing you can do about your work situation is starting to change a bit. Could you summarize what we've talked about today that's leading you to this conclusion?

Vanessa: Well, I realize that I haven't tried very many things to address the issue at work. I keep working hard hoping things will change but they haven't. I have past experiences plus the messages that I've received from my parents that influence me to believe that there's really nothing I can do about this kind of thing.

Therapist: Anything else?

Vanessa: Based on what you said about microaggressions and microinterventions, there may be a different approach I could take that I haven't tried yet.

Therapist: That's right, Vanessa. What else?

Vanessa: I'm not sure.

Therapist: Well, we also talked about how maybe you wouldn't feel so bad if you were able to redirect your thoughts in this situation and how you might even you feel more empowered.

Vanessa: That's right!

Therapist: Okay, so, given everything we've said, what's another way to focus your thoughts?

Vanessa: I think another way to focus my thoughts about this is that this situation is a common experience for many people of color, it's not me. I might feel like there's nothing I can do right now, but I can learn strategies that may help me point out these issues to my colleagues. Speaking out can help me feel better even if things don't change.

Therapist: So, how much do you believe this alternative thought to be true?

Vanessa: Well, I kind of believe it.

Therapist: Which parts?

Vanessa: I believe there are things I can learn that are supposed to help, I'm just not sure that I'll really feel better.

Therapist: You're right, Vanessa, we can't predict what will happen in the future, but what did you say would happen if you didn't change your approach to this situation?

Vanessa: I said everything would stay the same and I would continue to feel bad.

Therapist: So, could you adjust your alternative thought to include more of the benefits of speaking out as well as the risks of not speaking out so that the idea of feeling better seems more believable to you?

Vanessa: Yeah, I guess I would add that more specifically, speaking out could help me feel better even if things don't change because at least I would be standing up for myself. If I don't say anything, I'll continue to feel helpless.

Therapist: How believable does this sound?

Vanessa: A lot more believable.

Therapist: On a scale from 0 percent to 100 percent?

Vanessa: I'd say about 90 percent.

Therapist: Great! Based on this thought, what steps should you take between now and our next session?

Vanessa: I should learn more about microinterventions and remind myself of my new way of thinking when I start to feel discouraged at work.

Therapist: I think that's a great idea, Vanessa. At our next session, we could even roleplay some of the interventions to increase your comfort with using them at work.

Vanessa: Sounds good.

In this final aspect of Socratic questioning, the therapist demonstrates how one might approach helping Vanessa to make sense of what was learned throughout the discovery process. The therapist began by asking Vanessa to summarize how the information discussed throughout the process fits together to form a new conclusion. This included an initial statement of Vanessa's alternative thought, "This situation is a common experience for many people of color, it's not me. I might feel like there's nothing I can do right now, but I can learn strategies that may help me point out these issues to my colleagues. Speaking out can help me feel better even if things don't change," as well as a test of the believability of the alternative thought with the question, "So, how much do you believe this alternative thought to be true?" Based on Vanessa's response to the question of believability, the therapist was able to guide Vanessa in developing an alternative thought that would be even more effective by once again drawing in data from Vanessa's ideas about the utility of her thinking ("...what did you say would happen if you didn't change your approach to this situation?").

After developing an alternative thought, the therapist assisted Vanessa in identifying goal directed behavior to focus on, which consisted of reading a book on addressing microaggressions and roleplaying her ideas with her therapist at their next session. This offers the benefit of reducing cognitive fusion and experiential avoidance (Harris, 2019). It is also consistent with African-centered values such as *kujichagulia* (self-determination) and *imani* (faith). Other veins of exploration the therapist may have considered at this step of Socratic questioning include reconciling the new thought against the target cognition or core belief, exploring what was learned about the process of Socratic questioning, and incorporating imagery into the process using visualization or guided imagery techniques (Waltman et al., 2021).

Summary of Automatic Thoughts

To summarize, *automatic thoughts* refer to the negative, unintentional thoughts that occur during various situations in life (Matu, 2018). These thoughts may occur as words, images, or memories. During therapy, the goal is to identify the thoughts that are the most dysfunctional and emotionally charged. These thoughts are known as hot thoughts. Delineating hot thoughts from other less distressing automatic thoughts can be beneficial, as focusing on hot thoughts provides clients with the greatest psychological benefit. Working with automatic thoughts typically begins by asking clients to identify the situations and thoughts that contribute to their emotions, and then to rate the intensity of those emotions. This can be facilitated using tools such as thought records or Socratic questioning. When clients struggle to identify their negative automatic thoughts, there are several techniques therapists can employ including requesting that the client visualize themselves in the distressing situation, roleplaying the situation during therapy, and suggesting thoughts that are opposite to the automatic thoughts you suspect the client actually experienced during the situation (J. S. Beck, 2020).

Working With Core Beliefs

In CBT case formulation, core beliefs are considered the lens through which individuals process information received from their environment, and as such, serve as the basis of cognition that underlies automatic thoughts and leads to errors in thinking (Greenberger & Padesky, 2015). Recall from Chapter 1 that *core beliefs* are defined as an individual's most central ideas about themselves, other people, or the world (J. S. Beck, 2020). These beliefs may be negative or positive, and typically develop in response to early childhood experiences and societal messages about one's various social identities (Steele, 2020). In Chapter 6, I discussed core beliefs commonly associated with internalized racism, which is one psychological manifestation of racial oppression (Steele & Newton, 2022). As mentioned, these core beliefs highlight themes around inferiority, inadequacy, personal blame, powerlessness, and belief in a just world, and are often associated with avoidance or numbing coping strategies to compensate for the perceived deficits reflected in each core belief. Working with these beliefs typically involves culturally adapted use of traditional CBT interventions to help clients lessen the internalization of negative race-based messages (Williams et al., 2022). When integrating liberation and empowerment perspectives, this process should also include interventions designed to enhance resilience, encourage indigenous coping, foster critical consciousness, and encourage activism (Turner et al., 2022).

There are many ways to identify a client's core beliefs. The downward arrow technique presented earlier is one strategy therapists can use to identify a core belief when they suspect an automatic thought may reflect some deeper underlying meaning, but they do not have enough data to sufficiently hypothesize what the core belief may be. When therapists have noticed themes and patterns in a client's automatic thoughts over time and believe they do have sufficient data to suggest certain core beliefs may be contributing to the client's thoughts, the therapist can tentatively pose the core belief to the client, asking them to verify the accuracy of the therapist's hypothesis (J. S. Beck, 2020). Another similar strategy for identifying core beliefs would be to review a number of related automatic thoughts with clients and ask them to draw their own conclusions about what core beliefs may be present (J. S. Beck, 2020).

Once clients begin to become aware of their core beliefs, modification of these beliefs requires clients to have an understanding that their beliefs reflect subjective perceptions of themselves, others, or the world rather than immutable, unchangeable facts. This understanding can be facilitated through psychoeducation that emphasizes this and other important ideas about the nature of core beliefs such as the relationship between core beliefs and early childhood experiences and how over time, core beliefs can be changed so that clients come to view things in more adaptive and functional ways (J. S. Beck, 2020). As clients develop the understanding that core beliefs can be restructured to be more positive and functional, the process of modifying these beliefs typically begins by helping clients examine evidence that contradicts the old core belief and supports a new core belief using worksheets, continuums, credit lists, positive data logs, and historical tests of core beliefs (J. S. Beck, 2020; Padesky, 1994). According to J. S. Beck (2020), this evidence may include data that contradicts the old core belief, as well as data that seems to support the old core belief with a reframe. Table 7.2 presents data Vanessa used to challenge the negative core belief "I'm not good

Table 7.2 Core Beliefs Worksheet

Old core belief:	I'm not good enough.	
Current strength of the old core belief (0% to 100%):	60%	
New core belief:	I am good enough. The racism I experience as an African American is an obstacle but does not determine my value or ability to succeed.	
Current strength of the new core belief (0% to 100%):	50%	
Social Context Influencing the Old Belief	**Evidence that Supports the Old Belief with a Reframe**	**Evidence that Suggests the Old Core Belief is Not 100% True or Supports the New Belief**
Believing that I must conform to White cultural standards perpetuates White supremacy and limits my ability to be my best self. Even when I am aware of my worth, engaging in avoidance, conformity, or overperformance also reinforces dominant societal beliefs and causes me to internalize racism.	I may not always be recognized for my work, however, the trust and responsibility I am afforded prove I am a competent and valuable employee.	I am learning new strategies to address the microaggressions and discrimination I experience at work. I am being consistent with going to therapy and practicing the strategies I am learning. There are many recent examples of other Black women who have experienced racial discrimination in the workplace and been able to enact change.

enough," which was identified in the Socratic questioning excerpts presented above. To facilitate this process, the therapist asked Vanessa the following questions:

- What do your thoughts say about what you may believe about yourself, others, or the world?
- What societal messages may be influencing your negative view of yourself, others, or the world?
- How might your perceptions of your deficits change if they are placed in their social context?
- How might any internalization of racism and negative stereotypes about Black people be challenged when considered within the broader context of White supremacy and systemic oppression?
- How might your aspirations or beliefs about the future change when considered within the context of liberation and empowerment?

As shown in Table 7.2, Vanessa's old core belief was "I'm not good enough," while her new core belief was, "I am good enough. The racism I experience as an African American is an obstacle but does not determine my value or ability to succeed." With the old and new core beliefs in mind, Vanessa, with the assistance of her therapist, began to be intentional in looking for evidence to invalidate her old core belief and strengthen the new core belief. Table 7.2 shows examples of the initial evidence Vanessa collected to challenge her old core belief and support her new core belief during the week of her sixth counseling session. In the table, you will notice Vanessa's old and new core beliefs are written down, along with ratings of how much she accepted as true each belief at the time on a scale of 0 percent to 100 percent. Rating each belief on a weekly basis in this way allowed the therapist and Vanessa to monitor progress toward modifying her belief. You can see that when the table was completed, the strength of Vanessa's new core belief was increasing considerably, as she had collected several pieces of evidence to refute her old core belief and support the new core belief. First, Vanessa completed the enhanced psychoeducation on microaggressions and microinterventions (Sue et al., 2019a), which validated her experience at her place of employment, provided a framework to conceptualize her problems, and offered realistic and tangible strategies to address her issues. With these benefits, Vanessa began to feel more confident that there were steps she could take, and perhaps her future would not be overwhelmingly determined by the impacts of racism. Vanessa also reframed her interpretation of her problems at work, shifting her focus from the lack of acceptance she experiences because she is not White to a focus on her proven value and competence as an employee. In this way, Vanessa practiced cognitive defusion, which would increase her confidence in engaging in goal-driven behavior and lead to a sense of empowerment regardless of the outcomes of her actions (Williams et al., 2022).

According to J. S. Beck (2020), the quickest way to help clients feel and behave more adaptively is to work toward direct modification of their core beliefs as soon as possible. Yet, the decision to work with negative core beliefs should be made in consideration of the client's diagnosis and their cognitive conceptualization. According to Padesky (1994), negative core beliefs are most amenable to change when clients also have positive core beliefs that they believe about themselves when their negative core beliefs are not activated. People who do not have positive core beliefs when they are in a good state of mental health, or those who have chronic, severe depression may actually worsen when dealing with negative core beliefs. In these cases, it is typically more advisable to identify a new, more adaptive core belief and focus on shifting it little by little over time.

Summary of Core Beliefs

To summarize, core beliefs refer to central ideas about oneself, others, and the world (J. S. Beck, 2020). They may be negative or positive, and typically develop in response to early childhood experiences and societal messages about one's various social group identities (Steele, 2020). Core beliefs are significant because they serve as the underlying cognitions that lead to negative automatic thoughts and errors in thinking in daily situations. During therapy, the core beliefs that are of most interest to therapists initially are those that are negative in nature, as these beliefs shape how clients process information they receive from the environment and the negative automatic thoughts they develop. When working with core beliefs, however, therapists should seek to understand the client's alternatives to their negative core beliefs, as strengthening positive core beliefs is one of the most effective and affirming ways to help clients challenge negative views of themselves, others, and the world (J. S. Beck, 2020). When working with African American clients who are experiencing the effects of racism, this should include a focus on enhancing resilience, encouraging indigenous coping, fostering critical consciousness, and encouraging activism (Turner et al., 2022).

Working with Attitudes, Rules, and Assumptions

In order to adapt to their negative core beliefs, individuals develop a secondary class of underlying cognitions called intermediate beliefs. As defined in Chapter 6, *intermediate beliefs* refer to the attitudes, rules, and conditional assumptions clients develop in response to their negative core beliefs (J. S. Beck, 2020). Essentially, these cognitions describe the mindsets, guidelines, and if-then conditions clients develop to cope with their painful core beliefs.

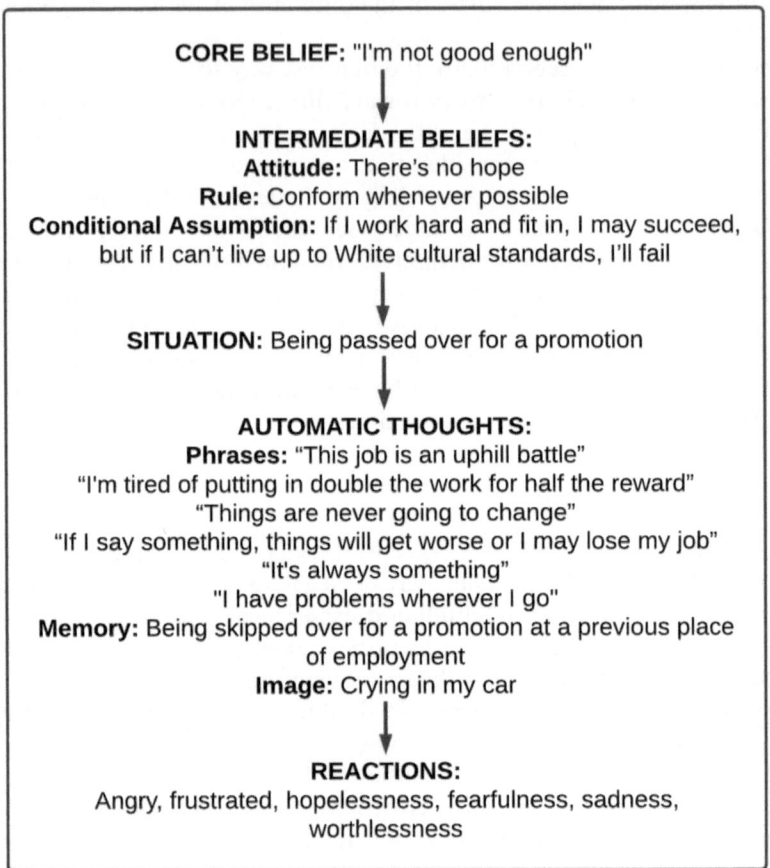

Figure 7.2 Vanessa's Hierarchy of Beliefs and Automatic Thoughts.

Helping clients modify their intermediate beliefs can be beneficial, as modifying these beliefs further assists clients with altering negative patterns in their perceptions and conclusions about events, which in turn, decreases the occurrence of negative automatic thoughts and makes clients less likely to relapse (J. S. Beck, 2020). A cognitive conceptualization inclusive of intermediate beliefs drawn from the case of Vanessa is presented in Figure 7.2. As shown in Figure 7.2, at the level of intermediate beliefs, Vanessa's attitude was, "There's no hope," her rule was "Conform whenever possible," and her conditional assumption was, "If I work hard and fit in, I may succeed, but if I can't live up to White cultural standards, I'll fail."

Strategies used to modify automatic thoughts and core beliefs can also be used to modify intermediate beliefs. The downward arrow technique, previously discussed, is commonly used to work with intermediate beliefs, as are the Socratic questioning, positive data log, and cognitive continuum strategies also mentioned previously. Another strategy to modify intermediate beliefs is *using other people as a reference point* (J. S. Beck, 2020). Looking at how negative beliefs operate in the lives of others often helps clients obtain psychological distance from their beliefs, allowing them to see the limits in their beliefs more clearly. Because Vanessa's intermediate beliefs were so deeply entrenched, the therapist decided to help Vanessa gain psychological distance from her problem by implementing the using others as a reference point strategy. To start, the therapist asked Vanessa to identify someone else she knows who experienced discrimination in their workplace. Vanessa reported that her father had worked his way up to become one of the first African American production supervisors at a large automotive manufacturing supplier. The therapist then helped Vanessa explore how accurate the belief "I'm not good enough" was for her father. Vanessa stated that the belief was "not accurate at all" and supplied examples illustrating how capable her father is in his life, especially at work. The therapist then asked Vanessa how she would view her father's difficulties prior to obtaining a promotion at his place of employment. Vanessa stated that her father has always been bright, competent, and a good leader. Difficulty obtaining a promotion is more of a reflection of racism than limitations in his ability or way of being. Knowing that her father was eventually able to obtain the promotion he deserved through the advocacy efforts of his union, Vanessa also stated that there are ways to address workplace discrimination other than hoping that people finally view you as good enough. To conclude the intervention, Vanessa and the therapist then did a roleplay where she tried to convince her father this was true and subsequently explored how this thinking might also apply to Vanessa in her current situation.

Prior to modification of intermediate beliefs, it is important that clients embrace two basic principles. The first principle is that just because a person believes something does not make it true. The second principle is that changing one's thinking so that it is more adaptive and functional can result in feeling better in the long run. CBT has a heavy emphasis on cognitions, however, upon examining the interrelationships among thoughts, feelings, and behaviors, it is apparent that intervention with any one of these factors will have an impact on the other two. Therefore, when clients do not respond well to cognitive interventions, or when it is in the therapist's best judgment, it may be beneficial to focus on behavioral strategies, knowing that when clients make behavioral changes in their lives that are consistent with new and healthier beliefs, they begin to see that these new beliefs have value and are associated with a better quality of life than the old, unhelpful beliefs (Wenzel et al., 2016).

One popular behavioral intervention that may be used to modify intermediate beliefs is called *acting as if*. Use of acting as if begins by identifying a belief and asking clients to rate how strong that belief is from 0 percent to 100 percent. Generally, acting as if works best with beliefs that are fairly weak and responsive to change (J. S. Beck, 2020). If the belief is stronger, acting as if should be used in conjunction with cognitive interventions. Because Vanessa's feelings of hopelessness were most directly related to her beliefs around powerlessness and her subsequent avoidance, conformity, or overperformance compensatory strategies (Steele & Newton, 2022), the therapist decided to target Vanessa's conditional assumption, "If I work hard and fit in, I may succeed, but if I can't live up to White cultural standards, I'll fail" which Vanessa rated at 95 percent. Once Vanessa rated the belief, the therapist then questioned her about what she would do if she were able to act as if she did not have the belief at all and what benefits she would experience as a result of acting this way. Vanessa talked about being free from dress and grooming rules rooted in Eurocentric beauty standards, as well as being more authentic in how she expresses herself and communicates with others. Vanessa also stated that she would be more assertive in addressing the microaggressions she experiences in the workplace. According to Vanessa, this would be positive because it would mitigate the psychological toll exacted due to pressure to outpace stereotypes, as well as reduce the depletion of cognitive resources required for code-switching (McCluney et al., 2019). It might also help with her relationships because she would be free to be herself rather than avoiding people.

With these benefits in mind, Vanessa and the therapist roleplayed how she might "act as if" throughout situations in a typical workday. To add cultural relevance to this exercise, the therapist suggested Vanessa think about a specific person, either a community leader or a person she personally knows and admires, to model her behavior after. As an example, the therapist shared a quote from writer and Civil Rights activist, James Baldwin, which says, "Not everything that can be faced can be changed, but nothing can be changed until it is faced" and discussed how Vanessa might focus on the feelings of empowerment and self-determination that might come along with use of specific microintervention strategies (Sue et al., 2019a) at work. During the roleplay, the therapist and Vanessa identified negative automatic thoughts she might experience in these situations and practiced restructuring these thoughts. A continued focus on cognitive interventions was crucial during this exercise given how highly Vanessa rated the strength of this belief (J. S. Beck, 2020). To help manage physiological distress, the therapist also implemented mindfulness-based strategies into this process, which burgeoning research suggests may also be effective when working with African Americans who experience race-based stressors (Bryant-Davis et al., 2021; Gutiérrez, 2022; Menakem, 2017; Watson-Singleton et al., 2019; Woods-Giscombé & Black, 2010).

Summary of Intermediate Beliefs

To summarize, intermediate beliefs are the attitudes, rules, and conditional assumptions clients develop in response to their negative core beliefs (J. S. Beck, 2020). Helping clients modify their intermediate beliefs can be beneficial, as modifying intermediate beliefs assists clients with altering negative patterns in their perceptions and conclusions about events, which in turn decreases the occurrence of negative automatic thoughts and makes clients less likely to relapse. Before beginning modification of intermediate beliefs, however, it is important that clients know that just because they believe something does not make it true, and that changing their thinking so that it is more adaptive and functional can help them feel better in the long run. Once clients have grasped this understanding, the same strategies used to modify automatic thoughts and core beliefs may also be used to modify intermediate beliefs. Additionally, behavioral strategies can also be of benefit, given that when clients make behavioral changes in their lives that are consistent with new and healthier beliefs, they begin to see that these new beliefs have value and are associated with a better quality of life than the old, unhelpful beliefs.

Finally, in concluding this chapter on working with automatic thoughts and underlying cognitions, it is important to keep in mind that a primary criticism of CBT has been its limited applicability to marginalized groups given its inattention to the role of environmental factors in the clients' lived experience (Iwamasa & Hays, 2019). This limitation is of particular relevance to healing from racism, as societal influences have a marked impact on life experiences that subsequently influence the development of stressors that lead to trauma as well as race-related beliefs that negatively affect one's view of self, others, and the world (Steele, 2020). Accordingly, the following chapter explores environmental interventions that therapists may implement in order to better address the impact of environmental factors on client cognitions and reactions to racism. Specific strategies and clinical examples are included throughout.

References

Beck, J. S. (2020). *Cognitive behavior therapy: Basics and beyond* (3rd ed.). Guilford Press.

Bryant-Davis, T., Fasalojo, B., Arounian, A., Jackson, K. L., & Leithman, E. (2021). Resist and rise: A trauma-informed womanist model for group therapy. *Women & Therapy*. Advance online publication. https://doi.org/10.1080/02703149.2021.1943114

Day-Vines, N. L., Cluxton-Keller, F., Agorsor, C., & Gubara, S. (2021). Strategies for broaching the subjects of race, ethnicity, and culture. *Journal of Counseling & Development*, 99(3), 348–357. https://doi.org/10.1002/jcad.12380

Day-Vines, N. L., Cluxton-Keller, F., Agorsor, C., Gubara, S., & Otabil, N. A. A. (2020). The multidimensional model or broaching behavior. *Journal of Counseling & Development*, *98*(1), 107–118. https://doi.org/10.1002/jcad.12304

Day-Vines, N.L., Wood, S. M., Grothaus, T., Craigen, L., Holman, A., Dotson-Blake, K., & Douglass, M. J. (2007). Broaching the subjects of race, ethnicity, and culture during the counseling process. *Journal of Counseling & Development*, *85*(4), 401–409. https://doi.org/10.1002/jcad.12069

Duncan, B. L., Miller, S. D., Wampold, B. E., & Hubble, M. A. (2010). *The heart & soul of change: Delivering what works in therapy* (2nd ed.). Washington, DC: American Psychological Association.

Graham, J. R., Sorenson, S., & Hayes-Skelton, S. A. (2013). Enhancing the cultural sensitivity of cognitive behavioral interventions for anxiety in diverse populations. *The Behavior Therapist*, *36*(5), 101–108.

Greenberger, D., & Padesky, C. A. (2015). *Mind over mood: Change how you feel by changing the way you think* (2nd ed.). Guilford Press.

Gutiérrez, N. Y. (2022). *The pain we carry: Healing from complex PTSD for people of color*. New Harbinger Publications, Inc.

Harris, R. (2019). *ACT made simple* (2nd ed.). New Harbinger.

Iwamasa, G. Y., & Hays, P. A. (Eds.). (2019). *Culturally responsive cognitive-behavioral therapy: Practice and supervision* (2nd ed.). American Psychological Association. https://doi.org/10.1037/0000119-000

Linehan, M. M. (1997). Validation and psychotherapy. In A. C. Bohart & L. S. Greenberg (Eds.), *Empathy reconsidered: New directions in psychotherapy* (pp. 353–392). American Psychological Association.

Mai, T., & Whitlock, J. (2022, November 28). *How to respond with compassion when someone is hurt by racism*. https://accelerate.uofuhealth.utah.edu/equity/how-to-respond-with-compassion-when-someone-is-hurt-by-racism

Matu, S. A. (2018). Cognitive therapy. In A. Vernon & K. A. Doyle (Eds.), *Cognitive behavior therapies: A guidebook for practitioners* (pp. 75–108). American Counseling Association.

McCluney, C. L., Robotham, K., Lee, S., Smith, R., & Durkee, M. (2019, November 15). The costs of code-switching. *Harvard Business Review*. https://hbr.org/2019/11/the-costs-of-codeswitching

Menakem, R. (2017). *My grandmother's hands: Racialized trauma and the pathway to mending our hearts and bodies*. Central Recovery Press.

Okeke-Adeyanju, N., Taylor, L. C., Craig, A. B., Smith, R. E., Thomas, A., Boyle, A. E., & DeRosier, M. E. (2014). Celebrating the strengths of Black youth: Increasing self-esteem and implications for prevention. *The Journal of Primary Prevention*, *35*(5), 357–369. https://doi.org/10.1007/s10935-014-0356-1

Overholser, J. C. (1993). Elements of the Socratic method: I. Systematic questioning. *Psychotherapy: Theory, Research, Practice, Training*, *30*(1), 67–74. https://doi.org/10.1037/0033-3204.30.1.67

Owen, J., Drinane, J. M., Tao, K. W., DasGupta, D. R., Zhang, Y. S. D., & Adelson, J. (2018). An experimental test of microaggression detection in psychotherapy: Therapist multicultural orientation. *Journal of Professional Psychology: Research and Practice*, *49*(1), 9–21. https://doi.org/10.1037/pro0000152

Padesky, C. A. (1993). *Socratic questioning: Changing minds or guiding discovery?* Keynote address delivered at the European Association for Behavioural and Cognitive Psychotherapies. London. https://padesky.com/newpad/wp-content/uploads/2012/11/socquest.pdf

Padesky, C. A. (1994). Schema change processes in cognitive therapy. *Clinical Psychology and Psychotherapy, 1*(5), 267–278. https://doi.org/10.1002/cpp.5640010502

Padesky, C. A. (2020, July 2021). *HOW DO WE TEST THIS THOUGHT? Padesky matches the level of thought with effective CBT interventions* [Video]. YouTube. https://youtu.be/xitheqH8Wxk?si=yZCNcjKOKQtj-rv3

Padesky, C. A., & Kennerley, H. (Eds.). (2023). *Dialogues for discovery: Improving psychotherapy's effectiveness.* Oxford University Press.

Palmer, R. T., & Walker, L. J. (2020, July 6). Proposing a concept of the Black tax to understand the experiences of Blacks in America. *Diverse Issues in Higher Education.* https://diverseeducation.com/article/182837/

Paul, R., & Elder, E. (2006). *The thinker's guide to the art of Socratic questioning.* Foundation for Critical Thinking Press.

Pierson, A. M., Arunagiri, V., & Bond, D. M. (2022). "You didn't cause racism, and you have to solve it anyways:" Antiracist adaptations to dialectical behavior therapy for White therapists. *Cognitive and Behavioral Practice, 29*(4), 796–815. https://doi.org/10.1016/j.cbpra.2021.11.001

Resick, P. A., Monson, C. M., & Chard, K. M. (2016). *Cognitive processing therapy for PTSD: A comprehensive manual.* Guilford Press.

Steele, J. M. (2020). A CBT approach to internalized racism among African Americans. *International Journal for the Advancement of Counselling, 42*(3), 217–233. https://doi.org/10.1007/s10447-020-09402-0

Steele, J. M., & Newton, C. S. (2022). Culturally adapted cognitive behavior therapy as a model to address internalized racism among African American clients. *Journal of Mental Health Counseling, 44*(2), 98–116. https://doi.org/10.17744/mehc.44.2.01

Sue, D. W., Alsaidi, S., Awad, M. N., Glaeser, E., Calle, C. Z., & Mendez, N. (2019a). Disarming racial microaggressions: Microintervention strategies for targets, White allies, and bystanders. *American Psychologist, 74*(1), 128–142. https://doi.org/10.1037/amp0000296

Sue, D. W., Calle, C. Z., Mendez, N., Alsaidi, S., & Glaeser, E. (2021). *Microintervention strategies: What you can do to disarm and dismantle individual and systemic racism and bias.* John Wiley & Sons, Inc.

Sue, D. W., Sue, D., Neville, H. A., & Smith, L. (2019b). *Counseling the culturally diverse: Theory and practice* (8th ed.). John Wiley & Sons, Inc.

Turner, E. A., Harrell, S. P., & Bryant-Davis, T. (2022). Black Love, Activism, and Community (BLAC): The BLAC model of healing and resilience. *Journal of Black Psychology, 48*(3–4), 547–568. https://doi.org/10.1177/00957984211018364

Waltman, S., Codd, R., III, McFarr, L., & Moore, B. (2021). *Socratic questioning for therapists and counselors: Learn how to think and intervene like a cognitive behavior therapist.* Routledge. https://doi.org/10.4324/9780429320392

Watson-Singleton, N. N., Black, A. R., & Spivey, B. N. (2019). Recommendations for a culturally-responsive mindfulness-based intervention for African Americans. *Complementary Therapy in Clinical Practice, 34,* 132–138. https://doi.org/10.1016/j.ctcp.2018.11.013

Wenzel, A. (2019). *Cognitive behavioral therapy for beginners*. Routledge.

Wenzel, A., Dobson, K. S., & Hays, P. A. (2016). Culturally responsive cognitive behavioral therapy. In A. Wenzel, K. S. Dobson, & P. A. Hays, *Cognitive behavioral therapy techniques and strategies* (pp. 145–160). American Psychological Association. https://doi.org/10.1037/14936-008

Williams, M. T., Holmes, S., Zare, M., Haeny, A., & Faber, S. (2022). An evidence-based approach for treating stress and trauma due to racism. *Cognitive and Behavioral Practice*. Advance online publication. https://doi.org/10.1016/j.cbpra.2022.07.001

Woods-Giscombé, C. L., & Black, A. R. (2010). Mind-body interventions to reduce risk for health disparities related to stress and strength among African American women: The potential of mindfulness-based stress reduction, lovingkindness, and the NTU therapeutic framework. *Complementary Health Practice Review*, *15*(3), 115–131. https://doi.org/10.1177/1533210110386776

Wright, J. H., Basco, M. R., & Thase, M. E. (2006). *Learning cognitive behavioral therapy: An illustrated guide*. American Psychiatric Publishing.

Chapter 8

Environmental Interventions

In terms of cultural responsiveness, one of the primary criticisms of CBT has been its lack of attention to environmental influences on client cognitions and reactions. In particular, scholars suggest that a focus on self without adequate attention to the role of environmental factors such as racism in client concerns may contribute to blaming clients for problems that are primarily environmentally based (Iwamasa & Hays, 2019). For this reason, many of these same scholars have developed culturally responsive approaches to CBT that integrate environmental considerations into all aspects of clinical practice including assessment, case conceptualization, and treatment planning (Iwamasa & Hays, 2019; Rathod et al., 2015). Kelly (2019), for example, suggested that use of a functional-analytic approach, which recognizes the significance of environmental interventions on symptom reduction, would allow therapists to modify CBT in ways that empower African American clients, expand their social support, and allow them to achieve their goals more effectively. Similarly, Rathod et al. (2015) suggested that working with clients to alter environmental factors that have a negative impact on their development reduces vulnerability and increases hope and resilience among members of diverse cultural groups. As such, environmental interventions, while not traditionally viewed in CBT as necessary in the remediation of client symptoms, should be considered when working with African American clients to address the psychological effects of racism.

In this chapter, I discuss specific environmental interventions therapists may implement in order to better address the impact of environmental factors on client cognitions and reactions to racism. Within Black psychology, critical awareness of one's racial group and racial oppression is emphasized as the foundation of psychological liberation and healing from racism (Freire, 1993; French et al., 2020; Turner et al., 2022; Watts, 2004). Accordingly, I begin this chapter with a discussion on psychological empowerment and strategies therapists may use to promote psychological empowerment

DOI: 10.4324/9781003196303-8

among African American clients. The specific psychological empowerment strategies discussed include exploring personal narratives, group therapy, counterspaces, and bibliotherapy. Next, I explore interventions therapists may use to assist their clients with making a direct impact on the environmental barriers that impinge on their mental health and wellness. These interventions include advocacy at micro-, meso-, and macro-levels (Lewis et al., 2003), as well as microinterventions clients may use when targeted by microaggressions (Sue et al., 2019). Examples and case illustrations are integrated throughout. I conclude the chapter by expanding the discussion of treatment planning described in Chapter 6 to include interventions focused on psychological empowerment and advocacy.

Psychological Empowerment

Psychological empowerment is considered a foundational component of healing from the effects of racism and racial trauma among African Americans for several reasons. First, psychological empowerment when viewed as liberated thought and committed action toward social change is consistent with the collectivistic orientation inherent to the Afrocentric worldview discussed in Chapter 3 (French et al., 2020; Turner et al., 2022). Recall that African-centered values, strengths, and ways of coping traditionally consist of variables such as positive racial socialization, interconnectedness, communalism, familism, unity, preparation for bias, and active resistance (Johnson & Carter, 2020; Okeke-Adeyanju et al., 2014). Interventions based on psychological empowerment exemplify these variables by helping individuals understand their experiences as part of a common collective struggle and through the promotion of empowered action (French et al., 2020). Recognition of a common struggle and empowered action, in turn, promote resistance, agency, and greater connectedness within the community (Bryant-Davis et al., 2021; French et al., 2020).

Within the counseling and psychology literature, several authors have described programs that build upon psychological empowerment and liberation frameworks in the African American community. Watts et al. (2002), for example, described the Young Warriors Program for young African American men, which used hip-hop to help participants increase consciousness of social factors that influence them and their communities. According to Watts and his colleagues (2002), this program not only helped participants increase their awareness of the cultural and political forces that shape their status in society, but it also cultivated growth in their analytical skills, emotional faculties, and capacity for action. In another example, Chioneso et al. (2020) developed the Community Healing and Resistance Through Storytelling (C-HeARTS) framework as a means to treat racial trauma and promote community healing. In this framework, storytelling, an African-centered tradition, was used as the means through which individuals were able to share their personal testimonies with others, which facilitates the reframing of negative cognitions to positive cognitions. Other benefits of this program and psychological empowerment through storytelling according to Chioneso et al. (2020) include resisting oppression, fostering healing, promoting spiritual communion, restoring cultural identities, building a sense of community, and identification of counterhegemonic narratives to refute negative stories about oppressed groups.

Beyond its consistency with Afrocentric forms of healing, another advantage of psychological empowerment is that it can reduce psychological distress and maladaptive behaviors associated with the effects of racism. For example, one study found that psychological empowerment in the form of Black activism provided several psychological benefits among Black womxn scholar-activists, including identity formation, self-love, connectedness, exposure to diverse representation, and greater perceptions of oneself as a change agent (Hickson et al., 2022). Another study among African American youth found that empowerment beliefs mediated the relationship between community involvement and adolescent sexual risk behaviors in that community involvement was associated with more positive empowerment beliefs, and empowerment beliefs, in turn, were associated with fewer sexual risk behaviors (Cooper & Conklin, 2015). Within the family system, research has also shown that family health programs focused on empowerment also provide substantial therapeutic effects including enhanced self-esteem, increased cultural pride and knowledge, enhanced conduct, increased intraracial community cohesion, and bolstered interracial community connection (McBride, 2011). Consequently, it is clear from these studies that interventions based on psychological empowerment offer substantial therapeutic effects in the treatment of racial trauma.

So, what exactly is psychological empowerment? In its broadest sense, *empowerment* may be defined as "the process of increasing personal, interpersonal, or political power so that individuals, families, and communities can take action to improve their situations" (L. M. Gutiérrez, 1995, p. 229). Accordingly, empowerment occurs across various levels and within several domains. *Psychological empowerment*, however, refers to the awareness of factors that impinge upon one's ability to structure their life and committed action to initiate change (Curtis-Tweed, 2003; Zimmerman, 1995). One of the primary sources of psychological empowerment is critical consciousness. *Critical consciousness* is defined as "the capacity of oppressed or marginalized people to critically analyze their social and political conditions, endorsement of societal equality, and action to change perceived inequities"

(Diemer et al., 2017, p. 461). According to L. M. Gutiérrez (1995), the development of critical consciousness consists of three primary psychological processes:

1. Group identification, which includes identifying areas of common experience and concern, a preference for one's own group culture and norms, and the development of feelings of shared fate
2. Group consciousness, which involves understanding the differential status and power of groups in society
3. Self- and collective efficacy, which broadly refers to beliefs that one is capable of effecting desired changes in one's life. More specifically, self- and collective agency involves perceiving oneself as a subject (rather than object) of social processes and as capable of working to change the social order

(p. 230)

Consistent with the research described previously, I have found that over time and with the support of the therapist, several interventions both in and outside of therapy can help clients increase their critical consciousness and sense of psychological empowerment. These interventions include telling one's story, group therapy, counterspaces, and bibliotherapy. A discussion of each intervention follows.

Telling One's Story

Because aspects of racial trauma such as self-alienation, self-loathing, and a diminished sense of self-worth are the result of negative societal messages, techniques that help clients realize and reconstruct the messages they have received about their racial/ethnic identities can be especially impactful. The Telling One's Story exercise allows individuals to tell their stories, find meaning in their stories, and tell themselves new stories. When considered within a CBT framework, this strategy more specifically allows African American clients to review and modify maladaptive core and intermediate beliefs in a way that is consistent with the community healing and resistance through storytelling approach advocated by Chioneso et al. (2020). To begin, instruct clients to imagine that their life was a story. Then, instruct clients to respond to the following prompts:

1. Write the title of your story
2. Write a minimum of seven chapter titles that describe defining events or themes related to your trauma or racial/ethnic identity. Then, write a one-line description of each chapter
3. Reflect on the messages given through these events and themes. What impact have these messages had on your sense of self and life overall?

4. Write at least one additional chapter title and description describing how you would like to view yourself in relation to your trauma or racial/ethnic identity in the future

Case Illustration: James

James was a 25-year-old African American man working as a data analyst at a computer manufacturing company. He initiated therapy due to anger associated with ongoing difficulties establishing himself in his workplace. According to James, African Americans in his field are generally perceived as having less intelligence. He further indicates there is also a perception that African Americans are only hired because of affirmative action or diversity, equity, and inclusion programs. As a result, James reports that despite his training and ability, he is often passed over for mentorship and promotions. James states that he has even trained individuals who have gone on to become his supervisor. Recently, James began to informally express his dissatisfaction with the lack of movement in his career, causing tension in the relationship with his supervisors and co-workers. Given the history of racism and exclusion in science and technology fields, James believes there is little hope for his problems to be addressed, which has not only resulted in anger, but anxiety and depression as well. During therapy, James and his therapist decided to complete the Telling One's Story exercise in order to help James articulate his story and identify and reframe any negative self-appraisals that may have developed as a result of his experiences at work. His completed exercise follows (Table 8.1).

In reviewing James's completed Telling One's Story exercise, psychological phenomena, schemas, intermediate beliefs, and compensatory strategies relevant to the African American experience are apparent. For example, several of the chapter titles and descriptions developed by James reflect the toll stereotypes and issues such as underrepresentation, Black tax, and John Henryism (see Chapter 2) have on the African American psyche. In particular, Chapter 1, "Black People Can't Be Professionals," suggests a story wherein stereotypes are understood to not only affect the way one is perceived by others, but also as a mechanism that limits the growth and development of those who are targeted. Chapter 2, "One is the Loneliest Number," expounds on these limitations by describing the sense of exclusion and alienation resulting from underrepresentation. Together, these chapters also suggest a powerlessness schema, wherein although not viewed as completely insurmountable, that state of racism in society is perceived by James to be enduring and unchangeable. From a clinical perspective, this schema is especially significant because of its accuracy; that is, the legacy of White supremacy and racism are deeply entrenched in U.S. society. While gains toward racial equality have and continue to be made, racism nevertheless remains

Table 8.1 James's Story

Title of your story:	*I Am Somebody*
Chapter 1:	**Black People Can't Be Professionals**: Throughout life, Black people are given the message that they can't be doctors, engineers, or other types of professionals.
Chapter 2:	**One is the Loneliest Number**: Black people do have the mental capacity to be at the highest levels of society, but we may be alone when we get there.
Chapter 3:	**Prove You Belong**: At work, Black people are often assigned the easiest tasks because people don't think they can handle challenging work. Eventually, they have to give you a chance and you can be an instant success.
Chapter 4:	**Fight to Stay**: Even once you show your value, you have to constantly prove you belong, each step from grade school into your career.
Chapter 5:	**The Struggle for Existence**: Throughout American history, Black people have struggled to exist, even after they've gained entry into spaces where they previously weren't wanted.
Chapter 6:	**You Can't Burn Down the Bridge**: You can't beat up everybody who says something inappropriate—that's a good way to get fired.
Chapter 7:	**I'm Not Your Negro**: Members of the dominant group may believe you're supposed to be subservient, but we're equal. "I am not your Negro."
Reflection: What impact have these messages had on your sense of self and life overall?	As Malcolm X said, "By any means necessary." You do what you have to do to get there. Things aren't equal and discrimination happens. These experiences hurt but they don't have to compel me to stay down. I have to mentally control my rage.
Chapter 8:	**Keep On Pushing**: Be aware of complacency—you may be living good but that doesn't mean racism and discrimination are over.

endemic. Accordingly, when processing these chapters and their implications with James, it would be important for the therapist to validate rather than challenge this perception and instead work toward modifying maladaptive rules and coping developed in response.

Chapters 3, 4, and 5, "Prove You Belong," "Fight to Stay," and "The Struggle for Existence," provide clues to what some of the maladaptive rules and compensatory strategies James has developed in response to racism may be. James's noted efforts to "constantly prove you belong" in particular suggest a rule of "being the best" and coping strategies grounded in working twice as hard and John Henryism. Again, because Black people often do have to be the best in their fields to achieve success, it would be important that the therapist validate this reality and focus on broadening James's coping strategies to include self-care and affirmation tools as well. Modification of the rule "be the best" should approached toward replacing it with something that would be more functional and relieve some of the pressure James likely experiences in response to this rule. Examples include being *his* personal best and following a set of self-defined rules and expectations.

Finally, beyond offering insight into the client's personal schemas, intermediate beliefs, and compensatory strategies, the Telling One's Story exercise provides an added benefit of identifying strengths and sources of support clients may draw on to counter the psychological effects of racism. While these strengths and sources of support are typically made evident in the final chapters of the exercise, Chapter 6, "You Can't Burn Down the Bridge" and Chapter 7, "I'm Not Your Negro," in the case of James also allude to personal qualities James may tap to manage his psychological distress. From these chapters, it is apparent that James understands the potential consequences of acting out and desires to find appropriate ways to channel his anger. His willingness to seek help in learning anger management and emotional regulation skills is a quality that can be affirmed by the therapist to instill hope and empowerment. Likewise, James's reference to Malcolm X and "I am not your Negro," the title of a documentary based on the work of civil rights activist James Baldwin, could be capitalized upon to facilitate further reading or other activities that promote critical consciousness.

Group Therapy

While the Telling One's Story exercise allows clients to explore their personal narratives, group therapy expands this opportunity by also building community, affording validation, providing a structure to support the psycho-education needed to increase critical consciousness, and teaching and strengthening coping skills to manage the effects of racism. In fact, several authors purport the efficacy of group therapy in facilitating these benefits (Bhambhani & Gallo, 2022; Bryant-Davis et al., 2021; Watson-Singleton et al., 2019). Bhambhani and Gallo (2022), for example, developed a mindfulness-based group for racially and ethnically diverse individuals in the Bronx and found that participants developed skills for coping with a variety of chronic environmental stressors, including health issues, financial stress, community violence, and family stress. Similarly, Bryant-Davis et al. (2021) developed a trauma-informed group based on the cultural traditions of Black women's experiences and identified outcomes such as increased agency, activism, and resistance to internalized oppression, as well as a positive racial/ethnic identity socialization experience. In yet another culturally responsive approach, Watson-Singleton et al. (2019) developed a mindfulness-based intervention with research findings that reinforced the essentiality of culturally-centered healing variables such as African American facilitators, salient cultural values, self-empowerment, interdependence, storytelling, culturally familiar terminology, and culturally tailored resources in mitigating mental health outcomes associated with racism.

As suggested by the research conducted by Watson-Singleton et al. (2019), many different factors, skills, and techniques are emphasized in consciousness-raising groups. Beyond the culturally-centered healing practices listed above, Watson-Singleton and her colleagues (2019) also identified several individual factors that influenced the extent to which the African Americans in their study were willing to participate in a mindfulness-based intervention. These factors included accentuating benefits, underscoring holistic health, and addressing religious concerns. In their work with African American women, Bryant-Davis and her colleagues (2021) also noted the significance of religious concerns in racial trauma groups. These researchers additionally identified specific skills and techniques necessary for cultivating connection and healing in these groups, including self-disclosure from facilitators, consciousness raising, psychoeducation, expressive arts, expressive writing, mindfulness, and activism. Other skills mentioned throughout the literature include acknowledgment of the client's broader sense of identity (Graham-LoPresti et al., 2017), internalized racism (Turner et al., 2022), colorism (Williams et al., 2022a), family and kinship (Turner et al., 2022), and racial identity (Williams et al., 2022a), as well as cognitive restructuring and defusion, in-vivo exposure, processing past racist events, and facilitating post-traumatic growth (Williams et al., 2022a).

According to the extant research described above, a variety of therapeutic elements must be considered in the development of group therapy interventions to address the psychological effects of racism. However, related research suggests that specific group discussion and problem-solving processes that contribute to the development of ethnic consciousness *must* be included in group therapy to truly facilitate psychological empowerment (L. M. Gutiérrez, 1995). In her research, L. M. Gutiérrez (1995) compared Latino individuals in ethnic consciousness, ethnic identity, and control groups finding that participants in the consciousness-raising group had a higher overall mean score on ethnic consciousness than those in the other two groups, with participants in the control group having the lowest levels of ethnic consciousness. Based on these results, L. M. Gutiérrez (1995) concluded that to develop a sense of ethnic consciousness, simple group contact or discussion concerning ethnic identity may not be as influential as discussion that involves a critical appraisal of the social situation and the generation of solutions to problems related to Latino status. Therefore, therapists working with African American clients should be sure to not only focus on the cultivation of racial pride and coping skills but should also focus on increasing awareness and action to address the social factors that influence them and their communities.

To summarize, group therapy supports psychological empowerment by providing a structure through which key aspects of psychological empowerment such as psychoeducation, critical consciousness, skill development, and empowered action may be facilitated. Chapter 2 briefly discussed a four-part trauma-focused CBT approach to the treatment of racial trauma. The stages of this model include: (1) assessment, (2) embodied healing, (3) adapted cognitive restructuring, and (4) empowerment. Table 8.2 provides an example racial trauma group outline that follows the stages of this approach.

As indicated in Table 8.2, group therapy focused on the healing of racial trauma should begin with an individualized assessment of client symptoms in order to measure the severity of their symptomatology and determine appropriateness for the group. During this assessment, the therapist should use a semi-structured interview protocol such as the Cultural Formulation Interview (American Psychiatric Association, 2013) in order to develop a broad understanding of the ways in which race and other cultural aspects influence how the client views and copes with their problems. Therapists may also utilize interview protocols that more specifically explore distress and trauma caused by racism, such as the University of Connecticut Racial Ethnic Stress and Trauma Survey (UnRESTS; Williams & Zare, 2022). This interview explores the client's experience with overt racism, racism by loved ones, vicarious racism, and covert racism. The interview protocol also includes questions to assess the extent to which the client's symptoms meet *DSM-5* criteria for PTSD, and a measure of ethnoracial identity. Further assessment may be conducted using a quantitative measure such as the Racial Trauma Scale (RTS; Williams et al., 2022b). Use of this type of assessment allows the therapist to obtain a baseline score of trauma and measure progress over time.

Once individual assessments have been completed, group sessions begin with a focus on embodied healing. *Embodied healing* refers to body-centric exercises designed to increase the client's awareness of their body's trauma responses, when and where they activate, the emotions they give rise to, and how to settle these emotions and physiological responses (N. Y. Gutiérrez, 2022; Menakem, 2017). Examples of these exercises include body scan, grounding, deep breathing, relaxation, and meditation (Steele & Newton, 2023). Through the psychoeducation provided during the Embodied Healing sessions of the group, participants learn how to define racial trauma and the ways in which this trauma lives in the body through symptoms such as increased somatic complaints, physical arousal, dissociation, and hypervigilance. This insight is significant, as trauma experts suggest that higher-order

Table 8.2 Group Outline

Stage	Session
Assessment	**Intake**: Participants are screened for inclusion in the group using culturally responsive interview and assessment tools such as the cultural formulation interview (American Psychiatric Association, 2013), the University of Connecticut Racial/Ethnic Stress & Trauma Survey (UnRESTS) interview (Williams & Zare, 2022), and the Racial Trauma Scale (Williams et al., 2022b)
Embodied Healing	**Session 1: Introduction to Racial Trauma**: Participants are provided with psychoeducation focused on understanding racial trauma and its impact.
	Session 2: Mindfulness-based Stress Reduction: Participants learn mindfulness-based strategies (Kabat-Zinn, 2013) designed to address somatic symptoms that result from racial trauma, emphasizing culture-centered practices such as song, touch, and movement (Menakem, 2017).
	Session 3: Self-care and Health: Participants learn about health complications that arise in response to race-based stress and identify personal self-care strategies to promote individual health and wellness.
Cognitive Restructuring	**Session 4: The More You Know...** Participants are provided with psychoeducation to further inform their understanding of racism and its effects. During this process, participants are provided with opportunities to explore how racist ideologies have influenced their perceptions of themselves and other people of color
	.**Session 5: I am Somebody!** Participants are provided with continued psychoeducation and activities designed to promote ethnic pride and cognitive restructuring. During this session, traditional CBT techniques such as Socratic questioning are integrated with culturally informed practices such as storytelling, expressive arts, and expressive writing (Bryant-Davis et al., 2021).
	Session 6: Mix It Up: Participants continue examination of racist ideologies that contribute to stereotypes and internalized racism and utilize cognitive restructuring techniques to challenge and reframe negative self-perceptions and anti-Black attitudes.

(Continued)

Table 8.2 (Continued)

Stage	Session
Empowerment	**Session 7: Cultivating Black Joy**: Participants engage in activities such as the development of self-definitions of joy, identification of self and community sources of strength, and the creation of a personal list of activities that enhance happiness and enjoyment in order to facilitate posttraumatic growth and appreciation of life. **Session 8: Strategies to Resist Racism**: Participants learn specific strategies to respond to racism and microaggressions in the environment including graduated exposure and microaggression microinterventions (Sue et al., 2019). **Session 9: Empowered Action**: Participants discuss various forms of social justice, political activism, and social transformation such as public storytelling, community engagement, and legislative action, and identify ways for personally becoming engaged in these activities (Bryant-Davis et al., 2021; Chioneso et al., 2020).
Closure	**Session 10: Reflections and Relapse Prevention**: Participants summarize insights gained as a result of group participation and develop a personal plan for self-care when confronted with racist events.

thought processing is not possible without first learning how to target the threat-processing networks of the brain using the body-centric strategies described above (van der Kolk, 2014). Consistent with the culturally responsive approach advocated in this text, these strategies are modified to include Afrocentric perspectives, for example, imagining being rooted by the ancestors during a grounding exercise and expanded to include culture-centered healing practices such as song, touch, and movement (Menakem, 2017). However, as mentioned previously, given cultural stigma surrounding the use of mindfulness and meditation practices in the Black community, therapists should be sure to introduce these strategies in culturally responsive ways that include the incorporation of cultural values, for example, helping participants draw connections between these practices and their own religious texts, as well as use of culturally-familiar terminology, for example, use of the terms "awareness" or "relaxation" (Watson-Singleton et al., 2019).

After participants develop an ability to regulate physiological responses that might interfere with higher-order processing, they then begin to learn cognitive restructuring strategies to reduce unhelpful thinking patterns that also contribute to their symptoms and ability to cope. Techniques used to accomplish these goals include psychoeducation and cognitive restructuring strategies such as Socratic questioning and modification of core beliefs. The psychoeducation throughout these sessions focuses on developing a greater understanding of societal forces that impinge on the mental health and well-being of African Americans, for example, stereotypes, legitimizing myths, and the social determinants of health discussed in Chapter 2. With this insight, participants are in turn encouraged to practice identifying and modifying negative automatic thoughts, core beliefs, and intermediate beliefs that have developed in response to negative societal messages about African Americans (Steele, 2020; Steele & Newton, 2022). As indicated in Table 8.2, this process involves the integration of traditional CBT techniques such as Socratic questioning with culturally informed practices such as storytelling, expressive arts, and expressive writing (Bryant-Davis et al., 2021). For example, in one modified expressive arts exercise known as the bridge drawing, participants are encouraged to draw an image that represents their core beliefs prior to psychoeducation received in the group on one side of a sheet of paper, an image of what they would like to believe about themselves on the other side of the paper, and a bridge representing the strategies they will use to get themselves from the old core beliefs to the new core beliefs across the middle of the paper (Hays & Lyons, 1981).

Finally, the last sessions of the group focus on ethnopolitical approaches participants may use to facilitate empowerment and reduce stress associated with the experience of racial discrimination. In these sessions, techniques known as microinterventions, which are discussed later in this chapter, are taught to help participants respond to microaggressions in their environment (Sue et al., 2019, 2021). Additionally, Black joy is explored as a form of resistance to anti-Black racism and as a means of healing and empowerment. In its most basic sense, Black joy refers to Black people enjoying recreation and celebrating life (Tichavakunda, 2022). Expounding on this definition, Black joy has been recognized as a form of resistance in that oppression is meant to limit one's happiness and wellbeing. Black people resist this aspect of oppression when they find joy anyhow (Packnett, 2017). As a newer construct within the Black community, Black joy has often been examined within the context of social media and the arts. Lu and Steele (2019), for example, explored the ways in which Black joy is demonstrated on social media platforms such as Twitter and Vine as a means to challenge dominant narratives that demean and dehumanize Black people. In their analysis of discourse on these platforms, the authors identified several themes which reflect this goal, including celebrating Black life in defiance of death and despair, asserting Black people's full humanity and range of emotion, and capturing Black life without concern for the White gaze. Accordingly, activities that capitalize on these themes are engaged to help participants thrive while affirming their Blackness, as described in Table 8.2, Session 7.

Counterspaces

Counterspaces are defined as "sites where deficit notions of people of color can be challenged and where a positive climate can be established and maintained" (Solórzano et al., 2000, p. 70). Essentially, counterspaces are the places where marginalized people experience an enhanced sense of wellbeing because they are able to express their frustrations with negative cultural messages about their social group and are supported by people who share the same group membership. According to research, there are many benefits associated with counterspaces. Some of these benefits beyond enhanced psychological wellbeing and social support include increased critical consciousness, greater cultural pride, a more positive sense of self, and more adaptive coping (Case & Hunter, 2012). A study of African American women student affairs workers, for example, found that participation in professional counterspaces had a positive impact on their physical, spiritual, and interpersonal wellness, and increased opportunities for mentoring and networking (West, 2019). Similarly, a different study of African American male high schoolers found that the counterspace of an all-male educational setting helped participants of the study experience greater academic success, personal validation, and opportunities to think critically about race and their racialized experiences (Terry et al., 2014).

Ethnic studies courses are a particular type of counterspace that allow individuals to explore the historical and contemporary experiences of various racial and ethnic groups (Chapman-Hilliard & Beasley, 2018). They can be formal classes taken through institutions such as colleges and universities, or they can be informal in nature, such as classes, workshops, or groups provided through various community organizations. Recently, Chapman-Hilliard and Beasley (2018) conducted research examining the effects of Black studies courses on the psychosocial experiences and identity development of Black students attending predominately White colleges. In their review of literature, these researchers found that ethnic studies courses offer several psychological benefits including encouragement of adaptive responding to systemic oppression, positive self-concept, the ability to challenge prior miseducation and introduce students to the contributions of African-descent individuals throughout world history, racial socialization that offers new ways to examine and understand one's identity, strategies for responding to racial issues within society, increased self-esteem and academic motivation, and development of critical thinking and conscious-nesses. In the results of their own study, Chapman-Hilliard and Beasley (2018) confirmed these broad psychological benefits, as findings from their research revealed that ethnic studies courses promoted psychological empowerment, self-determination, counterspaces, and community perpetu-ity. Concerning psychological empowerment, participants of the study noted that Black studies courses resulted in gaining a voice and shifting miseducation to reeducation by countering negative and biased historical nar-ratives presented in elementary and secondary education. Self-determination was experienced as participants explored the meanings associated with being Black and gained critical consciousness. Counterspaces were solidified as pro-fessors served as role models. Finally, community perpetuity was experienced as participants sensed a passing along of history and cultural values (Chapman-Hilliard & Beasley, 2018).

Examples of other counterspaces in the African American community include religious institutions such as the church or the mosque, civic organi-zations such as the NAACP, barbershops or beauty salons, local community centers, and formal spaces dedicated to the transmission of Black cultural knowledge such as museums, libraries, and historically Black colleges and universities (Steele & Newton, 2023). During therapy, therapists should help clients identify counterspaces local to their community as a source of sup-port and coping. This may be done by helping clients to first develop a list of the counterspaces in their community. Then, clients should create a list of their current needs and identify how the counterspaces they have identified can help meet these needs. For example, a client who is concerned about creating positive racial socialization experiences for their children who attend predominantly White schools may travel to museums such as the Smithsonian National Museum of African American History and Culture, which is devoted to the documentation of African American life, history, and culture (https://nmaahc.si.edu/about/about-museum). They might also enroll their children in Jack and Jill of America, Inc., which is a Black orga-nization devoted to providing social, cultural, and educational opportuni-ties for youth between the ages of 2 and 19 (https://www.jackandjillinc.org/about/).

Finally, when identifying counterspaces with African American clients, therapists should also be intentional in exploring any perceived barriers to entering these spaces. For example, some individuals may have experienced hurt in some institutions. *Church hurt*, which is defined as pain inflicted by religious institutions, has caused some individuals to turn away from partici-pation in formal religious institutions (Steele & Newton, 2023). In these cases, while the decision to remove oneself from the church may have been a protective effort, this action often has adverse side effects such as feeling cut off from a significant source of community and coping. Additionally, some African Americans may feel uncomfortable entering into certain Black spaces depending on their own racial identity or other life experiences. Accordingly, therapists should guide clients in a reflective discussion of challenges they may encounter when attempting to engage counterspaces, and work with the client to identify strategies and more adaptive ways of thinking to overcome these challenges.

Bibliotherapy

Generally, *bibliotherapy* is an intervention that uses storytelling or the reading of specific texts for the purpose of healing. As an intervention in the treatment of racial trauma, bibliotherapy uses narratives to consider personal dilemmas and teach cultural traditions in a process that can be either structured or unstructured (Byrd et al., 2021). In a structured approach, Byrd et al. (2021) combined bibliotherapy with critical race theory and developed guidelines for use with Black teen boys. These guidelines, based on an interactive process developed by Hynes and Hynes-Berry (2012), consist of the following steps:

1. **Recognition**: At this step, the client acknowledges a passage or phrase in the text that resonates with them
2. **Examination**: Next, the client explores personal feelings that arise from the passage
3. **Juxtaposition**: After exploring personal feelings, the client then describes how their understanding is expanding as a result of the reading and dialogue with the therapist
4. **Self-application**: Finally, the client ends the process by describing how what was learned may influence their future beliefs, attitudes, actions, and ways of being

According to Byrd and her colleagues (2021), beyond the steps identified in the list above, bibliotherapy as an intervention to address the psychological effects of racism among African Americans should also include the use of stories with protagonists that look like them, come from similar cultural backgrounds, and contend with familiar social/emotional issues and systemic barriers. Inclusion of these considerations in the selection of texts stimulates healthy discussions that increase self-awareness and understanding of the systemic barriers that clients navigate (Byrd et al., 2021). Moreover, when clients are able to read texts that include characters from similar racial backgrounds and cultural experiences, they are more able to see a reflection of their full humanity as opposed to the marginalized or demonized view of

African Americans espoused within dominant societal narratives. This offers the psychological benefit of challenging internalized anti-Black sentiments, facilitating individual growth, and identifying possible solutions to address adverse circumstances (Byrd et al., 2021; Ford et al., 2019).

Table 8.3 presents questions therapists may use at each step of the interactive process described by Hynes and Hynes-Berry (2012). Following Table 8.3, a brief list of suggested fiction and non-fiction books is provided.

Table 8.3 Questions to Guide Bibliotherapy by Using Hynes and Hynes-Berry's (2012) Interactive Process

Step	Questions
1. Recognition	• To which passages in the reading did you feel most connected? • Which passages helped you gain a deeper understanding of yourself and/or the world around you? • Which passages made you feel seen or validated? • Which passages felt triggering? • Which passages felt healing? • Of these passages, which one was most meaningful for you today?
2. Examination	• What specific thoughts did this passage evoke? • What specific feelings did this passage evoke? • When have you experienced situations similar to the situation connected to the passage you identified?
3. Juxtaposition	• What about your own life influences how you see this character or understand their situation? • What systems of oppression are connected to the passage you identified? • How are these systems of oppression reflected in your own life? • What beliefs or ideas are challenged by the passage you identified? • How have these beliefs or ideas influenced your own life?
4. Self-application	• What insights have you gained about yourself? • What insights have you gained about the world around you? • How do these insights change how see yourself? • How do these insights change how you see the world around you? • What will you start doing as a result of these insights? • What will you stop doing as a result of these insights?

List of Fiction Books

1. *Americanah* by Chimamanda Ngozi Adichie
2. *Children of Blood and Bone* by Tomi Adeyemi
3. *Monster: The Autobiography of an L.A. Gang Member* by Sanyika Shakur
4. *Pride: A Pride & Prejudice Remix* by Ibi Zoboi
5. *The Bluest Eye* by Toni Morrison
6. *The Hate U Give* by Angie Thomas
7. *Their Eyes Were Watching God* by Zora Neale Hurston
8. *Things Fall Apart* by Chinua Achebe
9. *Tristan Strong Punches a Hole in the Sky* by Kwame Mbalia
10. *Waiting to Exhale* by Terry McMillan

List of Non-Fiction Books

1. *Ain't I a Woman?* by bell hooks
2. *Between the World and Me* by Ta-Nehisi Coates
3. *Black Like Me* by John Howard Griffin
4. *I Know Why the Cage Bird Sings* by Maya Angelou
5. *Just Mercy* by Bryan Stevenson
6. *Long Walk to Freedom* by Nelson Mandela
7. *The Autobiography of Malcolm X* by Malcolm X and Alex Haley
8. *The Light We Carry* by Michelle Obama
9. *The Other Wes Moore: One Name, Two Fates* by Wes Moore
10. *The Souls of Black Folks* by W. E. B. Dubois

In conclusion, psychological empowerment can have significant therapeutic effects by helping to reduce depression, anxiety, and symptoms associated with other aspects of racial trauma. In order to experience a sense of psychological empowerment, clients must increase their critical consciousness. You can help clients increase their critical consciousness and sense of psychological empowerment using strategies such as exploring personal narratives, group therapy, counterspaces, and bibliotherapy. The next section explores efforts therapists and clients can take to make a direct impact on societal factors that impinge on mental health and wellbeing.

Advocacy

As discussed throughout this chapter, one of the primary goals of psychological empowerment is increased social action (Zimmerman, 1995). Within the counseling and psychology literature, several terms are used to describe this type of social action, including change agent, social justice action, and social justice advocacy (Baker & Hansen, 1972; Lee & Hipolito-Delgado, 2007; Steele, 2008). In sum, these terms describe practices that are designed to "facilitate the removal of external and institutional barriers to clients' well-being" (Toporek, 2000, p. 6). In their delineation of the American Counseling Association's advocacy competencies, Lewis et al. (2003) developed what is perhaps the most comprehensive framework of knowledge, attitudes, and skills necessary for mental health professionals to facilitate change within social and political contexts. They described advocacy as dynamic and complex, a task that occurs on multiple levels (i.e., acting with and acting on behalf of clients on micro and macrolevels) and across several domains. These domains include client/student empowerment, client/student advocacy, community collaboration, systems advocacy, collective action (formerly public information), and social/political advocacy and are discussed in the paragraph that follows (Toporek & Daniels, 2018).

In the client/student empowerment domain, therapists assist clients in becoming empowered to advocate for themselves (Toporek & Daniels, 2018). This is accomplished by helping clients to examine their lives, and the impact of social, political, economic, and cultural factors on their development. In the client/student advocacy domain, therapists implement environmental interventions that help clients acquire access to needed services. Community collaboration involves working with community organizations to alert them to clients' issues and help them identify ways to be involved in the advocacy process. In the systems advocacy domain, therapists lead the advocacy process in school or community systems by working collaboratively to develop plans for implementing social change. In the collective action domain, therapists inform the public about the role of environmental factors in human development through written publications or other forms of public media. Finally, in the social/political advocacy domain, therapists work to influence public policy in large public arenas by taking social or political action such as lobbying legislators and other policymakers (Toporek & Daniels, 2018).

Within the African American community, advocacy and social activism have been a significant source of healing in response to the traumatic effects of racism. Al'Uqdah and Adomako (2018), for example, described advocacy for social reform as a catalyst in transforming grief and pain experienced by African American mothers whose children had been murdered because of their race. In particular, through the lives of women such as Mamie Bradley Till and other present day African American mothers who formed a coalition known as "Mothers of the Movement," we see the power of social justice advocacy to bring about several processes that aid healing from the loss of a loved one. These processes include meaning making, political mourning, and empowerment. For example, Al'Uqdah and Adomako (2018) noted that African American women who engage in behaviors such as political participation and organizational membership mentoring in response to the loss of their children find ways to personally cope, make meaning of their lives, and continue their roles as mothers. These behaviors, in turn, not only provide these women with ways to transform their grief, but they also ultimately transform the education, social, political, and economic welfare of their communities.

In the broader African American community, the personal and communal healing power of activism is also evidenced through the various sociopolitical movements aimed at eradicating anti-Black racism that have occurred over the past several decades. For example, the Black is Beautiful Movement of the 1960s led to a nationwide phenomenon that not only embraced the physical beauty of people of African descent, but their cultural and intellectual strengths as well, resulting in some healing of aspects of the African American psyche that had internalized the ideal of White beauty as superior (Steele & Newton, 2023; Workneh, 2022). More recently, the Black Lives Matter Movement has also sought to increase critical consciousness and address anti-Black racism. In their study of 12 Black Lives Matter activists, Mosley and her colleagues (2021) found that while involvement in the Black Lives Matter Movement had actually led to some experiences of racial trauma, activism had also led to the development of qualities that allowed the participants of their study to better process anti-Black racism. These qualities included cognitive growth, intersectional growth, and behavioral growth. According to Mosley and her colleagues (2021), cognitive growth is defined as increased awareness of anti-Black racism as a systemic rather than singularly interpersonal phenomenon. Intersectional growth includes greater awareness of the ways in which Black, religious and/or spiritual, gender, and sexual identities intersect and create differential positions of privilege and oppression. Behavioral growth consists of increased coping with racial trauma and the desire to enhance their agency as activists.

Beyond highlighting the ways in which African Americans learn to process anti-Black racism through advocacy efforts such as the Black Lives Matter Movement, the results of Mosley et al.'s (2021) study also provide a taxonomy of activism that describes the types of action individuals, including therapists, may engage to fight systemic racial oppression. These actions encompass a variety of epistemologies and culture-centered practices, including storying survival, artivism, physical resistance, organizing, teaching, coalition-building, modeling/mentoring, scholar-activism, and space-making. The Black racial justice activist approaches upon which this taxonomy is built include having urgency, being self-reflective, specifying focus, being actively intersectional, being resourceful, contextualizing, being present, and maintaining a future orientation. In terms of implications for clinical practice, the taxonomy and Black racial justice activist approaches together provide an indication of the culturally congruent interventions therapists may utilize as they engage advocacy efforts in the various domains described by Lewis and her colleagues (2003). The following section illustrates the application of Mosley et al.'s (2021) framework within the advocacy domains (Toporek & Daniels, 2018) by exploring the case of Matt, a psychologist who works in a university college counseling center.

Case Illustration: Matt

Matt is a novice psychologist who was hired at a university college counseling center approximately two years ago. Throughout his tenure in the counseling center, Matt has noticed certain themes reflected in the stories of many of the African American students he counsels. In particular, Matt has observed racial disparities in the overall student experience of these clients, especially as it relates to feeling integrated and accepted on their university's campus. For example, several African American students have reported stress and anxiety associated with their involvement in student activities, with these students noting racial differences in the amount of university funding student organizations receive and the types of vendors invited to campus events, as well as poor acknowledgment of events and celebrations significant to members of the African American community. Matt admits that while the inability to do things like buy Black Greek-letter paraphernalia at campus welcome activities or attend university sponsored Black History Month events may seem trivial, these deficits in campus culture send messages of exclusion and inferiority to the students they affect. Beyond this, Matt has additionally heard complaints about racial disparities in the academic aspects of campus life, including low numbers of African American faculty outside of the Black American Studies program, few African American advisors, and low retention of African American students in science, technology, engineering, and mathematics (STEM) programs. It is clear that these academic issues further contribute to the sense of isolation and lack of belonging African American students feel on the university's campus.

With his background in college student development, Matt understands that the difficulties African American students experience as it relates to poor social and academic integration not only affect their mental health, but their academic persistence and achievement as well (Tinto, 1975). Broadly, the student development literature suggests that the more integrated students are, the more likely they are to remain and do well in college (Morley, 2003). Unfortunately, African American students who attend predominantly White institutions (PWIs) tend to have less favorable interactions with faculty, especially when compared to African American students who attend historically Black colleges and universities (HBCUs), according to research (Allen, 1992). Moreover, research further suggests that these students, many of whom are accustomed to being part of smaller communities, also have concerns about themes that include fitting into the social landscape of their campuses, separation from family life, being placed socially by race/ethnicity, racial/ethnic accountability, the pervasiveness of White culture, the pursuit of a color-blind society, and the overrepresentation of minority students among weaker students (Morley, 2003, p. 168).

Given what he knows, Matt believes that part of his professional role as a psychologist in his university counseling center is to support the academic and social integration of his African American students by advocating for changes in the aspects of their college environment that contribute to negative racial dynamics in student integration. To do so, Matt began by first gathering data from his African American students concerning their perceptions of racial inequities on campus and the impact of these inequities on their mental health. After compiling this data, Matt presented his findings to the university counseling center's clinical director and sought permission to lead a consciousness-raising group focused on healing racial trauma and advocacy. Because Matt is not African American, he also sought permission to invite one of the African American doctoral students in counseling psychology to co-facilitate the group.

Once permission was granted, Matt worked with his co-facilitator to devise an initial outline of the group, identifying interventions for the client/ student and school/community levels of advocacy (Toporek & Daniels, 2018). At the client/student level, Matt and the co-facilitator implemented culturally-centered practices that provided participants with the space needed to examine environmental factors that impinge on their wellbeing and to also process and heal from racial trauma (Ratts & Hutchins, 2009). For example, consistent with the taxonomy of activism described by Mosley and her colleagues (2021), Matt and the co-facilitator guided the group participants in exercises that allowed them to share their stories, increase their coping skills, identify their strengths, learn more about anti-Black racism, and facilitate individual and collective empowerment. This resulted in the group's self-identification of actions they could take to organize and educate the broader campus community on anti-Black racism. Some of these actions included an art-hop event where African American students submitted graphic and mixed media pieces depicting their lived experiences on campus, a symposia series, and the formation of a special interest group consisting of African American students, faculty, and staff to study the problem and develop recommendations.

At the school/community level, Matt, his co-facilitator, the group's participants, and the other relevant stakeholders who had joined their advocacy efforts continued their coalition building, working with various university officials such as the head of registered student organizations, STEM program department chairs, and the university's diversity, equity, and inclusion officer to enact the recommendations developed by the special interest group. The group recognized that some of the recommendations, such as the inclusion of Black interests in campus event planning would be easy to implement; however, other efforts to bring about more systemic changes to faculty representation and student retention would take more time. Therefore, part of the group's planning at the school/community level included the development of an ongoing alliance between students and university officials, as well as regularly scheduled meetings to assess the effects of the group's work (Lopez-Baez & Paylo, 2009).

As illustrated in the case of Matt, advocacy is an activity that occurs with and on behalf of individuals affected by inequitable social policies and practices. Matt began his advocacy efforts on behalf of his students by collecting data and broaching the students' issues with his clinic director. However, as soon as possible, Matt engaged those directly affected by the systems of oppression evident in his concerns—that is, his students. This approach reflects further consistency with the philosophy of liberation psychology referenced throughout this chapter (e.g., Freire, 1993; French et al., 2020). Freire (1993), for example, argued that when students are given material based on real problems that are related to them as they live in the world as opposed to theoretical contexts, students "feel increasingly challenged and obliged to respond to that challenge" (p. 81). As therapists, it is important that we remember this key aspect of advocacy in order to avoid paternalism or other behaviors that may ultimately interfere with lasting change in inequitable environments.

Reflection 8.1: Dissecting the Role of Social Justice Advocacy in Clinical Practice

The topic of social justice advocacy has been somewhat controversial in the mental health profession. Some of this controversy surrounds the perceived liberal political agenda of social justice advocates, the marginalization of conservative counselors, and the inappropriate use of resources from professional organizations for social activism (Canfield, 2007, 2008a, 2008b; Harrist & Richardson, 2012; Hunsaker, 2008, 2011; King, 2010; Smith et al. 2009). Yet, research I previously conducted found that mental health professionals generally have positive attitudes toward social justice advocacy when it is broken down into its component attitudes and behaviors (Steele et al., 2014). If you are struggling to understand the place of social justice advocacy in your own professional role, exploration of its component attitudes and behaviors of social justice advocacy may help. You can begin by downloading your profession's description of advocacy from your code of ethics, relevant articles, or the ACA Advocacy Competencies (Toporek & Daniels, 2018), which are found here: (https://www.counseling.org/docs/default-source/competencies/aca-advocacy-competencies-updated-may-2020.pdf). Then, respond to the following questions:

1. What are the primary values of your profession as defined by your code of ethics, training, or membership in professional organizations?
2. What are your own professional values, personally?
3. How are your professional and personal values consistent with the task of social justice advocacy in your professional role?
4. How do your professional and personal values diverge with social justice advocacy in your professional role?
5. Think about the clients who are currently on your caseload. How might they be better supported through advocacy efforts on your part?
6. What other professionals or organizations can you partner with to meet client needs that you believe are outside of your professional role?

Anti-bias Strategies

Recall from Chapter 2 our discussion on microaggressions. They refer to subtle, often unintentional, put-downs that reflect prejudiced or discriminatory messages about minority groups (Sue et al., 2019). Recently, Sue and his colleagues (2019) introduced a specific type of anti-bias strategy, microinterventions, into the literature as a way to confront microaggressions. According to Sue and his colleagues (2019), *microinterventions* are defined as

> the everyday words or deeds, whether intentional or unintentional, that communicate to targets of microaggressions (a) validation of their experiential reality, (b) value as a person, (c) affirmation of their racial or group identity, (d) support and encouragement, and (e) reassurance that they are not alone.
>
> (p. 134)

More recently, these interventions were categorized into three distinct modes of action that include: (1) microaffirmations, (2) microprotections, and (3) microchallenges (Sue et al., 2021). *Microaffirmations* are small acts that affirm an individual's identity, experiential reality, or worth. Examples of microaffirmations include statements designed to support targets of discrimination, such as the anti-racist statements put out by many organizations in the wake of recent social unrest and police brutality, or words of validation commonly shared among targets and allies such as "I see you." *Microprotections* refer to proactive measures taken by influential figures to teach others about the reality of racism, promote cultural pride, and equip others to challenge bias and discrimination. These interventions occur between members of the same social identity and include traditional empowerment strategies such as consciousness-raising and teaching skills to deal with racism. Finally, *microchallenges* are direct actions taken to challenge biased and oppressive behaviors, policies, and practices. They may include directly confronting perpetrators, social advocacy, and civil disobedience such as protests or boycotts (Sue et al., 2021).

Microinterventions may be implemented by targets, bystanders, or allies (Sue et al., 2019, 2021). *Targets* are the individuals to whom microaggressions are directed. When microinterventions are implemented by targets, they not only challenge and disrupt ongoing bias and discrimination in the environment but also provide targets with a sense of psychological relief by better equipping targets to defend themselves. In sum, these defenses take the form of: (1) making the "invisible" visible, (2) disarming the microaggression, (3) educating the offender about the messages they send, and (4) including external support when needed (Sue et al., 2019). The strategies used to accomplish these objectives vary in their degree of subtlety and directness, ranging from simply naming the microaggression with a statement such as "That's a stereotype," to helping the perpetrator differentiate between intent and impact with a statement such as "You probably didn't mean it this way, but stereotypes like that hurt members of this group" (Sue et al., 2019, 2021). Other strategies include asking for clarification of a statement (e.g., "Do you really believe drug use is more accepted in the African American community?"), interrupting the communication (e.g., "Let's not go there"), or using a short exclamatory statement (e.g., "Ouch!"). For a complete discussion of microintervention tactics, the reader is referred to Sue et al. (2021); however, in this chapter, I return to the case of Jessica found in Chapter 6 to illustrate how a therapist may roleplay the use of microinterventions to address microaggressions experienced in the environment.

Case Illustration: Jessica

Jessica is a 45-year-old African American woman who was referred to therapy by her primary care physician for psychological evaluation after an unlawful arrest. Jessica completed her assessment and was diagnosed with PTSD. Due to the racial aspects of the case, Jessica's therapist believes a specifier of racial trauma more accurately describes her condition, although this is not an option with the current iteration of the *DSM*. Nevertheless, Jessica and the therapist have discussed racial trauma and developed an initial treatment plan focused on addressing her symptoms and facilitating empowerment. Throughout the course of therapy, Jessica has made significant progress, however, she continues to experience microaggressions when working with the attorney in her lawsuit against the police department. For example, Jessica reports that the attorney regularly makes glib statements such as asking if "the fathers" of her children are available for childcare during court appearances. Jessica says that she does not look down on women with multiple fathers of their children; however, assuming that she is one of these women is a stereotype.

Jessica feels stuck in her situation. She has already invested a significant amount of time and money in her attorney. Moreover, few attorneys were willing to take her case when she initiated the lawsuit. Recognizing that Jessica may be limited in her choice of attorneys, the therapist decided to teach Jessica about microinterventions. The session excerpt below illustrates psychoeducation on this topic as well as a roleplay of responses Jessica might give when targeted by microaggressions. Table 8.4 shows an updated treatment

Table 8.4 Jessica's Treatment Plan

Problem List
1. Depression, especially social withdrawal, fatigue, and poor concentration
2. Anger, especially irritability, humiliation, and resentment toward others
3. Reliving the trauma, including flashbacks and distressing memories
4. Difficulty leaving the house
5. Panic, including chest pain and shortness of breath
6. Microaggressions perpetrated by personal attorney in the wrongful arrest lawsuit

Treatment Goals:
1. Reduce the amount of emotional and mental distress experienced when thinking about or discussing the trauma (modify the negative self-appraisals in response to the event)
2. Reduce the occurrence of intrusive thoughts, arousal, and avoidance associated with the trauma
3. Increase the use of self-regulation skills and other positive coping strategies such as diaphragmatic breathing, mindfulness, self-compassion, prayer, positive racial identity development, and connections with social supports
4. Increase her sense of power in addressing the legal aspects of her unlawful arrest
5. Increase use of microinterventions to disarm microaggressions

Interventions
1. Psychoeducation focused on consciousness-raising and the nature of racial trauma
2. Relaxation and mindfulness training including the use of breathing exercises and loving-kindness meditations
3. Cognitive restructuring including the use of Socratic questioning, thought records, and modification of core beliefs
4. Participation in community support groups
5. Microintervention training

plan that includes additional goals and interventions to address the difficulties she experiences in her environment.

Therapist: Jessica, I hear that you often feel put down by some of the statements your attorney makes, is that correct?

Jessica: Absolutely. And it's hard to deal with because every time he makes these statements it's a reminder that some people will always assume things about me based on stereotypes—even people who are supposed to help me.

Therapist: I understand what you mean, Jessica. In fact, many people who experience what you describe feel the same way. There's even a term for these putdowns called *microaggressions*. Have you heard this term before?

Jessica: Actually, I have. It's exactly how I would describe what's happening to me.

Therapist: Well, as you stated, microaggressions can be hard to deal with because they accumulate and contribute to the stress you feel. Microaggressions can also be difficult to deal with because sometimes we don't know if the person understands what they are saying. At other times, what was said may even have been meant as a compliment. A common example of this is when someone is surprised that a Black person "speaks well." This suggests that "normally" Black people are unintelligent and inarticulate. Do you have any examples of microaggressions you've experienced besides those from your attorney?

Jessica: Yes, I do. People often say that natural hair looks good "on me," as if natural Black hairstyles usually look ugly.

Therapist: That's a great example, Jessica. Statements like that suggest that in most cases, people should strive toward Eurocentric standards of beauty. I imagine it can be hard to know what to say to that type of compliment because while the person who said it may have meant well, it's actually quite offensive.

Jessica: Exactly.

Therapist: Fortunately, there are certain strategies called microinterventions you can use to respond to microaggressions. Some of these strategies include making the "invisible" visible, disarming the microaggression, and educating the offender about the messages they send.

Jessica: Okay, I've never heard this before.

Therapist: Yeah, it's a recent addition to the literature. Maybe we could roleplay using some of these strategies today. Then, you could begin reading a book about microaggressions and we could do some more roleplaying at our next session. Does this sound okay?

Jessica: Sure.

Therapist: Great. So, one of the strategies I named was called making the invisible visible. One of the ways you can do this is by simply naming the stereotype behind what was said. For example, in response to a statement that a Black person speaks well, I might say something like, "I know you might not mean it this way, but when people make statements like that it implies that it's not normal for Black people to speak well."

Jessica: Okay, I get it.

Therapist: Good. Why don't you give it a try? How would you respond to a person who compliments you for wearing natural hair?

Jessica: Hmm...I guess I could say something like, "I know you might not mean it this way, but when people make statements like that it implies that Afro-textured hair isn't normally beautiful. It actually feels like an insult to people who have hair like mine."

Therapist: Great job, Jessica! How did it feel to give that response?

Jessica: It actually felt good. I guess I am worried that I would be too nervous to say something like that to my attorney, though.

Therapist: That's completely normal. Can I give you this book to borrow until our next session? It's called *Microintervention Strategies*. Why don't you read through Chapters 6, 7, and 8. This will give you more strategies and examples you can use. Then, at our next session, we can roleplay how you might respond to your attorney and examine any negative thoughts you might have about using these strategies. Would this be ok?

Jessica: Sounds good.

Therapist: Great.

As shown in the session excerpt between Jessica and her therapist, environmental interventions are often used in combination with each other. For example, in order for Jessica to be able to implement microinterventions, psychoeducation and roleplay were necessary to help increase Jessica's understanding of microaggressions and skillfully apply the interventions. In the remaining chapters, I combine all of the major ideas presented in this text thus far to explore how CBT including environmental interventions may be used to empower healing among African Americans experiencing racial issues while receiving treatment for depression, anxiety, and posttraumatic stress disorder.

References

Allen, W. R. (1992). The color of success: African-American college student outcomes at predominantly White and historically Black public colleges and universities. *Harvard Educational Review, 62*(1), 26–44. https://doi.org/10.17763/haer.62.1.wv5627665007v701

Al'Uqdah, S., & Adomako, F. (2018). From mourning to action: African American women's grief, pain, and activism. *Journal of Loss and Trauma, 23*(2), 91–98. https://doi.org/10.1080/15325024.2017.1393373

American Psychiatric Association. (2013). *Diagnostic and statistical manual of mental disorders* (5th ed.). American Psychiatric Association. https://doi.org/10.1176/appi.books.9780890425596

Baker, S., & Hansen, J. C. (1972). School counselor attitudes on a status quo-change agent measurement scale. *The School Counselor, 19*(2), 243–248.

Bhambhani, Y., & Gallo, L. (2022). Developing and adapting a mindfulness-based group intervention for racially and economically marginalized patients in the Bronx. *Cognitive and Behavioral Practice, 29*(4), 771–786. https://doi.org/10.1016/j.cbpra.2021.04.010

Bryant-Davis, T., Fasalojo, B., Arounian, A., Jackson, K. L., & Leithman, E. (2021). Resist and rise: A trauma-informed womanist model for group therapy. *Women & Therapy.* Advance online publication. https://doi.org/10.1080/02703149.2021.1943114

Byrd, J. A., Washington, A. R., Williams, J. M., & Lloyd, C. (2021). Reading woke: Exploring how school counselors may use bibliotherapy with adolescent Black boys. *Professional School Counseling.* Advance online publication. https://doi.org/10.1177/2156759X211040031

Canfield, B. S. (2007, December). Back to the future of counseling [From the President]. *Counseling Today*, p. 5.

Canfield, B. S. (2008a, January). Valuing diversity of thought [From the President]. *Counseling Today*, p. 5.

Canfield, B. S. (2008b, May). The informed counselor [From the President]. *Counseling Today*, p. 5.

Case, A. D., & Hunter, C. D. (2012). Counterspaces: A unit of analysis for understanding the role of settings in marginalized individuals' adaptive responses to oppression. *American Journal of Community Psychology, 50*(1–2), 257–270. https://doi.org/10.1007/s10464-012-9497-7

Chapman-Hilliard, C., & Beasley, S. T. (2018). "It's like power to move": Black students' psychosocial experiences in Black studies courses at a predominantly white institution. *Journal of Multicultural Counseling and Development, 46*(2), 129–151. https://doi.org/10.1002/jmcd.12097

Chioneso, N. A., Hunter, C. D., Gobin, R. L., McNeil Smith, S., Mendenhall, R., & Neville, H. A. (2020). Community healing and resistance through storytelling: A framework to address racial trauma in Africana communities. *Journal of Black Psychology, 46*(2–3), 95–121. https://doi.org/10.1177/0095798420929468

Cooper, A. A., & Conklin, L. R. (2015). Dropout from individual psychotherapy for major depression: A meta-analysis of randomized clinical trials. *Clinical Psychology Review, 40*, 57–65. https://doi.org/10.1016/j.cpr.2015.05.001

Curtis-Tweed, P. (2003). Experiences of African American empowerment: A Jamesian perspective on agency. *Journal of Moral Education, 32*(4), 397–409. https://doi.org/10.1080/0305724032000161295

Diemer, M. A., Rapa, L. J., Park, C. J., & Perry, J. C. (2017). Development and validation of the Critical Consciousness Scale. *Youth & Society, 49*(4), 461–483. https://doi.org/10.1177/0044118X14538289

Ford, D. Y., Walters, N. M., Byrd, J. A., & Harris, B. N. (2019). I want to read about me: Engaging and empowering gifted Black girls using multicultural literature and bibliotherapy. *Gifted Child Today*, *42*(1), 53–57. https://doi.org/10.1177/107621 7518804851

Freire, P. (1993). *Pedagogy of the oppressed*. The Continuum International Publishing Group.

French, B. H., Lewis, J. A., Mosley, D. V., Adames, H. Y., Chavez-Dueñas, N. Y., Chen, G. A., & Neville, H. A. (2020). Toward a psychological framework of radical healing in communities of color. *The Counseling Psychologist*, *48*(1), 14–46. https://doi.org/10.1177/0011000019843506

Graham-LoPresti, J. R., Gautier, S. W., Sorenson, S., & Hayes-Skelton, S. A. (2017). Culturally sensitive adaptations to evidence-based cognitive behavioral treatment for social anxiety disorder: A case paper. *Cognitive and Behavioral Practice*, *24*(4), 459–471. https://doi.org/10.1016/j.cbpra.2016.12.003

Gutiérrez, L. M. (1995). Understanding the empowerment process: Does consciousness make a difference? *Social Work Research*, *19*(4), 229–237.

Gutiérrez, N. Y. (2022). *The pain we carry: Healing from complex PTSD for people of color*. New Harbinger Publications, Inc.

Hays, R. E., & Lyons, S. J. (1981). The bridge drawing: A projective technique for assessment in art therapy. *The Arts in Psychotherapy*, *8*(3–4), 207–217. https://doi.org/10.1016/0197-4556(81)90033-2

Harrist, S., & Richardson, F. C. (2012). Disguised ideologies in counseling and social justice work. *Counseling and Values*, *57*(1), 38–44. https://doi.org/10.1002/j.2161-007X.2012.00006.x

Hickson, J. M., Paul, R. J., Perkins, A. C., Anderson, C. R., & Pittman, D. M. (2022). Sankofa: A testimony of the restorative power of Black activism in the self-care practices of Black activists. *Journal of Black Psychology*, *48*(3–4), 448–474. https://doi.org/10.1177/00957984211015572

Hunsaker, R. (2008, April). Social justice: An inconvenient irony [Opinion]. *Counseling Today*, pp. 21, 43.

Hunsaker, R. C. (2011). Counseling and social justice. *Academic Questions*, *24*(3), 319–340.

Hynes, A. M., & Hynes-Berry, M. (2012). *Bibliotherapy—The interactive process: A handbook*. North Star Press.

Iwamasa, G. Y., & Hays, P. A. (Eds.). (2019). *Culturally responsive cognitive-behavioral therapy: Practice and supervision* (2nd ed.). American Psychological Association. https://doi.org/10.1037/0000119-000

Johnson, V. E., & Carter, R. T. (2020). Black cultural strengths and psychosocial well-being: An empirical analysis with Black American adults. *Journal of Black Psychology*, *46*(1), 55–89. https://doi.org/10.1177/0095798419889752

Kabat-Zinn, J. (2013). *Full catastrophe living: How to cope with stress, pain and illness with mindfulness meditation*. Piatkus Books.

Kelly, S. (2019). Cognitive behavior therapy with African Americans. In G. Y. Iwamasa & P. A. Hays (Eds.), *Culturally responsive cognitive behavior therapy: Practice and supervision* (pp. 105–128). American Psychological Association. https://doi.org/10.1037/0000119-005

King, J. H. (2010, June). Are professional counselors becoming social workers? [Opinion]. *Counseling Today*, p. 51.

Lee, C. C., & Hipolito-Delgado, C. P. (2007). Introduction: Counselors as agents of social justice. In C. C. Lee (Ed.), *Counseling for social justice* (2nd ed., pp. xiii–xxviii). American Counseling Association.

Lewis, J., Arnold, M., House, R., & Toporek, R. (2003). *ACA advocacy competencies*. American Counseling Association. https://www.counseling.org/Resources/Competencies/Advocacy_Competencies.pdf

Lopez-Baez, S. I., & Paylo, M. J. (2009). Social justice advocacy: Community collaboration and systems advocacy. *Journal of Counseling & Development*, 87(3), 276–283. https://doi.org/10.1002/j.1556-6678.2009.tb00107.x

Lu, J. H., & Steele, C. K. (2019) 'Joy is resistance': Cross-platform resilience and (re)invention of Black oral culture online. *Information, Communication & Society*, 22(6), 823–837. https://doi.org/10.1080/1369118X.2019.1575449

McBride, D. F. (2011). Manifesting empowerment: How a family health program can address racism. *Journal of Black Psychology*, 37(3), 336–356. https://doi.org/10.1177/0095798410390690

Menakem, R. (2017). *My grandmother's hands: Racialized trauma and the pathway to mending our hearts and bodies*. Central Recovery Press.

Morley, K. M. (2003). Fitting in by race/ethnicity: The social and academic integration of diverse students at a large predominantly white university. *Journal of College Student Retention: Research, Theory and Practice*, 5(2), 147–174. https://doi.org/10.2190/K1KF-RTLW-1DPW-T4CC

Mosley, D. V., Hargons, C. N., Meiller, C., Angyal, B., Wheeler, P., Davis, C., & Stevens-Watkins, D. (2021). Critical consciousness of anti-Black racism: A practical model to prevent and resist racial trauma. *Journal of Counseling Psychology*, 68(1), 1–16. https://doi.org/10.1037/cou0000430

Okeke-Adeyanju, N., Taylor, L. C., Craig, A. B., Smith, R. E., Thomas, A., Boyle, A. E., & DeRosier, M. E. (2014). Celebrating the strengths of Black youth: Increasing self-esteem and implications for prevention. *The Journal of Primary Prevention*, 35(5), 357–369. https://doi.org/10.1007/s10935-014-0356-1

Packnett, B. (2017, August 21). I'm an activist, and joy is my resistance. *Self*. https://www.self.com/story/charlottesville-joy-is-resistance

Rathod, S., Kingdon, D., Pinninti, N., Turkington, D., & Phiri, P. (2015). *Cultural adaptation of CBT for serious mental illness: A guide for training and practice*. Wiley Blackwell. https://doi.org/10.1002/9781118976159

Ratts, M. J., & Hutchins, A. M. (2009). ACA advocacy competencies: Social justice advocacy at the client/student level. *Journal of Counseling & Development*, 87(3), 269–275. https://doi.org/10.1002/j.1556-6678.2009.tb00106.x

Smith, S. D., Reynolds, C. A., & Rovnak, A. (2009). A critical analysis of the social advocacy movement in counseling. *Journal of Counseling & Development*, 87(4), 483–491. https://doi.org/10.1002/j.1556-6678.2009.tb00133.x

Solórzano, D., Ceja, M., & Yosso, T. (2000). Critical race theory, racial microaggressions, and campus racial climate: The experiences of African American college students. *Journal of Negro Education*, 69(1–2), 60–73.

Steele, J. M. (2008). Preparing counselors to advocate for social justice: A liberation model. *Counselor Education and Supervision*, 48(2), 74–85. https://doi.org/10.1002/j.1556-6978.2008.tb00064.x

Steele, J. M. (2020). A CBT approach to internalized racism among African Americans. *International Journal for the Advancement of Counselling, 42*(3), 217–233. https://doi.org/10.1007/s10447-020-09402-0

Steele, J. M., Bischof, G. H., & Craig, S. E. (2014). Political ideology and perceptions of social justice advocacy among members of the American Counseling Association. *International Journal for the Advancement of Counselling, 36*(4), 450–467. https://doi.org/10.1007/s10447-014-9217-0

Steele, J. M., & Newton, C. S. (2023). *Black lives are beautiful: 50 tools to heal from trauma and promote positive racial identity*. Routledge.

Steele, J. M., & Newton, C. S. (2022). Culturally adapted cognitive behavior therapy as a model to address internalized racism among African American clients. *Journal of Mental Health Counseling, 44*(2), 98–116. https://doi.org/10.17744/mehc.44.2.01

Sue, D. W., Alsaidi, S., Awad, M. N., Glaeser, E., Calle, C. Z., & Mendez, N. (2019). Disarming racial microaggressions: Microintervention strategies for targets, White allies, and bystanders. *American Psychologist, 74*(1), 128–142. https://doi.org/10.1037/amp0000296

Sue, D. W., Calle, C. Z., Mendez, N., Alsaidi, S., & Glaeser, E. (2021). *Microintervention strategies: What you can do to disarm and dismantle individual and systemic racism and bias*. John Wiley & Sons, Inc.

Terry, C. L., Sr., Flennaugh, T. K., Blackmon, S. M., & Howard, T. C. (2014). Does the "Negro" "still" need separate schools? Single-sex educational settings as critical race counterspaces. *Urban Education, 49*(6), 666–697.

Tichavakunda, A. A. (2022). Taking Black joy seriously in higher education. *Change: The Magazine of Higher Learning, 54*(5), 52–56. https://doi.org/10.1080/00091383.2022.2101868

Tinto, V. (1975). Dropout from higher education: A theoretical synthesis of recent research. *Review of Educational Research, 45*(1), 89–125. https://doi.org/10.3102/00346543045001089

Toporek, R. L. (2000). Developing a common language and framework for understanding advocacy in counseling. In J. Lewis & L. Bradley (Eds.), *Advocacy in counseling: Counselors, clients & community* (pp. 5–14). ERIC Clearinghouse on Counseling and Student Services.

Toporek, R. L., & Daniels, J. (2018). *American Counseling Association advocacy competencies* (updated 2018). American Counseling Association. https://www.counseling.org/docs/default-source/competencies/aca-advocacy-competencies-updated-may-2020.pdf

Turner, E. A., Harrell, S. P., & Bryant-Davis, T. (2022). Black Love, Activism, and Community (BLAC): The BLAC model of healing and resilience. *Journal of Black Psychology, 48*(3–4), 547–568. https://doi.org/10.1177/00957984211018364

van der Kolk, B. A. (2014). *The body keeps the score: Brain, mind, and body in the healing of trauma*. Penguin Random House.

Watson-Singleton, N. N., Black, A. R., & Spivey, B. N. (2019). Recommendations for a culturally-responsive mindfulness-based intervention for African Americans. *Complementary Therapy in Clinical Practice, 34*, 132–138. https://doi.org/10.1016/j.ctcp.2018.11.013

Watts, R. J. (2004). Integrating social justice and psychology. *The Counseling Psychologist, 32*(6), 855–865. https://doi.org/10.1177/0011000042692

Watts, R. J., Abdul-Adil, J. K., & Pratt, T. (2002). Enhancing critical consciousness in young African American men: A psychoeducational approach. *Psychology of Men & Masculinity, 3*(1), 41–50. https://doi.org/10.1037/1524-9220.3.1.41

West, N. M. (2019). In the company of my sister-colleagues: Professional counter-spaces for African American women student affairs administrators. *Gender and Education, 31*(4), 543–559. https://doi.org/10.1080/09540253.2018.1533926

Williams, M. T., Holmes, S., Zare, M., Haeny, A., & Faber, S. (2022a). An evidence-based approach for treating stress and trauma due to racism. *Cognitive and Behavioral Practice.* Advance online publication. https://doi.org/10.1016/j.cbpra.2022.07.001

Williams, M. T., Osman, M., Gallo, J., Pereira, D. P., Gran-Ruaz, S., Strauss, D., Lester, L., George, J. R., Edelman, J., & Litman, L. (2022b). A clinical scale for the assessment of racial trauma. *Practice Innovations, 7*(3), 223–240. https://doi.org/10.1037/pri0000178

Williams, M., & Zare, M. (2022). A psychometric investigation of racial trauma symptoms using a semi-structured clinical interview with a trauma checklist (UnRESTS). *Chronic Stress, 6*, 1–11. https://doi.org/10.1177/24705470221145126

Workneh, L. (2022, January/February). The rise of the Black is Beautiful revolution. *Essence*, 80–83.

Zimmerman, M. A. (1995). Psychological empowerment: Issues and illustrations. *American Journal of Community Psychology, 23*(5), 581–599. https://doi.org/10.1007/BF02506983

Chapter 9

Putting It All Together

Major Depressive Disorder

Depression is a significant issue in the African American community. While the overall lifetime prevalence of Major Depressive Disorder (MDD) is lower for African Americans than it is for White Americans, 10.4 percent compared to 17.9 percent, respectively, the chronicity of MDD has been found to be higher for African Americans than it is for White Americans, 56.0 percent compared to 38.6 percent, according to one report (Bailey et al., 2019). Yet, although MDD is more chronic in the African American community, some research suggests that less than half seek treatment for depression despite rating their condition as severe or disabling (D. R. Williams et al., 2007). Statistics from the Substance Abuse and Mental Health Services Administration (2022), for example, show that among adults who had a past year Major Depressive Episode (MDE) with severe impairment, Black adults were less likely than White adults to receive treatment for depression (52.5 vs. 68.6 percent).

For African Americans, perceived racial discrimination is a common precipitant to depression. Broadly, *perceived racial discrimination* may be defined as one's felt experience of unjust, prejudicial treatment on the basis of their racial status (D. R. Williams, 2018). While an in-depth review of how perceived racial discrimination functions as a chronic stressor within various stress and coping frameworks is beyond the scope of this chapter, the integrated framework developed by Vines et al. (2017) based on their review of the literature provides insight into the ways in which perceived racial discrimination diminishes psychological wellbeing. According to their model, the persistent and unpredictable nature of exposure to discrimination can diminish one's protective psychological resources over time, which, in turn, can lead to maladaptive behaviors and weaken emotional control, worsening mental health. Conversely, in their model, mental health also has the potential to negatively affect health behaviors, creating an adverse cyclical pattern. This process, however, is influenced by factors such as family context, for example, socialization or parenting practices, as well as demographic variables, for example, socioeconomic status, which all influence the

DOI: 10.4324/9781003196303-9

degree to which an individual perceives discrimination as a stressor and its subsequent effect on mental health (Vines et al., 2017).

This chapter and those that follow culminate this text with case example application of the concepts discussed throughout the earlier chapters of the book. The current chapter applies culturally adapted CBT to the treatment of depression among African Americans who experience stress from racial discrimination. The chapter begins with a review of depression and its primary features, followed by further exploration of depression and the role of racial discrimination. Cognitive conceptualization and treatment planning are then discussed, with client dialogues integrated as appropriate. Each stage of therapy is explored, starting with assessment and rapport building in the first session of therapy, followed by a discussion of the working and termination phases of therapy.

Understanding Depression

According to the *Diagnostic and Statistical Manual of Mental Disorders, Fifth Edition* (*DSM-5*), depressive disorders refer to several clinical conditions, including Disruptive Mood Dysregulation Disorder, Major Depressive Disorder, Persistent Depressive Disorder, Premenstrual Dysphoric Disorder, and Substance/Medication-Induced Depressive Disorder (American Psychiatric Association, 2013). This chapter focuses on Major Depressive Disorder (MDD).

Individuals must experience five or more symptoms of depression during the same two-week period to be diagnosed with MDD (American Psychiatric Association, 2013). The primary feature of MDD is a depressed mood and/or loss of interest or pleasure in daily activities. In addition to depressed mood and/or loss of interest or pleasure in daily activities, individuals may also experience significant weight changes, sleep disturbances, psychomotor difficulties, fatigue or loss of energy, feelings of worthlessness or inappropriate guilt, poor concentration or indecisiveness, or recurrent thoughts of death, suicidal ideation without a specific plan, or a suicide attempt or a specific plan for suicide (American Psychiatric Association, 2013). These symptoms must cause significant distress in one's social, occupational, or psychological functioning and not be attributable to the effects of a substance or medical condition.

Criteria provided in the *DSM-5* describe the diagnostic features of MDD; however, extant research offers additional insight into culture-related issues in the diagnosis of MDD in African American clients. Research conducted by Payne (2014), for example, found that study participants who were presented with videos of a male client with depressive symptoms influenced by social determinants were less accurate in their diagnoses than were participants presented with videos of a male client exhibiting classic depressive symptoms. To derive this finding, Payne (2014) developed two cases of a man with more than five of the criteria necessary for diagnosis of MDD, one with classic depressive symptoms and another with symptoms affected by social determinants. Socially determined symptoms were defined as those that develop in response to social factors like invisibility or microaggressions, and included irritable mood or hostility, decreased verbalization of symptoms, and psychomotor retardation, which may be interpreted as indifference or laziness in African Americans. One White and one Black actor who were of similar age and physical build, wore identical attire, and used standardized verbal and nonverbal behaviors read both the classic and socially determined cases and participants were randomly assigned to one of the four treatment conditions.

As stated, results of Payne's (2014) study showed that participants were less able to accurately diagnose the client with socially determined clinical symptoms. Specifically, participants provided diagnoses that were more behavioral in nature for the clients who presented with socially determined symptoms than they did for clients with classic depression symptoms. Participants additionally considered personality disorders with a poor prognosis, as well as psychotic disorders, even in the absence of hallucinations, delusions, or other psychotic symptoms for the client with symptoms influenced by social determinants. This suggests that when working with African American clients, therapists should be aware of the different ways in which depression symptoms present among African Americans due to their marginalized identities. As discussed in Chapter 4, the findings of Payne's (2014) study further suggest that therapists who work with African American clients should also be cognizant of the role implicit bias may play in the diagnosis of MDD in this population and be proactive in developing awareness of and bracketing this bias.

Depression in African Americans and the Role of Racial Discrimination

While the previously mentioned study conducted by Payne (2014) highlights the unique ways depressive symptoms may present in response to socially determined factors, a substantial body of research provides additional insight into the relationship between racial discrimination and depression (Britt-Spells et al., 2018; Pascoe & Smart Richman, 2009; Pieterse et al., 2012). In terms of suicidality, one study of African Americans found that perceived racial discrimination was both directly and indirectly associated with suicide ideation in a sample of African American men and women (Walker et al., 2014). In another study, researchers found that experienced, anticipated, and vicarious racial and ethnic discrimination were associated with an increased risk of depression and suicidal behavior among African

American and Hispanic youth living in Chicago neighborhoods (Zimmerman & Miller-Smith, 2022). Associations between racial discrimination and depression beyond classic symptoms have also been found as it relates to emotional eating (Hoggard et al., 2019), somatic symptoms (Holden et al., 2015), a sense of straddling two worlds (Walton, 2022), and decreased resilience (Keith et al., 2010). Furthermore, the effects of racial discrimination may additionally put African Americans at risk for increased alcohol use and related problems through depressive symptoms (Su et al., 2021). In sum, these findings highlighting the need for depression treatment that is sensitive to the experience of racial discrimination within this population and considerate of their unique, culturally derived approaches to healing.

Beyond direct experiences with racism, vicarious trauma associated with witnessing racial discrimination has also been found to result in depression among African Americans. This fact is perhaps illustrated most impactfully through the African American response to the several incidents of police brutality highlighted throughout the media over the past decade. A study conducted by Das et al. (2021), for example, found that recent publicized police killings of unarmed African Americans resulted in an 11 percent increase in emergency department visits related to depression among African Americans in the concurrent month and three months following the exposure. Similarly, another report found that according to Gallup data, in the week following the murder of George Floyd, anger and sadness increased to unprecedented levels in the U.S. population, with more than a third of individuals surveyed reporting these emotions (Eichstaedt et al., 2021). For African Americans, these increases were even more pronounced, with nearly half reporting feelings of anger and sadness. The authors of the report further indicated that according to U.S. Census Household Pulse data, in the week following Floyd's death, depression and anxiety severity increased among Black Americans at significantly higher rates than that of White Americans, corresponding to an additional 900,000 Black Americans who would have screened positive for depression.

Within the African American population, internalized racism is yet another aspect of racial oppression with significant correlates to depression. As discussed in Chapter 2, *internalized racism* refers to a negative view of oneself based on the perceived inferiority of one's own cultural or racial group (Bailey et al., 2014). Researchers such as Bivens (1995, 2005) differentiate this construct from other similar psychological issues such as low self-esteem in that internalized racism results in ideas and behaviors that reinforce racial oppression. While one of the more significant outcomes of internalized racism is that it results in feelings of shame, alienation, and powerlessness that limit one's perceived ability to enact change in their environments, another significant consequence of internalized racism is the psychological distress that occurs when African Americans internalize messages about the superiority of White culture and accept negative stereotypes about their own racial/ethnic group (Bailey et al., 2014). A study conducted by Mouzon and McLean (2017), for example, found a significant relationship between measures of internalized racism and depression among a sample of 4,573 African American and Caribbean Black adults. Likewise, other studies have also found significant relationships between internalized racism and depression among college students (Fuller-Rowell et al., 2021), as well as in other large samples of African American and Caribbean Blacks (Molina & James, 2016).

From a CBT perspective, internalized racism may be conceptualized as an outcome of life experiences and societal influences that have a negative impact on race-related aspects of an individual's core beliefs. In Chapter 2, I discussed a cognitive developmental model of internalized racism that describes cognitive processes that occur once internalized racist beliefs are activated, as well as contextual factors that influence the development and maintenance of these beliefs (J. M. Steele, 2020). In this model, societal influences, along with individual childhood experiences, affect the core beliefs African Americans develop about themselves, other people, and their world, as well as the assumptions and rules they establish to guide their behavior in consideration of these beliefs. Once developed, this hierarchy of beliefs is reinforced through interactions that strengthen the sense of inferiority, shame, and powerlessness experienced within this group. Resulting race-related beliefs and continued exposure to racist interactions, in turn, act as an additional lens through which everyday situations are interpreted, leading to subsequent emotional, behavioral, and physiological reactions.

Recently, James (2021) offered additional empirical support to delineate the underlying mechanisms contributing to the association between internalized racism and poor mental health. To conduct his study, James (2021) explored the relationship between core self-evaluation traits, internalized racism, and poor mental health among 780 Black/African American adults. In the study, core self-evaluation traits included self-esteem, emotional stability, generalized self-efficacy, and locus of control. Results of the study indicate that self- and group focused internalized racism predicted greater depression symptoms and lower self-esteem and emotional stability among participants, while both forms of internalized racism were associated with increased internal locus of control and were not associated with generalized self-efficacy. According to the researcher, this suggests that internalized racism may be related to depression via the more affective aspects of core self-evaluation relative to its motivational components. When considered within the context of using CBT to empower healing from racism, this may further suggest a need to prioritize managing the emotional impacts of internalized racism during the initial phases of treatment.

Besides the affective aspects of core self-evaluation, several cultural factors also moderate the relationship between racist experiences and depression. A study conducted by Graham et al. (2015), for example, found that valued living was significantly negatively correlated with depressive symptoms. In this study, valued living was defined as "attending to and making choices based on one's values (i.e., the things that are meaningful and matter to an individual)" (Graham et al., 2015, p. 49). As such, the researchers concluded that engaging in actions consistent with what matters to the individual may buffer the negative emotional impact of racist experiences.

Somewhat relatedly, Powell et al. (2017) explored the role of forgiveness in coping with everyday racial discrimination and found that letting go of negative emotion or letting go of negative emotion combined with embracing positive emotion were directly related to lower depressive symptoms. Similar results were found in a study conducted by Brooks et al. (2021). This suggests that CBT approaches that integrate spirituality or other value systems that emphasize forgiveness may enhance treatment. Other cultural factors that reduce depressive symptoms include Africentric coping (i.e., cognitive-emotive coping, ritual-centered coping, emotional debriefing, and communalistic coping; Gaylord-Harden & Cunningham, 2009), racial identity (Jones et al., 2021), social support (i.e., friends, family, support groups), religion (i.e., prayer, church, spirituality), avoidance (i.e., attempting to avoid stressors), and problem-focused coping (i.e., confronting the situation directly) (Jacob et al., 2023).

At the community level, research has also shown that perceptions of neighborhood social cohesion may protect against racial discrimination for African American adolescents (Saleem et al., 2018). Additionally, this research furthers indicates that when boys perceive less neighborhood disorganization, racial discrimination has a greater influence on their depressive symptoms. As such, attention to the role of both intraindividual and environmental factors may be necessary for effective treatment within this population.

The Cognitive Triad

The cognitive triad is part of a larger cognitive theory of depression originally developed by Aaron T. Beck in 1976. In this theory, depression is conceptualized within a vulnerability-stress framework comprised of four vulnerabilities: depressogenic schemata, cognitive errors, the cognitive triad, and automatic thoughts (Sacco et al., 2023). *Depressogenic schemata* refer to relatively enduring stored representations of meaning used to organize information in ways that determine how new experiences are perceived and conceptualized. These schemas are characterized by heightened sensitivity to negative stimuli as well as internal structures that refer exclusively to the self and are therefore self-referent (Clark et al., 1999). Moreover, depresso-genic schemata may be described as containing chronic misconceptions, dis-torted attitudes, invalid premises, and unrealistic goals that are dominated by themes of personal deficiency, self-blame, and negative expectations. The second aspect of Beck's theory, *cognitive errors*, refer to distorted percep-tions of reality that among depressed individuals are applied in a systemic manner resulting in bias against the self. According to Beck (1963, 1976), these distortions tend to reflect arbitrary inference, selective abstraction, overgeneralization, magnification/minimization, dichotomous thinking, and personalization thinking errors.

During an activating event, depressogenic schemata trigger cognitive errors that lead to negative shifts in how an individual perceives self, the world, and the future (Clark et al., 1999). These negative views about self, the world, and the future are known as the *cognitive triad*. Negative self-appraisals refer to views of oneself as inadequate, unworthy, or unlovable, which, according to Sacco et al. (2023), contributes to an inability to attain goals and adequately perform tasks (e.g., "All of my difficulties are my own fault," J. M. Steele & Newton, 2022). Negative views of the world involve perceived limitations due to one's social context (e.g., "Everyone is against me, nothing I can do will matter" J. M. Steele & Newton, 2022). Finally, negative views of the future involve pessimistic predictions that the future will consist of continued hardships, as well as beliefs that current difficulties are hopeless (e.g., "Things will always stay the same," J. M. Steele & Newton, 2022). When activated, the negative views of the cognitive triad manifest into negative automatic thoughts, leading to subsequent depressive symp-toms (Sacco et al., 2023).

Berghuis et al. (2020) noted that without stress activating depressogenic schemata, individuals who hold such schemata are no more likely to become depressed than those who do not hold such schemata. Accordingly, "depres-sogenic schemata are thought to remain inactive until activated in response to stressful events, which subsequently leads to depressive symptoms" (Berghuis et al., 2020, p. 649). This may explain the chronic nature of depres-sion among African Americans referenced in the introduction to this chap-ter, given the ongoing and insidious nature of racism. In fact, one recent study of perceived discrimination as a stressor in Beck's cognitive theory of depression found that everyday experiences with discrimination is a statisti-cally significant predictor of negative views of self, the world, and the future among one sample of college students (Sacco et al., 2023). Moreover, the results of this study further suggested that perceived everyday discrimina-tion more strongly predicts negative views of the world than the negative views of the self and future, which the study's researchers argue is consistent with conceptualizations of perceived everyday discrimination as a stressor that is primarily social in nature. Similarly, another recent study of perceived everyday discrimination, the cognitive triad, and depressive symptoms among 9th grade students at an inner-city public high school also found that perceived everyday discrimination was a significant predictor of the cognitive triad, although the cognitive triad only partially mediated the relationship between perceived everyday discrimination and depressive symptoms (Berghuis et al., 2020).

Assessment

There are several formalized assessments of depression. The Beck Depression Inventory-II (BDI-II; A. T. Beck et al., 1996) is one of the more commonly used assessments. This inventory is a 21-item self-report scale that measures the severity of depression in adults and adolescents aged 13 years and older. Total scores from 0 to 13 points are considered to reflect a minimal level of depression; scores of 14 to 19 indicate mild depression; scores of 20 to 28 reflect moderate depression; and scores of 29 to 63 indicate severe depression. Symptoms assessed on the BDI-II are consistent with depression criteria identified in the most recent version of the *DSM* at the time of the measure's development, the *DSM-IV* (A. T. Beck et al., 1996).

Another assessment of depression more theoretically grounded in CBT is the Cognitive Triad Inventory (Beckham et al., 1986). This assessment was developed as a quantification of Beck's cognitive triad. As such, this 36-item instrument consists of three factors: self, world, and future. Broadly, the scale showed good internal consistency in its initial development (Beckham et al., 1986), as well as in versions translated into different languages, including German (Pössel, 2009), Polish (Śliwerski, 2014), and Turkish (Erarslan & Işikli, 2019).

Children's versions of the Beck (J. S. Beck et al., 2005) and Cognitive Triad (Kaslow et al., 1992) inventories are also available. The Beck Depression Inventory-Youth (BDI-Y) is a 20-item self-report scale that measures the severity of depression in children and adolescents. Unlike its adult counterpart, the BDI-Y measures children's negative thoughts about themselves, their world, and their future. Items 3, 11, 13, and 15 measure a negative view of self. Item 1 measures a negative view of the world. Item 20 measures hopelessness or a negative view of the future. Items 5 and 9 measure vegetative and somatic symptoms. Items 2, 4, and 16 measure motivational aspects of depression. The remaining items measure emotional symptoms of depression. Total raw scores may range from 0 to 60; however, these scores are converted to *T* scores. *T* scores of 70 or more are extremely elevated, 60 to 69 moderately elevated, 55 to 59 mildly elevated, and *T* scores of 54 or below average. The other measure of Beck's cognitive triad for children and adolescents, the Cognitive Triad Inventory-Children (CTI-C), is also widely used, although test-retest reliability scores for the future subscale of the assessment were significantly lower for African American than for White adolescents in one analysis of the measure (Greening et al., 2005). According to the researchers who conducted this analysis, this finding may be a function of African American adolescents' cognitions about their future within the context of discrimination and limited opportunities, emphasizing the need for culturally responsive assessment and case conceptualization.

Activity Scheduling

Activity scheduling, also known as *behavioral activation*, is an intervention designed to have a positive impact on mood by increasing client engagement in activities that offer a sense of pleasure and accomplishment (J. S. Beck, 2020). Within the literature, behavioral activation is often considered a standalone treatment for depression due to its ability to help clients become more actively engaged in their environments, which acts as an anti-depressant through the positive reinforcement received from the environment (Wenzel, 2019). To use behavioral activation, therapists should first ask clients to monitor how they currently spend their time. This includes recording the activities they engage in on a daily basis and rating the amount of *pleasure* and *accomplishment* they feel as a result of completing each activity on a scale of 1 to 10. After gaining a baseline of their current activity levels, therapists should then ask clients to draw conclusions from what they have recorded and identify activities that would introduce more pleasure and accomplishment in their lives. Next, the client and therapist work together to strategically schedule activities throughout each day to increase the number of opportunities clients have to feel good. For clients who have difficulty identifying activities they enjoy, it may be beneficial to help clients devise a list of activities prior to implementing the intervention.

Culturally Adapted Cognitive Restructuring

In the previous section, behavioral activation was identified as the primary treatment for depression; however, this intervention may be enhanced by additionally integrating restructuring of the client's negative automatic thoughts and underlying cognitions (M. M. Carter, 1999). This includes the integration of strategies that help clients identify, evaluate, and modify negative thoughts such as thought records and Socratic questioning, as well as behavioral experiments that help clients directly test their thoughts in the environment. Among African Americans, extant research shows that this type of integrated approach to depression treatment is effective. One single-case study of an African American female veteran, for example, found that integrated CBT treatment inclusive of psychological symptom and behavioral monitoring, thought stopping, cognitive restructuring, deep breathing, calming thoughts, social support, sleep hygiene, and problem-solving skills was effective in reducing depressive symptoms according to scores on the Patient Health Questionnaire-8 (Trahan et al., 2016). Similarly, a study of African American women participating in an integrated substance abuse and HIV program also found that an approach that includes cognitive restructuring may be effective in the reduction of depression symptoms according to scores on the Beck Depression Inventory (Nobles et al., 2009). The program, which was based on a conceptual framework called "culture-cology" and an African-centered behavioral change model, utilized cognitive restructuring as one aspect of a process called culturalization, "wherein the person minimizes negative social conditions and maximizes conditions that are prosocial and life affirming" (Nobles et al., 2009, p. 231). According to the study's authors, this approach had the effect of reconfiguring how one thinks about self and the world, which, in turn, allowed participants to gain a better understanding of their rightful place of rulership and self-governance from the African-centered perspective.

Case Illustration: Savion

Savion is a 23-year-old African American man in his first year of enrollment at a predominantly White medical school. He initiated therapy approximately three months after beginning classes, endorsing both mood and interpersonal difficulties. At intake, Savion reported that he has struggled to form connections with his peers and faculty, sharing as an example one recent experience where he was the only student left out of a group assignment. Savion admitted feeling slightly embarrassed but also irritated in response to the situation, thinking, "Am I really that different?" Beyond increased irritability, other symptoms endorsed by Savion at intake included sadness, withdrawal, insomnia, anxiety, fatigue, poor concentration, and weight loss. Savion denied past or present thoughts, plan, or attempts to die by suicide.

Savion scored a 25 on the BDI-II, which is in the moderate range. Based on his score on the BDI-II, data obtained in his initial evaluation session, as well as his report of difficulties in his academic and social functioning, he was diagnosed by his therapist with F32.1 Major Depressive Disorder, Single Episode, Moderate, with Anxious Distress. His difficulties with anxiety did not appear to meet criteria for an anxiety disorder. He had no previous history of diagnosed psychiatric disorder and had never received mental health services.

In discussing his relevant social history, Savion reported being raised in New York City in a household headed by a single mother. Savion, who is an only child, described his relationship with his mother as "close," expressing deep admiration and appreciation for the sacrifices she made for him while he was growing up. According to Savion, his mother worked and attended university classes during most of his early grade school years. Upon graduating with a bachelor's degree in elementary education when Savion was in the 7th grade, his mother went on to earn a master's degree in education administration and now works as a middle school principal in New York City's public school system. Savion stated that having a mother in education taught him the importance of learning. He also recalled that one of his mother's most common sayings while he was growing up was, "Your mind is the only thing they can't take from you," explaining that his mother tried to prepare him for the real world by warning him about disparate treatment and underrepresentation of African Americans at the higher echelons of society, and teaching him how to overcome it through hard work and excelling at school.

Given the explicit messages he received about the importance of education, Savion worked hard to earn good grades, regularly appearing on the honor roll during grade school and on the dean's list in college. Yet, despite his academic record, Savion has had difficulty adjusting to medical school, stating, "I guess I'm swimming in a much bigger pond now." Savion notes that while studying used to come easy, much more concentration and time is required for him to master the concepts discussed in his medical courses, causing Savion to have thoughts such as "Maybe I'm not as smart as I thought" and "Maybe I'm not as smart as everybody else." Savion additionally admitted to worrying about confirming negative stereotypes about African Americans while at school, stating, "Everyone already assumes you're only there because of affirmative action. I have to prove I belong."

Case Formulation

Since intake, Savion has continued to experience instances of racial discrimination in his classes that trigger depressogenic schemata and lead to negative shifts in his view of self, the world, and the future. In one situation, Savion described attending an informational session for students considering a specialization in neurosurgery. He recalled that while there were only a few students who attended the meeting, the majority were White, and none were African American. His automatic thought in the situation was, "There's no one here who looks like me." Emotionally, Savion felt a sense of loneliness and his behavior was to stay to himself in one corner of the room. In another situation, Savion reported being challenged by an instructor concerning his ability to succeed in medical school after receiving a poor grade on an exam. Savion explained to his therapist that he did not have sufficient time to prepare for the exam due to a family emergency; however, he had received above average scores on all assignments and exams until that time. Savion recalled being upset that the instructor had ascribed his low score to his intelligence or ability to succeed rather than atypical circumstances. He identified his automatic thoughts in this situation as, "Here's another White man expecting to see me fail" and "He won't catch me slipping again." His emotion was anger, and his behavior was to resolve within himself to work hard in order to prove the instructor wrong.

Savion closely identified with his mother as the only child of a single parent household. In this relationship, Savion's mother emphasized the importance of education both as a family value as well as a means to overcome barriers to upward mobility due to racism. While these messages were delivered as an attempted to prepare Savion for the racial bias he would face throughout his life, it had the unintended effect of leading to depressogenic schemata that were dominated by themes of self-blame and negative expectations, consistent with the sense of being an outsider reported in extant research by other Black medical students (Liebschutz et al., 2006), and expressed in core beliefs such as "The world is against me" (world) and "I don't fit in" (self). In response to these beliefs, Savion developed the conditional assumption, "If I work hard, I can prove myself," the rule, "I must outperform everyone," and the attitude, "Life will always be hard but the only thing that can stop me, is me" (future). Compensatory strategies used in response to these core and intermediate beliefs include overperforming to meet perceived expectations greater than those expected for White students, taking the blame even when prejudice and discrimination are factors, and being vigilant for mistakes or obstacles. A diagram presenting cross-sectional and longitudinal views of Savion's cognitions and behaviors is shown in Figure 9.1.

Activity 9.1: Case Formulation in the Case of Savion

Review the diagram of Savion's cognitions and behaviors presented in Figure 9.1, then respond to the following questions:

- Based on the case presented, what other core or intermediate beliefs appear evident?
- What socially determined psychological phenomena and stressors may be relevant?
- What other culture-specific factors might you want to explore?

Treatment Plan

In the case of Savion, several psychological phenomena related to the African American experience are evident; namely, stereotype threat (C. M. Steele & Aronson, 1995), working twice as hard/John Henryism (Hudson et al., 2016; Palmer & Walker, 2020), and imposter syndrome (Bernard et al., 2018).

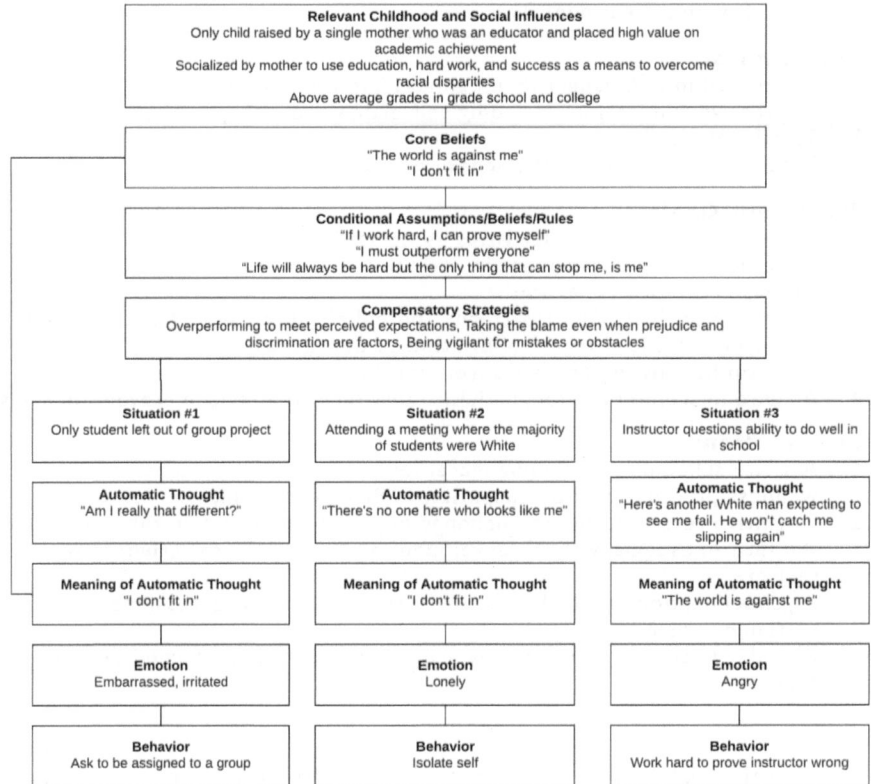

Figure 9.1 Cross-Sectional and Longitudnal Views of Savion's Cognitions and Behaviors. Adapted from Beck, J. S. (2020). *Cognitive behavior therapy: Basics and beyond* (3rd ed.). Guilford Press.

Additionally, his current issues with depression appear to be precipitated by stressors consistent with everyday experiences with racial discrimination, including environmental microaggressions (M. T. Williams, 2019) and micro-insults (Sue et al., 2007). In light of these considerations, the problem list, treatment goals, and interventions used to formulate Savion's initial treatment plan are presented in Table 9.1 and discussed in the sections that follow.

Problem List

Information provided by Savion in his evaluation session provides the data used to develop his initial problem list, shown in Table 9.1. Savion initiated therapy due to a decline in his mood, as well as interpersonal difficulties with his peers and the faculty at his medical school. Discussing these problems

Table 9.1 Savion's Treatment Plan

Problem List
1. Depressed mood, especially loneliness and irritability
2. Depressive rumination, including self-blame and worry
3. Social isolation
4. Race-based stressors in the school environment

Treatment Goals:
1. Increase engagement in activities associated with pleasure or mastery, while decreasing engagement in activities that maintain depression or increase risk for depression
2. Develop healthy thinking patterns and beliefs about self, the world, and the future that lead to the alleviation of depression
3. Develop healthy interpersonal relationships
4. Acquire microintervention, activism, advocacy, and relapse prevention skills

Interventions
1. Activity scheduling, including increased use of culturally centered wellness practices and participation in Black community spaces
2. Cognitive restructuring to challenge negative views of self, the world, and the future, especially those developed in response to experiences with racism
3. Psychoeducation and bibliotherapy focused on microaggressions and systemic racism
4. Roleplay microintervention, advocacy, and other skills learned during therapy

revealed the socially determined nature of his presenting concerns, namely, the impact of everyday experiences with discrimination on Savion's mood, relationships, and academic experience. Accordingly, problems included in the problem list not only reflect Savion's current symptomatology, but also acknowledge the need to address environmental race-based stressors in his treatment.

Treatment Goals

According to M. T. Williams (2019), there are several reasons why racial problems continue to exist in university settings despite changes in legal statues codifying racial discrimination and the egalitarian values typically espoused across many university campuses. Broadly, M. T. Williams (2019) suggests that White people tend to underestimate the degree and severity of racism; thus, when targets of racism attempt to address racial discrimination, these individuals are often socially punished by being dismissed, ridiculed, or met with defensive and avoidant reactions. Moreover, the very nature of racism suggests that those at the top of the racial hierarchy will continue to act in ways that maintain oppressive societal structures, whether intentionally or in response to unconscious programming by White supremacy, which limits change in these environments. Relatedly, aversive racism, a phenomenon wherein individuals who explicitly support racial equality have conflicted or unconscious negative attitudes toward people of color, also contributes to ongoing racial tension on university campuses when people of color violate social expectations based on the traditional racial hierarchy and are consequently subjected to various microaggressions and prejudicial behavior from faculty and administrators.

Among Black physicians specifically, barriers to success have been identified as discrimination, especially being punished more harshly for the same transgressions as White students, lower expectations, social isolation, and consequences including emotional dysregulation, hypervigilance, and exiting the medical profession or one's field of practice (Khubchandani et al., 2022; Liebschutz et al., 2006). Given the systemic nature of racial discrimination experienced by students of color broadly in university settings and specifically in medical school settings, treatment goals in the case of Savion were developed in consideration of his unique cognitive conceptualization, as well as his lived experienced with racial discrimination and the need for social change. These treatment goals, which emphasize providing Savion with a safe space to verbalize his experience with racism, explore and modify negative views of self, the world, and the future that develop as a result of racism, and identify actions that can be taken to increase his sense of empowerment, are presented in Table 9.1.

Activity 9.2: Treatment Goals in the Case of Savion

Table 9.1 identifies treatment goals in the case of Savion. Based on the areas of focus for treatment goals discussed in Chapter 6 (i.e., self-regulation, insight, processing strong emotions, and resilience) and Savion's problem list, what other goals would you identify?

Interventions

Earlier, I identified behavioral activation and cognitive restructuring as two of the primary interventions used in the treatment of depression. Accordingly, interventions listed on Savion's treatment plan (see Table 9.1) include activity scheduling, emphasizing increased use of culturally centered wellness practices and participation in Black community spaces, as well cognitive restructuring to challenge negative views of self, the world, and the future, especially those developed in response to experiences with racism. Throughout this text, the importance of the African-centered worldview and culturally derived healing practices in the process of healing from racism among African Americans have been highlighted. In the case of Savion, there is an apparent need for strategies that promote community and kinship given the sense of isolation he experiences in his school environment (French et al., 2020), storytelling to develop counternarratives to negative views of self, the world, and the future (Chioneso et al., 2020), critical consciousness (French et al., 2020), and activism/advocacy to address the microaggressions and other encounters with racism he experiences in his environment (Turner et al., 2022). Culturally derived activities that promote physical activity and Black joy (Tichavakunda, 2022) may also be of benefit in the implementation of the behavioral activation intervention.

Course of Treatment

As discussed in Chapter 1, session structure in CBT is heavily dependent upon each client's unique case formulation; however, CBT generally adheres to specific objectives for the beginning, middle, and end of sessions (J. S. Beck, 2020). At the beginning of a session, CBT therapists typically pay close attention to building rapport, conducting a mood check, reviewing action plans, and collaborating with the client to develop an agenda for the session. For clients who have experienced issues related to race and racism, broaching (Day-Vines et al., 2007, 2021) and validation (Walling et al., 2012) are critical skills at this point in the session as failures to implement these skills may lead to ruptures to the therapeutic relationship, contributing to negative outcomes such as (a) limitations to client disclosure level, (b) early termination of the therapy session, (c) increased self-doubt and decreased self-esteem, (d) feelings of embarrassment, worthlessness, shame, and anger in the client, and (e) reinforcement of the client's presenting problems (Miles et al., 2021). During the middle portion of the session, the therapist spends time gathering information about the problems identified on the agenda and implementing the interventions identified on the client's treatment plan. Near the end of the session, the therapist also collaborates with the client to develop an action plan identifying skills or activities to implement outside of the session. As the session draws to a close, the therapist invites the client to offer a summary of the session, finalizes the action plan, and encourages the client to identify any obstacles, including thoughts and feelings, that might interfere with completion of the action plan and how they might respond to these obstacles.

Like sessions in traditional CBT, the course of treatment in culturally adapted CBT also consists of beginning, middle, and end phases. During the beginning phase, therapy typically focuses on orienting the client to treatment, developing a good therapeutic alliance, providing psychoeducation, establishing goals, and obtaining information needed for initial case formulation (Matu, 2018). For depression, this would include teaching the client the structure of sessions in CBT and educating the client on the generic cognitive model (J. S. Beck, 2020) and the cognitive triad (A. T. Beck, 1963,

1976). During the beginning phase of therapy, the therapist should also be intentional in broaching race, ethnicity, and culture across the various dimensions of the counseling process in order to establish a sense of safety and normality around discussing these issues within the context of the therapy (Day-Vines et al., 2007, 2021).

In the middle phase of treatment, clients should be actively engaged in the application of cognitive and behavioral techniques to help them restructure their thoughts (Matu, 2018). As previously mentioned, the primary technique implemented during this process when treating depression is behavioral activation (Wenzel, 2019), which may be enhanced for use with African American clients by integrating African-centered principles and cultural practices (Turner et al., 2022). Similarly, cognitive restructuring during this process should also be approached with sensitivity to the client's lived experience with race. This includes validation of the client's experience, as well as the integration of culture into the client's unique cognitive conceptualization. The client's specific conceptualization should also evolve during the process as the therapist obtains additional data describing the client's automatic thoughts and underlying beliefs (Matu, 2018).

Finally, the last phase of treatment in CBT focuses on continued modification of thoughts and preparing clients for termination (Matu, 2018). Preparing for termination may include reviewing skill development and progress, tapering sessions, connecting clients to resources, and discussing possible relapses and how to prevent them. Given the chronicity of depression and the lower odds of obtaining depression care among African Americans (González et al., 2010) in response to racial discrimination, emphasis should be placed on problem-solving and reengaging services if necessary.

The sections below describe the course of treatment in the case of Savion. Note the therapist's attention to the various cultural considerations described throughout this chapter. As you read, write down any further cultural factors, interventions, or case formulation hypotheses you might consider during treatment with this client.

Beginning Phase of Treatment: Sessions 2 and 3

Earlier in this chapter, a summary of the case of Savion was presented, which described Savion's presenting concerns, symptoms, and scores on the BDI-II. Recall that Savion was a 23-year-old African American man in his first year at a predominantly White medical school who initiated therapy approximately three months after beginning classes, endorsing both mood and interpersonal difficulties. Symptoms Savion reported at intake included irritability, sadness, withdrawal, insomnia, anxiety, fatigue, poor concentration, and weight loss without past or present thoughts, plans, or attempts to die by suicide. His score on the BDI-II was 25, which is in the moderate range.

At Session 2, Savion scored a 27 on the BDI-II, which was slightly elevated from the previous week, but still in the moderate range. After setting an agenda, the therapist reviewed his score using a mood check and obtained an update, illustrated in the dialogue that follows.

Therapist: Savion, I noticed the score on your depression inventory was slightly higher than it was at your previous session. Could you tell me in a few sentences how you've been feeling for most of the week?

Savion: Yeah, I've just been so irritated with people at school.

Therapist: Okay. What else is important for me to know about how you've been feeling?

Savion: I don't know. I'm just so overwhelmed by everything.

Therapist: It sounds like things continue to be difficult at the school. What's gone on between last week and now that's important for me to know?

Savion: Well, I didn't do well on a test in one of my classes and the professor suggested that I might not be able to succeed in medical school.

Therapist: That sounds pretty upsetting. Is this something we should add to our agenda?

Savion: Yeah.

After finalizing the agenda, the therapist then conducted a review of Savion's presenting concerns and diagnosis. Due to the history of mental health stigma in the African American community (Taylor & Kuo, 2019), the therapist was intentional in broaching (Day-Vines et al., 2007, 2021) Savion's attitudes toward his diagnosis as well as his attitudes toward professional help-seeking during the review. As you read the dialogue that follows, notice the therapist's attention to the intraindividual dimensions of Savion's background given the intersectionality of his African American male identity, as well as the therapist's attention to inter-racial, ethnic, and cultural dimensions of Savion's case through her acknowledgment of the racism he experiences in his environment.

Therapist: Savion, your initial evaluation shows you've been experiencing problems with depression, which sounds consistent with what you reported today during the check of your mood and in the updates you shared.

Savion: Okay.

Therapist: As a medical student, you may have some understanding that the way we diagnose depression is by determining how closely the symptoms you describe match the symptoms described in our diagnostic manual of mental health concerns. Some of the symptoms of depression you reported included irritability, sadness, withdrawal, insomnia, anxiety, fatigue, poor concentration, and weight loss. While most people experience these symptoms at times, they become significant when they cause difficulties in our ability to function at school, socially, or at work. Does this make sense so far?

Savion: Yes.

Therapist: Good. Fortunately, cognitive behavioral therapy is very effective in helping people overcome depression and I am confident that we'll find a way to help you manage your problems with depression.

Savion: That's good to hear. I was nervous about coming here.

Therapist: You know what, Savion? That's completely normal. Most people are at least a little nervous when starting therapy for the first time. Could you share some of what you were nervous about?

Savion: Well, the way I was raised, we just really didn't talk to strangers about our problems.

Therapist: I hear what you're saying. This is a common way many families protect themselves. From what I understand, this is especially true in the African American community, is that correct?

Savion: Yes, at least where I'm from.

Therapist: Thank you for sharing that. Knowing about your cultural background helps me have a better understanding of who you are and what your life experiences have been like. I appreciate your willingness to discuss what it's like to be African American with me, especially given the racism you're currently experiencing at school.

Savion: Yeah, things there have been pretty intense. I'm trying to keep my cool, but it seems like no matter what I do people are going to have a certain image of me and the next few years are going to be pretty miserable.

Therapist: And when you say, "a certain image of me," do you mean stereotypes about you as an African American man?

Savion: Yes, exactly.

Activity 9.3: Broaching Race, Ethnicity, and Culture

In the preceding dialogue, the therapist in the case of Savion broached race, ethnicity, and culture by taking opportunities to acknowledge cultural beliefs that may influence Savion's attitudes toward therapy (e.g., "This is a common way many families protect themselves. From what I understand, this is especially true in the African American community, is that correct?"), the role of racism in his presenting concerns (e.g., "I appreciate your willingness to discuss what it's like to be African American with me, especially given the racism you're currently experiencing at school"), and the unique pressure stereotyped images of African American men contribute to his experience (e.g., "And when you say, "a certain image of me," do you mean stereotypes about you as an African American man?").

Recall from Chapter 4 that a multicultural orientation in therapy consists of taking opportunities to discuss culture with clients, as well as exhibiting humility and comfort when taking these opportunities. *Humility* refers to a way of being that seeks to understand how culture influences the worldviews of both the counselor and the client, as well as dynamics within the counseling relationship, while *comfort* refers to the level of comfort one has while discussing issues related to diversity, power, and oppression during therapy (Owen et al., 2011). When therapists are comfortable discussing these issues during therapy, they experience the emotional state of feeling at ease, open, calm, and relaxed (Hook et al., 2017).

- What additional opportunities to discuss culture do you see in the dialogue presented above?
- In what ways did the therapist exhibit humility?
- In what other ways could the therapist show humility?
- What do you believe the therapist's level of comfort was during the dialogue?
- What evidence supports your belief?

After reviewing his diagnosis, Savion and the therapist took time in Session 2 to create problem and goal lists for his treatment plan, and discussed the interventions that would be used to address his treatment goals (see Table 9.1). The therapist also educated Savion on the generic cognitive model and the cognitive triad, using the situation where his professor suggested he may not succeed in medical school as an example. During this process, the therapist utilized a partial thought record to help Savion understand the connection between his automatic thoughts and emotions. The therapist also explained the connection between activity and mood and introduced activity scheduling during Session 2, assigning Savion the task of monitoring his activity on a daily basis and rating the amount of pleasure and accomplishment each activity provided on a scale from 1 to 10, along with rating his mood on a scale from 0 to 100 percent (M. M. Carter, 1999). Session 2 ended with final summaries provided by Savion and the therapist and finalizing of the action plan, which consisted of continuing the partial thought record and activity scheduling.

In Session 3, Savion scored a 25 on the BDI-II, indicating continued depression in the moderate range, although with a slight improvement. After setting an agenda, conducting the mood check, and discussing updates, Savion and the therapist reviewed the behavioral activation (see Table 9.2) and thought record assignments written on his homework list at the conclusion of the previous session. In reviewing the activities on his daily schedule, Savion observed that while he was frequently engaged in school-related activities which contributed to a sense of mastery in his life, he spent limited time engaged in activities that gave him a sense of pleasure. He was also somewhat socially isolated. In response, the therapist worked with Savion to identify activities that would be fun, increase social contact, and draw upon culturally derived wellness practices. Savion was generally open to the idea of making changes in his schedule; however, he expressed concern about the impact these changes would have on his academic performance. Sensing that this thought may inhibit Savion's motivation to institute change, the therapist decided to inquire about setting up a behavioral experiment to test the thought, which they explored as part of the agenda they set for the session (J. S. Beck, 2020).

Therapist: Savion, you say that as a result of monitoring your daily schedule over the past week, you've concluded that you're not spending enough time engaged in activities that give you a sense of pleasure, is that correct?

Savion: Yes.

Therapist: What ideas do you have about how you could introduce more pleasurable activities into your schedule?

Savion: I'm not really sure.

Therapist: Hmm. Sometimes it's helpful to think about activities you've enjoyed in the past. Activities that have provided a sense of community can be especially beneficial.

Savion: Well, when I was in undergrad, I was active in my fraternity. I suppose I could look into the graduate chapter here.

Therapist: I sense some reluctance about this.

Savion: Yeah, I guess I am just worried about not having enough time to study.

Therapist: Is there any way to test this out to see if this is true?

Savion: Umm, I could attend a few meetings before committing to anything to see how it would affect my study time.

Therapist: What would be the advantage of doing that?

Savion: Well, I might have more fun, which could help me feel better. I could also meet other Black people on campus or in the community who might understand what I am going through at school.

At the conclusion of the session, Savion included the behavioral experiment into his action plan for the week and additionally agreed to continue using his thought record and monitoring his daily activity. The therapist hoped

Table 9.2 Savion's Weekly Activity Schedule: Week 1

Time	Monday	Tuesday	Wednesday	Thursday	Friday	Saturday	Sunday
5–6am	Sleep	Sleep	Sleep	Sleep	Sleep	Sleep	Sleep
6–7am	Morning Routine A=2; P=0; M=50	Morning Routine A=2; P=0; M=50	Morning Routine A=2; P=0; M=50	Morning Routine A=2; P=0; M=50	Morning Routine A=2; P=0; M=50	Sleep	Sleep
7–8am	Travel to School A=2; P=2; M=55	Morning Routine A=2; P=0; M=55	Morning Routine A=2; P=0; M=50	Morning Routine A=2; P=0; M=50	Travel to School A=2; P=2; M=55	Sleep	Sleep
8–9am	Team Learning A=8; P=3; M=60	Morning Routine A=2; P=0; M=50	Travel to Therapy A=2; P=0; M=50	Morning Routine A=2; P=0; M=50	Team Learning A=8; P=3; M=60	Sleep	Sleep
9–10am	Team Learning A=8; P=3; M=60	Travel to School A=2; P=2; M=55	Therapy A=7; P=5; M=50	Travel to School A=2; P=2; M=55	Team Learning A=8; P=3; M=60	Chores A=6; P=4; M=40	Study A=7; P=3; M=65
10–11am	Study A=7; P=3; M=50	Pathology Lecture A=7; P=5; M=55	Travel from Therapy A=2; P=0; M=50	Anatomy Lecture A=7; P=5; M=55	Break A=2; P=7; M=40	Study A=7; P=3; M=65	Study A=7; P=3; M=65
11–12pm	Study A=7; P=3; M=55	Pathology Lecture A=7; P=5; M=55	Break A=2; P=7; M=40	Anatomy Lecture A=7; P=5; M=55	Study A=7; P=3; M=65	Study A=7; P=3; M=65	Study A=7; P=3; M=65
12–1pm	Study A=7; P=3; M=50	Break A=2; P=7; M=50	Break A=2; P=7; M=50	Break A=2; P=7; M=50	Study A=7; P=3; M=65	Break A=2; P=7; M=50	Break A=2; P=7; M=50
1–2pm	Study A=7; P=3; M=60	Pathology Lab A=7; P=3; M=60	Practice of Medicine A=8; P=8; M=30	Anatomy Lab A=7; P=3; M=60	Study A=7; P=3; M=65	Break A=2; P=7; M=50	Break A=2; P=7; M=50
2–3pm	Travel Home A=2; P=5; M=40	Pathology Lab A=7; P=3; M=60	Practice of Medicine A=8; P=8; M=30	Anatomy Lab A=7; P=3; M=60	Travel Home A=2; P=5; M=40	Study A=7; P=3; M=65	Study A=7; P=3; M=65

3–4pm	Laundry A=6; P=5; M=40	Pathology Lab A=7; P=3; M=60	Practice of Medicine A=8; P=8; M=30	Anatomy Lab A=7; P=3; M=60	Break A=0; P=5; M=40	Study A=7; P=3; M=65
4–5pm	Break A=0; P=5; M=40	Pathology Lab A=7; P=3; M=60	Practice of Medicine A=8; P=8; M=30	Anatomy Lab A=7; P=3; M=60	Break A=0; P=5; M=40	Study A=7; P=3; M=65
5–6pm	Dinner A=2; P=7; M=40	Travel Home A=2; P=5; M=40	Travel Home A=2; P=5; M=40	Travel Home A=2; P=5; M=40	Dinner A=2; P=7; M=40	Study A=7; P=3; M=65
6–7pm	TV A=0; P=6; M=40	Dinner A=2; P=7; M=40	Dinner A=2; P=7; M=40	Dinner A=2; P=7; M=40	TV A=0; P=6; M=40	Dinner A=2; P=7; M=40
7–8pm	TV A=0; P=6; M=50	Study A=7; P=3; M=60	Chores A=6; P=4; M=40	Study A=7; P=3; M=65	TV A=0; P=6; M=50	TV A=0; P=6; M=70
8–9pm	TV A=0; P=6; M=60	Study A=7; P=3; M=65	TV A=0; P=6; M=60	Study A=7; P=3; M=70	TV A=0; P=6; M=60	TV A=0; P=6; M=70
9–10pm	TV A=0; P=6; M=70	TV A=0; P=6; M=75	TV A=0; P=6; M=70	TV A=0; P=6; M=75	TV A=0; P=6; M=70	TV A=0; P=6; M=70
10–11pm	Sleep	Sleep	Sleep	Sleep	Sleep	Sleep
11–12am	Sleep	Sleep	Sleep	Sleep	Sleep	Sleep
12–1am	Sleep	Sleep	Sleep	Sleep	Sleep	Sleep
1–2am	Sleep	Sleep	Sleep	Sleep	Sleep	Sleep
2–3am	Sleep	Sleep	Sleep	Sleep	Sleep	Sleep
3–4am	Sleep	Sleep	Sleep	Sleep	Sleep	Sleep
4–5am	Sleep	Sleep	Sleep	Sleep	Sleep	Sleep

that by focusing on activities that not only provided a sense of pleasure but also offered a sense of community, Savion might experience the added benefit of increasing his sense of belonging and mattering (J. M. Steele & Newton, 2023). According to Goodenow and Grady (1993), *belongingness* can be defined as how much an individual feels personally accepted, respected, included, and supported by others in their social environment, while *mattering* refers to the experience of feeling significant to others (Tucker et al., 2010). When an individual is low on belongingness and mattering, reactions to prejudice and discrimination may be intensified, and individuals may experience adverse impacts to their academic, occupational, or social functioning (Adejumo, 2021; Boston & Warren, 2017). Conversely, a high sense of belongingness and mattering can serve as a protective factor, as these constructs result in more positive racial identity (Yap et al., 2011), self-determination, self-definition, self-acceptance, and self-love (Johnson, 2016). The therapist made a note to explore these factors more intentionally at a future session.

Middle Phase of Treatment: Sessions 4 through 7

At Session 4, Savion scored a 23 on the BDI-II. During updates, Savion reported that he had attended a meeting of the graduate chapter of his fraternity, completing the behavioral experiment designed at the prior session. Savion stated that he was happy to learn the chapter only met once a month and focused primarily on community service activities Savion may attend as he is able. Savion additionally reported continued monitoring of his daily activities and use of this thought record, which had helped him to notice that he tended to feel more depressed when at home alone. The therapist gave Savion credit for making this observation, and the two agreed to spend the remainder of the session exploring what else he had learned from his activity schedule and addressing the thoughts on his thought record.

To facilitate exploration of learning from his weekly activity schedule, the therapist asked Savion questions developed by Greenberger and Padesky (2015) such as, "What activities helped you feel better?" "What activities helped you feel worse?" "What activities could you do instead?" "Were there certain times of the day or week when you felt worse?" and "What could you do instead?" Savion reported that he had been intentional about exercising on Tuesday, Wednesday, Thursday, and Saturday mornings, which had a positive impact on his mood. He also reported, however, that he felt worse in the evenings while spending time alone studying or watching TV, as mentioned during the update. Using data obtained from his thought record, Savion and the therapist explored the automatic thoughts contributing to his low mood during these times. While studying, Savion would often ruminate on his difficulties in the program, having thoughts such as "Everyone judges me," "What if I can't prove them wrong?" and "Things will never be fair for a Black man in America." As a result of these thoughts, Savion spent most evenings feeling sad, angry, and hopeless.

Given the salience of race in Savion's automatic thoughts, the therapist decided to explore his level of racial identity development. Recall from Chapter 2 that term *racial identity* refers to an individual's sense of belonging to a particular racial group, while *racial identity development* refers to the process through which individuals develop a healthy view of themselves, members of their racial group, and members of other racial groups (Constantine et al., 1998). To learn more about Savion's level of racial identity development, the therapist asked questions reflective of the Immersion-Emersion and Internalization (Cross & Vandiver, 2001) stages of Black racial identity development (see Table 2.1). Through this exploration, the therapist hoped to attain additional insight into Savion's ability to cope with racial discrimination and race-based stress. Broadly, research suggests a positive racial identity can serve as a protective factor against racial discrimination; however, studies have also found that individuals with higher Internalization attitudes tend to experience less race-based stress, while individuals with Immersion-Emersion attitudes may experience more stress (R. T. Carter et al., 2017). An excerpt from the dialogue of the therapist's discussion on racial identity development follows.

Therapist: Savion, your thought record seems to highlight how difficult your experience in your med program is as a Black man.

Savion: Yeah.

Therapist: You've previously shared that your mother was very intentional in preparing you to deal with racial bias throughout your childhood. If it's okay with you, I'd like to spend a little more time exploring the impact of race on your life and how you see the world. Is that okay?

Savion: Yes.

Therapist: Great. Besides the lessons you received from your mother, what events have clarified your understanding of what it means to a Black person in the United States?

Savion: Well, I think growing up in New York was really positive for me as a Black person. Yeah, it was tough, but I also got to see so much of the beauty of Black culture because there were Black people everywhere, you know what I mean? And not just African American people, but Dominicans, Jamaicans, Haitians, Nigerians, *Black people*.

Therapist: It sounds like you developed a real love and appreciation for Black culture while growing up. What else can you tell me about your interest in Black culture and history?

Savion: I guess I've always had an interest in Black culture, but I didn't start to learn about real Black history until college. You know, they don't really teach us much about our history in public schools except slavery and people like Martin Luther King and Rosa Parks. In my last couple of years of college, I decided to minor in Africana Studies, which helped me learn much more about the Black experience, here and in Africa. Even though I've graduated, I still love learning about Black history and culture.

Therapist: That's awesome. Based on your studies, what is your sense of the contributions your ancestors have made over the years?

Savion: This country, really the world, wouldn't exist the way it is today without us. And I'm not just talking about slavery. Black people have been critical to developments made in every field. Take medicine for example. Charles Drew invented the methods necessary to safely store blood for blood transfusions. Vivien Thomas helped invent cardiac surgery. Solomon Carter Fuller was a pioneer in the study of Alzheimer's disease. And there are so many more people that I could name. So, the fact that people in this medical program treat me as if I am inferior just because I am Black is infuriating.

Therapist: Yes, racism is wrong, and it makes sense that you would feel anger in this situation. Given your feelings, what's it like working with mostly White professors and students?

Savion: Well, it's not like I hate White people or anything like that. It's just that this specific situation is difficult to deal with because of all the racism, microaggressions, implicit bias, or whatever you want to call it. To be honest, I'm not really trying to think too much about White people. I'm more interested in understanding who I am as a Black man and becoming a doctor so that at least Black patients won't have to experience discrimination in the healthcare system when they come to see me.

Therapist: I see. So, how comfortable are you with being a Black man?

Savion: You know, until I minored in Africana Studies, I never really thought too intentionally about it. Since then, I've realized that I still have some growing to do as it relates to connecting with the part of my identity that was stolen during slavery.

Based on the preceding dialogue, the therapist determined that Savion's level of racial identity was most closely aligned with the Intense Black Involvement attitudes at the Immersion-Emersion stage of development (Cross & Vandiver, 2001). For example, Savion's interest in Africana Studies, as well as his assertion, "I still have some growing to do as it relates to connecting with the part of my identity that was stolen during slavery," were consistent with what Vandiver et al. (2001) described as the eager desire to embrace Black culture and learn more about Africa and African Americans observed at the Immersion-Emersion stage of Black racial identity development. Given this assessment and the saliency of race at this stage, the therapist determined that Savion may be more susceptible to overwhelming emotions associated with race-based stress at this time of his life, necessitating increased emphasis on this aspect of his depression (R. T. Carter et al., 2017).

In Sessions 5 and 6, Savion scored 20 on the BDI-II in both weeks. Due to the therapist's understanding of his current stage of racial identity development and the overwhelming emotions people at the Immersion-Emersion stage of racial identity development have because of their heightened awareness of the historic hardships faced by members of their racial group (R. T. Carter et al., 2017), time was spent helping Savion more clearly identify and label his emotions. Savion often labeled his emotion as anger on his weekly thought records; however, when discussing his feelings with the therapist during sessions, they more accurately reflected feelings of alienation and at times, humiliation. Correctly labeling these feelings increased Savion's satisfaction with therapy (J. S. Beck, 2020). It also helped increase the sense of validation Savion experienced in the counseling relationship, which in turn strengthened the therapeutic bond (M. T. Williams et al., 2022).

In Session 7, Savion scored a 17 on the BDI-II, which indicated that his depression was now in the mild range. While discussing this score and offering feedback, Savion attributed his improvement in mood to developing relationships with local members of his fraternity, increased exercise, and the therapist's ability to accurately reflect and validate his emotions. With the improvement in mood experienced through the therapeutic relationship and behavioral activation, Savion and the therapist placed greater emphasis on cognitive restructuring. During this process, the therapist was careful with her use of questions examining the evidence for Savion's thoughts, recognizing that they may invalidate his experience of discrimination and other race-related concerns (Graham et al., 2013). Instead, the therapist took a differentiated approach to examining various aspects of the cognitive triad. Extant research suggests perceived everyday discrimination predicts all three aspects of the cognitive triad, but more strongly predicts negative views of the world when compared to negative views of the self and future (Sacco et al., 2023). This research also finds that both negative views of self and the world mediate perceived everyday discrimination and depressive symptoms, although negative views of the world do not have a stronger mediational effect on this relationship. Accordingly, while the therapist worked with all three aspects of the cognitive triad, she more intensely targeted negative thoughts about self and the world. For negative thoughts of self, the therapist focused on self-compassion, mindfulness, and placing experiences in their sociohistorical context (M. T. Williams et al., 2022), which was helpful for Savion because his negative views of himself tended to reflect self-blame and criticism (e.g., "I should've done better").

For negative thoughts about the world, which in the case of Savion were often true, the therapist focused on psychoeducation, investigating invalid conclusions, and problem-solving (J. S. Beck, 2020). For example, in Session 7, Savion discussed attending an informational session for students considering a specialization in neurosurgery. On his thought record he noted that while there were only a few students who attended the meeting, the majority were White, and none were African American. His automatic thought in the situation was, "There's no one here who looks like me." His emotion in response to the thought was loneliness, which he rated at 85 percent, and his behavior was to stay by himself in one corner of the room. Using psycho-education, the therapist helped Savion to identify this situation as an environmental microaggression, which was defined as aspects of the environment that send messages of invalidation to a marginalized group (Sue et al., 2007, 2019). In this case, the invalidating aspect of the environment was the underrepresentation of African Americans and the message communicated was "you don't belong." Through Socratic questioning, the therapist learned that the meaning of this message for Savion was, "I won't have support." For problem-solving, the therapist worked with Savion to identify other potential sources of support through professional networking, friends and family, and the community. The therapist also addressed Savion's self-isolating behaviors which he had developed in response to fears of rejection and embarrassment, roleplaying the use of microintervention skills as an alternative to these behaviors (Sue et al., 2019) and discussing ways he might advocate for changes in his environment.

Final Phase of Treatment: Sessions 8 through 12

In Session 8, Savion scored a 15 on the BDI-II. By this time, the therapist hypothesized some of Savion's core and intermediate beliefs based on patterns observed in his automatic thoughts. For example, the automatic thought, "I should have done better" seemed to reflect the intermediate belief, "If I do better, I can protect myself." To explore her hypotheses, the therapist elicited the full assumption by responding to the first half of it that was reflected in Savion's automatic thought (J. S. Beck, 2020).

Therapist: So, you've had the automatic thought, "I should've done better."

Savion: Yes.

Therapist: What happens as a result of not "doing better?"

Savion: Then I can't protect myself from their accusations. They can accuse me of not deserving to be here, and there's nothing I can say about it.

Therapist: So, it sounds like you've developed the belief "If I do better, I can protect myself," is that correct?

Savion: I guess it is.

The therapist then utilized the downward arrow technique to learn more about Savion's core beliefs (J. S. Beck, 2020).

Therapist: And if that's true, that you can't protect yourself from their accusations, what does that mean?

Savion: I don't know, it's hard to explain. As a Black man, I don't fit into what my mom used to call the "good ole' boys club." That world is against me. So, I'm vulnerable.

In response to Savion's core and intermediate beliefs, the therapist took time to confirm her conceptualization and then provided education on the nature of these underlying beliefs and their connection to his automatic thoughts. During this process, the therapist was careful to situate Savion's beliefs in their sociohistorical context, discussing concepts such as working twice as hard and its psychological effects (DeSante, 2013; Palmer & Walker, 2020). For example, the therapist talked to Savion about a study conducted by McGee et al. (2019) that explored the effect of working twice as hard on African American doctoral students in engineering and computing programs. According to the results of that study, these students often felt pressure to prove they were worthy of full and unbiased participation in their departments, for example, maintaining a constant presence in the research activities of the department and lab and sacrificing weekends and holidays to a greater extent than White or Asian students in the program. As a result of these efforts, the students also reported experiencing a significant amount of distress, leading to a sort of survival mode and a worsening of symptoms over time. Savion related to this research and could see through the examples in the research and his own life the way these beliefs contributed to his depression and ways of coping. Accordingly, Savion and the therapist agreed to explore ways to develop and strengthen new core beliefs at the next session.

In Session 9, Savion experienced a relapse in his depression symptoms, which was reflected in a BDI-II score of 23. Savion explained that an instructor questioned his ability to succeed in medical school after receiving a poor grade on an exam, which Savion attributed to not having enough time to prepare for the exam due to a family emergency. Savion noted that he had received above average scores on all assignments and exams prior to that time and recalled being upset that the instructor ascribed his low score to Savion's intelligence or ability to succeed rather than atypical circumstances. He identified his automatic thoughts in this situation as, "Here's another White man expecting to see me fail" and "He won't catch me slipping again." His emotion was anger, and his behavior was to focus on studying in order to prove the instructor wrong. Responding to his report, the therapist helped Savion connect these thoughts, feelings, and behaviors to the core and intermediate beliefs discussed at the prior session, using a cognitive conceptualization diagram (J. S. Beck, 2020) to illustrate the connections. Savion and the therapist then used this situation to accomplish the task of developing new core beliefs. Specifically, Savion replaced the old belief "The world is against me" with the new belief "Some people are racist." He also replaced the old core belief "I don't fit in" with the new core belief "I'm a trailblazer." According to Savion, these new beliefs were helpful because they challenged the rigid, distorted view that everyone was against him and reframed his position in the program as one preparing the way for African Americans who would come after him.

Once they were identified, the therapist initiated the process of strengthening the new beliefs by helping Savion to devise a criteria continuum for each belief (Padesky, 1994). Initially, Savion had difficulty identifying behavioral criteria to include in the continuum "Some people are racist." Through discussion, Savion realized that this was because he was assigning racism to a personality trait rather than specific attitudes and behaviors that had the impact of maintaining systems of oppression through the use of power directed against members of racially marginalized groups (R. T. Carter, 2007) and subsequently developed the following criteria: (a) committed to exploration of one's racial worldview vs. lacks awareness, (b) is a racial ally vs. stays silent in the face of racism, (c) is respectful and open to other cultures vs. uses racist language/espouses racist beliefs, and (d) committed to diversity, equity, and inclusion vs. actively discriminates against others.

After focusing on specific attitudes and behaviors, Savion was able to develop criteria that broadened his view of the world and allowed him to more accurately process information that was contrary to the old core belief. Specifically, by conceptualizing his experiences with racism according to his criteria, Savion was able to personalize and internalize these experiences less and view them as a systemic result of White supremacy instead. This had the additional effect of helping Savion to become a more confident advocate, as he was able to more clearly articulate problematic attitudes and behaviors to others.

By Session 10, Savion reported a significant reduction in his depression symptoms, obtaining a BDI-II score of 13, which was in the minimal range. Savion attributed his reduction in symptoms to a shift in his worldview, which was previously characterized by a sense of powerlessness and personal blame. Now, Savion had a greater understanding that his difficulties were not the result of his inability to "do better," but rather a consequence of a system of oppression designed to marginalize others by assigning moral and intellectual justifications to social inequalities among racial groups (Sidanius et al., 1996). He further understood that a standard of perfection was unrealistic and no amount of "doing better" would eliminate racial prejudices. Moreover, through interventions such as psychoeducation, behavioral activation, and criteria continuums, Savion also realized he was not completely without support and there were certain microintervention and emotional regulation strategies he could use when he did encounter racism.

Given his progress, Savion and the therapist decided to reduce the frequency of sessions from weekly to bi-weekly and worked together to develop a relapse prevention plan with the goal of terminating therapy by Session 12 (J. S. Beck, 2020). To prepare for the tapering of sessions and eventual termination of therapy, the therapist and Savion discussed the advantages of both, with Savion stating that he would have more time to engage himself academically or socially. Savion also acknowledged that nearing the completion of therapy meant that he had made progress toward his therapy goals and had developed adequate skills to manage his depression and cope with his life stressors. Although Savion generally had a positive attitude toward tapering and terminating therapy, he also expressed some reservations, including worries about relapsing (e.g., "What if I get depressed again?") and not being able to manage his emotions on his own (e.g., "What if I need someone to talk to?"). Accordingly, the therapist utilized decatastrophizing questions such as "What's the worst that could happen?" and "What could you do then?" to help Savion respond to his worries (J. S. Beck, 2020). Savion stated that he could read his therapy notes, maintain use of his behavioral activation and cognitive restructuring activities, and seek support from friends, family, and trusted community members. Savion additionally acknowledged that he could return to therapy if his symptoms became severe.

At Sessions 11 and 12, Savion scored a 9 and 7 on the BDI-II. In Session 11, Savion and the therapist continued work on his relapse prevention plan, with Savion identifying risk factors for relapse that included increased racial stressors in his school environment, social isolation, and poor activity scheduling. Savion described the strategies discussed at the previous session as methods for managing these factors, as well as increased prayer and giving back to his community. In the final session, Savion and the therapist focused on summarizing progress made toward his treatment goals and what he had learned from therapy. Overall, Savion was satisfied with the results of therapy, and he looked forward to completing the remainder of his medical program with a new outlook on both himself and the future.

References

Adejumo, V. (2021). Beyond diversity, inclusion, and belonging. *Leadership, 17*(1), 62–73. https://doi.org/10.1177/1742715020976202

American Psychiatric Association. (2013). *Diagnostic and statistical manual of mental disorders* (5th ed.). American Psychiatric Association. https://doi.org/10.1176/appi.books.9780890425596

Bailey, T.-K. M., Williams, W. S., & Favors, B. (2014). Internalized racial oppression in the African American community. In E. J. R. David (Ed.), *Internalized oppression: The psychology of marginalized groups* (pp. 137–162). Springer Publishing Company, Inc.

Bailey, R. K., Mokonogho, J., & Kumar, A. (2019). Racial and ethnic differences in depression: current perspectives. *Neuropsychiatric Disease and Treatment, 15*, 603–609. https://doi.org/10.2147/NDT.S128584

Beck, A. T. (1963). Thinking and depression: I. Idiosyncratic content and cognitive distortions. *Archives of General Psychiatry, 9*(4), 324–333. https://doi.org/10.1001/archpsyc.1963.01720160014002

Beck, A. T. (1976). *Cognitive therapy and the emotional disorders*. International Universities Press.

Beck, A. T., Steer, R. A., & Brown, G. K. (1996). *Manual for the Beck Depression Inventory-II*. Pearson.

Beck, J. S. (2020). *Cognitive behavior therapy: Basics and beyond* (3rd ed.). Guilford Press.

Beck, J. S., Beck, A. T., & Jolly, J. B. (2005). *Manual for the Beck Youth Inventories* (2nd ed.). Pearson.

Beckham, E. E., Leber, W. R., Watkins, J. T., Boyer, J. L., & Cook, J. B. (1986). Development of an instrument to measure Beck's cognitive triad: The cognitive triad inventory. *Journal of Consulting and Clinical Psychology, 54*(4), 566–567. https://doi.org/10.1037/0022-006x.54.4.566

Berghuis, K. J., Pössel, P., & Pittard, C. M. (2020). Perceived discrimination and depressive symptoms: Is the cognitive triad a moderator or mediator? *Child & Youth Care Forum, 49*(4), 647–660. https://doi.org/10.1007/s10566-019-09537-1

Bernard, D. L., Hoggard, L. S., & Neblett, E. W., Jr. (2018). Racial discrimination, racial identity, and impostor phenomenon: A profile approach. *Cultural Diversity and Ethnic Minority Psychology, 24*(1), 51–61. https://doi.org/10.1037/cdp0000161

Bivens, D. (1995). *Internalized racism: A definition*. https://www.racialequitytools.org/resourcefiles/bivens.pdf

Bivens, D. K. (2005). What is internalized racism? *Flipping the Script: White Privilege and Community Building, 1*, 43–51.

Boston, C., & Warren, S. R. (2017). The effects of belonging and racial identity on urban African American high school students' achievement. *Journal of Urban Learning, Teaching, and Research, 13*, 26–33.

Britt-Spells, A. M., Slebodnik, M., Sands, L. P., & Rollock, D. (2018). Effects of perceived discrimination on depressive symptoms among Black men residing in the United States: A meta-analysis. *American Journal of Men's Health, 12*(1), 52–63. https://doi.org10.1177/1557988315624509

Brooks, J. R., Hong, J. H., Madubata, I. J., Odafe, M. O., Cheref, S., & Walker, R. L. (2021). The moderating effect of dispositional forgiveness on perceived racial discrimination and depression for African American adults. *Cultural Diversity and Ethnic Minority Psychology, 27*(3), 511–520. https://doi.org/10.1037/cdp0000385

Carter, M. M. (1999). Ethnic awareness in the cognitive behavioral treatment of a depressed African American female. *Cognitive and Behavioral Practice, 6*(3), 273–278. https://doi.org/10.1016/S1077-7229(99)80089-3

Carter, R. T. (2007). Racism and psychological and emotional injury: Recognizing and assessing race-based traumatic stress. *The Counseling Psychologist, 35*(1), 13–105. https://doi.org/10.1177/0011000006292033

Carter, R. T., Johnson, V. E., Roberson, K., Mazzula, S. L., Kirkinis, K., & Sant-Barket, S. (2017). Race-based traumatic stress, racial identity statuses, and psychological functioning: An exploratory investigation. *Professional Psychology: Research and Practice, 48*(1), 30–37. https://doi.org/10.1037/pro0000116

Chioneso, N. A., Hunter, C. D., Gobin, R. L., McNeil Smith, S., Mendenhall, R., & Neville, H. A. (2020). Community healing and resistance through storytelling: A framework to address racial trauma in Africana communities. *Journal of Black Psychology, 46*(2–3), 95–121. https://doi.org/10.1177/0095798420929468

Clark, D. A., Beck, A. T., & Alford, B. A. (1999). *Scientific foundations of cognitive theory and therapy of depression.* John Wiley & Sons Inc.

Constantine, M. G., Richardson, T. Q., Benjamin, E. M., & Wilson, J. W. (1998). An overview of Black racial identity theories: Current limitations and considerations. *Applied and Preventive Psychology, 7*(2), 95–99. https://doi.org/10.1016/S0962-1849(05)80006-X

Cross, W. E., Jr., & Vandiver, B. J. (2001). Nigrescence theory and measurement: Introducing the Cross Racial Identity Scale (CRIS). In J. G. Ponterotto, J. M. Casas, L. A. Suzuki, & C. M. Alexander (Eds.), *Handbook of multicultural counseling* (2nd ed., pp. 371–393). Sage.

Das, A., Singh, P., Kulkarni, A. K., & Bruckner, T. A. (2021). Emergency department visits for depression following police killings of unarmed African Americans. *Social Science & Medicine, 269*, 1–6. https://doi.org/10.1016/j.socscimed.2020.113561

Day-Vines, N. L., Cluxton-Keller, F., Agorsor, C., & Gubara, S. (2021). Strategies for broaching the subjects of race, ethnicity, and culture. *Journal of Counseling & Development, 99*(3), 348–357. https://doi.org/10.1002/jcad.12380

Day-Vines, N.L., Wood, S. M., Grothaus, T., Craigen, L., Holman, A., Dotson-Blake, K., & Douglass, M. J. (2007). Broaching the subjects of race, ethnicity, and culture during the counseling process. *Journal of Counseling & Development, 85*(4), 401–409. https://doi.org/10.1002/jcad.12069

DeSante, C. D. (2013). Working twice as hard to get half as far: Race, work ethic, and America's deserving poor. *American Journal of Political Science, 57*(2), 342–356. https://doi.org/10.1111/ajps.12006

Eichstaedt, J. C., Sherman, G. T., Giorgi, S., Roberts, S. O., Reynolds, M. E., Ungar, L. H., & Guntuku, S. C. (2021). The emotional and mental health impact of the murder of George Floyd on the U.S. population. *Proceedings of the National Academy of Sciences of the United States of America, 118*(39), e2109139118. https://doi.org/10.1073/pnas.2109139118

Erarslan, Ö., & Işikli, S. (2019). Adaptation of the Cognitive Triad Inventory into Turkish: A validity and reliability study. *Noro Psikiyatri Arsivi, 56*(1), 32–39. https://doi.org/10.29399/npa.19390

French, B. H., Lewis, J. A., Mosley, D. V., Adames, H. Y., Chavez-Dueñas, N. Y., Chen, G. A., & Neville, H. A. (2020). Toward a psychological framework of radical healing in communities of color. *The Counseling Psychologist*, *48*(1), 14–46. https://doi.org/10.1177/0011000019843506

Fuller-Rowell, T. E., Nichols, O. I., Burrow, A. L., Ong, A. D., Chae, D. H., & El-Sheikh, M. (2021). Day-to-day fluctuations in experiences of discrimination: Associations with sleep and the moderating role of internalized racism among African American college students. *Cultural Diversity & Ethnic Minority Psychology*, *27*(1), 107–117. https://doi.org/10.1037/cdp0000342

Gaylord-Harden, N. K., & Cunningham, J. A. (2009). The impact of racial discrimination and coping strategies on internalizing symptoms in African American youth. *Journal of Youth and Adolescence*, 38(4), 532–543. https://doi.org/10.1007/s10964-008-9377-5

González, H. M., Tarraf, W., Whitfield, K. E., & Vega, W. A. (2010). The epidemiology of major depression and ethnicity in the United States. *Journal of Psychiatric Research*, *44*(15), 1043–1051. https://doi.org/10.1016/j.jpsychires.2010.03.017

Goodenow, C., & Grady, K. E. (1993). The relationship of school belonging and friends' values to academic motivation among urban adolescent students. *Journal of Experimental Education*, *62*(1), 60–71. https://doi.org/10.1080/00220973.1993.9943831

Graham, J. R., Calloway, A., & Roemer, L. (2015). The buffering effects of emotion regulation in the relationship between experiences of racism and anxiety in a Black American sample. *Cognitive Therapy and Research*, *39*(5), 553–563. https://doi.org/10.1007/s10608-015-9682-8

Graham, J. R., Sorenson, S., & Hayes-Skelton, S. A. (2013). Enhancing the cultural sensitivity of cognitive behavioral interventions for anxiety in diverse populations. *The Behavior Therapist*, *36*(5), 101–108.

Greenberger, D., & Padesky, C. A. (2015). *Mind over mood: Change how you feel by changing the way you think* (2nd ed.). Guilford Press.

Greening, L., Stoppelbein, L., Dhossche, D., & Martin, W. (2005). Psychometric evaluation of a measure of Beck's negative cognitive triad for youth: Applications for African-American and Caucasian adolescents. *Depression and Anxiety*, *21*(4), 161–169. https://doi.org/10.1002/da.20073

Hoggard, L. S., Volpe, V., Thomas, A., Wallace, E., & Ellis, K. (2019). The role of emotional eating in the links between racial discrimination and physical and mental health. *Journal of Behavioral Medicine*, *42*(6), 1091–1103. https://doi.org/10.1007/s10865-019-00044-1

Holden, K. B., Belton, A. S., Hall, S. P. (2015). Qualitative examination of African American women's perspectives about depression. *Health, Culture and Society*, *8*(1), 44–57. https://doi.org/10.5195/hcs.2015.182

Hook, J. N., Davis, D., Owen, J., & DeBlaere, C. (2017). *Cultural humility: Engaging diverse identities in therapy*. American Psychological Association. https://doi.org/10.1037/0000037-000

Hudson, D. L., Neighbors, H. W., Geronimus, A. T., & Jackson, J. S. (2016). Racial discrimination, John Henryism, and depression among African Americans. *Journal of Black Psychology*, *42*(3), 221–243. https://doi.org/10.1177/0095798414567757

Jacob, G., Faber, S. C., Faber, N., Bartlett, A., Ouimet, A. J., & Williams, M. T. (2023). A systematic review of Black people coping with racism: Approaches, analysis, and empowerment. *Perspectives on Psychological Science*, *18*(2), 392–415. https://doi.org/10.1177/17456916221100509

James, D. (2021). Self- and group-focused internalized racism, anxiety, and depression symptoms among African American adults: A core self-evaluation mediated pathway. *Group Processes & Intergroup Relations*, *24*(8), 1335–1354. https://doi.org/10.1177/1368430220942849

Johnson, P. D. (2016). Somebodiness and its meaning to African American men. *Journal of Counseling & Development*, *94*(3), 333–343. https://doi.org/10.1002/jcad.12089

Jones, M. S., Womack, V., Jérémie-Brink, G., & Dickens, D. D. (2021). Gendered racism and mental health among young adult U.S. Black women: The moderating roles of gendered racial identity centrality and identity shifting. *Sex Roles: A Journal of Research*, *85*(3–4), 221–231. https://doi.org/10.1007/s11199-020-01214-1

Kaslow, N. J., Stark, K. D., Printz, B., Livingston, R., & Tsai, S. L. (1992). Cognitive Triad Inventory for Children: Development and relation to depression and anxiety. *Journal of Clinical Child Psychology*, *21*(4), 339–347. https://doi.org/10.1207/s15374424jccp2104_3

Keith, V. M., Lincoln, K. D., Taylor, R. J., & Jackson, J. S. (2010). Discriminatory experiences and depressive symptoms among African American women: Do skin tone and mastery matter? *Sex Roles: A Journal of Research*, *62*(1–2), 48–59. https://doi.org/10.1007/s11199-009-9706-5

Khubchandani, J. A., Atkinson, R. B., Ortega, G., Reidy, E., Mullen, J. T., Smink, D. S., & PACTS Trial Group (2022). Perceived discrimination among surgical residents at academic medical centers. *The Journal of Surgical Research*, *272*, 79–87. https://doi.org/10.1016/j.jss.2021.10.029

Liebschutz, J. M., Darko, G. O., Finley, E. P., Cawse, J. M., Bharel, M., & Orlander, J. D. (2006). In the minority: Black physicians in residency and their experiences. *Journal of the National Medical Association*, *98*(9), 1441–1448.

Matu, S. A. (2018). Cognitive therapy. In A. Vernon & K. A. Doyle (Eds.), *Cognitive behavior therapies: A guidebook for practitioners* (pp. 75–108). American Counseling Association.

McGee, E. O., Griffith, D. M., & Houston Stacey, L. III. (2019). "I know I have to work twice as hard and hope that makes me good enough:" Exploring the stress and strain of Black doctoral students in engineering and computing. *Teachers College Record*, *121*(4), 1–38. https://doi.org/10.1177/01614681191210040

Miles, J. R., Anders, C., Kivlighan, D. M. III, & Belcher Platt, A. A. (2021). Cultural ruptures: Addressing microaggressions in group therapy. *Group Dynamics: Theory, Research, and Practice*, *25*(1), 74–88. https://doi.org/10.1037/gdn0000149

Molina, K. M., & James, D. (2016). Discrimination, internalized racism, and depression: A comparative study of African American and Afro-Caribbean adults in the US. *Group Processes & Intergroup Relations*, *19*(4), 439–461. https://doi.org/10.1177/1368430216641304

Mouzon, D. M., & McLean, J. S. (2017). Internalized racism and mental health among African-Americans, US-born Caribbean Blacks, and foreign-born

Caribbean Blacks. *Ethnicity & Health, 22*(1), 36–48. https://doi.org/10.1080/13557 858.2016.1196652

Nobles, W., Goddard, L., & Gilbert, D. (2009). Culturecology, women, and African-centered HIV prevention. *Journal of Black Psychology, 35*(2), 228–246. https://doi.org/10.1177/0095798409333584

Owen, J., Imel, Z., Tao, K. W., Wampold, B., Smith, A., & Rodolfa, E. (2011). Cultural ruptures in short-term therapy: Working alliance as a mediator between clients' perceptions of microaggressions and therapy outcomes. *Counselling & Psychotherapy Research, 11*, 204–212. https://doi.org/10.1080/14733145.2010.491551

Padesky, C. A. (1994). Schema change processes in cognitive therapy. *Clinical Psychology and Psychotherapy, 1*(5), 267–278. https://doi.org/10.1002/cpp.5640010502

Palmer, R. T., & Walker, L. J. (2020, July 6). Proposing a concept of the Black tax to understand the experiences of Blacks in America. *Diverse Issues in Higher Education.* https://diverseeducation.com/article/182837/

Pascoe, E. A., & Smart Richman, L. (2009). Perceived discrimination and health: A meta-analytic review. *Psychological Bulletin, 135*(4), 531–554. https://doi.org/10.1037/a0016059

Payne, J. S. (2014). Social determinants affecting major depressive disorder: Diagnostic accuracy for African American men. *Best Practices in Mental Health, 10*(2), 78–95.

Pieterse, A. L., Todd, N. R., Neville, H. A., & Carter, R. T. (2012). Perceived racism and mental health among Black American adults: A meta-analytic review. *Journal of Counseling Psychology, 59*(1), 1–9. https://doi.org/10.1037/a0026208

Pössel, P. (2009). Cognitive Triad Inventory (CTI): Psychometric properties and factor structure of the German translation. *Journal of Behavior Therapy and Experimental Psychiatry, 40*(2), 240–247. https://doi.org/10.1016/j.jbtep.2008.12.001

Powell, W., Banks, K. H., & Mattis, J. S. (2017). Buried hatchets, marked locations: Forgiveness, everyday racial discrimination, and African American men's depressive symptomatology. *American Journal of Orthopsychiatry, 87*(6), 646–662. https://doi.org/10.1037/ort0000210

Sacco, A., Pössel, P., & Roane, S. J. (2023). Perceived discrimination and depressive symptoms: What role does the cognitive triad play? *Journal of Clinical Psychology, 79*(4), 985–1001. https://doi.org/10.1002/jclp.23452

Saleem, F. T., Busby, D. R., & Lambert, S. F. (2018). Neighborhood social processes as moderators between racial discrimination and depressive symptoms for African American adolescents. *Journal of Community Psychology, 46*(6), 747–761. https://doi.org/10.1002/jcop.21970

Sidanius, J., Levin, S., & Pratto, F. (1996). Consensual social dominance orientation and its correlates within the hierarchical structure of American society. *International Journal of Intercultural Relations, 20*(3–4), 385–408. https://doi.org/10.1016/0147-1767(96)00025-9

Śliwerski, A. (2014). Psychometric properties of the Polish version of the Cognitive Triad Inventory (CTI)—Preliminary study. *Archives of Psychiatry and Psychotherapy, 16*(1), 47–54. https://doi.org/10.12740/APP/21444

Steele, C. M., & Aronson, J. (1995). Stereotype threat and the intellectual test performance of African-Americans. *Journal of Personality and Social Psychology, 69*(5), 797–811. https://doi.org/10.1037/0022-3514.69.5.797

Steele, J. M. (2020). A CBT approach to internalized racism among African Americans. *International Journal for the Advancement of Counselling, 42*(3), 217–233. https://doi.org/10.1007/s10447-020-09402-0

Steele, J. M., & Newton, C. S. (2022). Culturally adapted cognitive behavior therapy as a model to address internalized racism among African American clients. *Journal of Mental Health Counseling, 44*(2), 98–116. https://doi.org/10.17744/mehc.44.2.01

Steele, J. M., & Newton, C. S. (2023). *Black lives are beautiful: 50 tools to heal from trauma and promote positive racial identity.* Routledge.

Su, J., Seaton, E. K., Williams, C. D., Spit for Science Working Group, & Dick, D. M. (2021). Racial discrimination, depressive symptoms, ethnic-racial identity, and alcohol use among Black American college students. *Psychology of Addictive Behaviors: Journal of the Society of Psychologists in Addictive Behaviors, 35*(5), 523–535. https://doi.org/10.1037/adb0000717

Substance Abuse and Mental Health Services Administration. (2022). *Key Substance Use and Mental Health Indicators in the United States: Results from the 2021 National Survey on Drug Use and Health.* https://www.samhsa.gov/data/report/2021-nsduh-annual-national-report

Sue, D. W., Alsaidi, S., Awad, M. N., Glaeser, E., Calle, C. Z., & Mendez, N. (2019). Disarming racial microaggressions: Microintervention strategies for targets, White allies, and bystanders. *American Psychologist, 74*(1), 128–142. https://doi.org/10.1037/amp0000296

Sue, D. W., Capodilupo, C. M., Torino, G. C., Bucceri, J. M., Holder, A. M. B., Nadal, K. L., & Esquilin, M. (2007). Racial microaggressions in everyday life: Implications for clinical practice. *American Psychologist, 62*(4), 271–286. https://doi.org/10.1037/0003-066X.62.4.271

Taylor, R. E., & Kuo, B. C. H. (2019). Black American psychological help-seeking intention: An integrated literature review with recommendations for clinical practice. *Journal of Psychotherapy Integration, 29*(4), 325–337. https://doi.org/10.1037/int0000131

Tichavakunda, A. A. (2022) Taking Black joy seriously in higher education. *Change: The Magazine of Higher Learning, 54*(5), 52–56. https://doi.org/10.1080/00091383.2022.2101868

Trahan, L. H., Carges, E., Stanley, M. A., & Evans-Hudnall, G. (2016). Decreasing PTSD and depression symptom barriers to weight loss using an integrated CBT approach. *Clinical Case Studies, 15*(4), 280–294. https://doi.org/10.1177/1534650116637918

Tucker, C., Dixon, A., & Griddine, K. (2010). Academically successful African American male urban high school students' experiences of mattering to others at school. *Professional School Counseling, 14*(2), 135–145. https://doi.org/10.1177/2156759X1001400202

Turner, E. A., Harrell, S. P., & Bryant-Davis, T. (2022). Black Love, Activism, and Community (BLAC): The BLAC model of healing and resilience. *Journal of Black Psychology, 48*(3–4), 547–568. https://doi.org/10.1177/00957984211018364

Vandiver, B. J., Fhagen-Smith, P. E., Cokley, K. O., Cross, W. E., Jr., & Worrell, F. C. (2001). Cross's Nigrescence model: From theory to scale to theory. *Journal of Multicultural Counseling and Development, 29*(3), 174–200. https://doi.org/10.1002/j.2161-1912.2001.tb00516.x

Vines, A. I., Ward, J. B., Cordoba, E., & Black, K. Z. (2017). Perceived racial/ethnic discrimination and mental health: A review and future directions for social epidemiology. *Current Epidemiology Reports*, *4*(2), 156–165. https://doi.org/10.1007/s40471-017-0106-z

Walker, R. L., Salami, T. K., Carter, S. E., & Flowers, K. (2014). Perceived racism and suicide ideation: Mediating role of depression but moderating role of religiosity among African American adults. *Suicide & Life-threatening Behavior*, *44*(5), 548–559. https://doi.org/10.1111/sltb.12089

Walling, S. M., Suvak, M. K., Howard, J. M., Taft, C. T., & Murphy, C. M. (2012). Race/ethnicity as a predictor of change in working alliance during cognitive behavioral therapy for intimate partner violence perpetrators. *Psychotherapy*, *49*(2), 180–189. https://doi.org/10.1037/a0025751

Walton, Q. L. (2022). Living in between: A grounded theory study of depression among middle-class Black women. *Journal of Black Psychology*, *48*(2), 139–172. https://doi.org/10.1177/00957984211036541

Wenzel, A. (2019). *Cognitive behavioral therapy for beginners*. Routledge.

Williams, D. R. (2018). Stress and the mental health of populations of color: Advancing our understanding of race-related stressors. *Journal of Health and Social Behavior*, *59*(4), 466–485. https://doi.org/10.1177/0022146518814251

Williams, D. R., González, H. M., Neighbors, H., Nesse, R., Abelson, J. M., Sweetman, J., & Jackson, J. S. (2007). Prevalence and distribution of major depressive disorder in African Americans, Caribbean blacks, and non-Hispanic whites: Results from the National Survey of American Life. *Archives of General Psychiatry*, *64*(3), 305–315. https://doi.org/10.1001/archpsyc.64.3.305

Williams, M. T. (2019). Adverse racial climates in academia: Conceptualization, interventions, and call to action. *New Ideas in Psychology*, *55*, 58–67. https://doi.org/10.1016/j.newideapsych.2019.05.002

Williams, M. T., Holmes, S., Zare, M., Haeny, A., & Faber, S. (2022). An evidence-based approach for treating stress and trauma due to racism. *Cognitive and Behavioral Practice*. Advance online publication. https://doi.org/10.1016/j.cbpra.2022.07.001

Yap, S. C. Y., Settles, I. H., & Pratt-Hyatt, J. S. (2011). Mediators of the relationship between racial identity and life satisfaction in a community sample of African American women and men. *Cultural Diversity and Ethnic Minority Psychology*, *17*(1), 89–97. https://doi.org/10.1037/a0022535

Zimmerman, G. M., & Miller-Smith, A. (2022). The impact of anticipated, vicarious, and experienced racial and ethnic discrimination on depression and suicidal behavior among Chicago youth. *Social Science Research*, *101*, 102623. https://doi.org/10.1016/j.ssresearch.2021.102623

Chapter 10

Putting It All Together

Anxiety Disorders

Anxiety disorders are some of the most common mental health challenges experienced in the United States, with a lifetime prevalence rate of up to 34 percent among the general U.S. population (Bandelow & Michaelis, 2015) and 22 percent among African Americans (Alvarez et al., 2019). While the exact cause of any anxiety disorder varies by individual, there is evidence that biological factors, family background, and life experiences, particularly stressful ones, play a role.

According to the fifth edition of the *Diagnostic and Statistical Manual of Mental Disorders* (*DSM-5*), anxiety disorders include mental health conditions such as Separation Anxiety Disorder, Selective Mutism, Specific Phobia, Social Anxiety Disorder, Panic Disorder, Agoraphobia, and Generalized Anxiety Disorder (American Psychiatric Association, 2013). Within CBT, there are a number of models that explain the connections among the thoughts, feelings, and behaviors that lead to these disorders. D. A. Clark and A. T. Beck (2011), for example, theorized that anxiety occurs when individuals overestimate the probability and severity of danger and underestimate their resources to cope with the danger. This is called the *risk/resource model* (Beck Institute, n.d.). Once this model is activated, people who suffer from anxiety become overly focused on the things they perceive as threats. This is called *hypervigilance*. Hypervigilance is driven by the belief that being attentive to potential threats can help one avoid these threats or cope with them better. Unfortunately, being overly focused on potential threats actually has the opposite effect. It prevents individuals from being able to accurately perceive how much danger there actually is in a situation, causes them to view neutral situations as threatening, makes them ignore signs of safety in their environment, interferes with their performance, and leads to physiological symptoms like an upset stomach, rapid heart rate, nausea, dizziness, or difficulty breathing.

In this chapter, I explore one anxiety disorder, Social Anxiety Disorder (SAD), and one cognitive model of SAD, the Rapee-Heimberg (1997) model, during treatment with an African American client who experiences

DOI: 10.4324/9781003196303-10

SAD within the context of racialized social interactions. In the section that follows, key features of SAD are described, proceded by a discussion of the experience of social anxiety among African Americans and the role of racial discrimination. The Rapee-Heimberg (1997) model of social anxiety is then discussed, followed by a review of common cognitive restructuring and exposure approaches utilized in the treatment of SAD. I then illustrate a course of treatment using a case example.

Understanding Social Anxiety Disorder

Social Anxiety Disorder, previously known as Social Phobia, is one of the most common types of anxiety disorders (Asnaani et al., 2015). To be diagnosed with SAD, individuals must meet the following criteria: (A) marked fear or anxiety in social situations in which the person may be exposed to scrutiny by others; (B) fear of anxiety symptoms being judged by others; (C) social situations almost always provoke fear or anxiety; (D) social situations are almost always avoided; (E) fear or anxiety is disproportionate to the actual threat posed; (F) the fear, anxiety, or avoidance is persistent; (G) the fear, anxiety, or avoidance causes clinically significant distress or impairment in functioning; (H) the fear, anxiety, or avoidance is not attributable to substance use or a medical condition; (I) the fear, anxiety, or avoidance is not better explained by another mental health condition; and (J) the fear, anxiety, or avoidance is not related to another medical condition (American Psychiatric Association, 2013).

As defined by the *DSM-5* criteria presented above, individuals with SAD fear being negatively evaluated, judged, or humiliated by others (American Psychiatric Association, 2013). For many individuals, these fears are linked to the individual's core beliefs. Recall from Chapter 7 that *core beliefs* are the specific thoughts individuals have about themselves (J. S. Beck, 2020). When these beliefs are negative, they tend to focus on being unlovable, helpless, or worthless. Because of these beliefs, individuals with social anxiety experience social interactions with intense dread or attempt to avoid them altogether. This process consists of five primary elements (Beck Institute, n.d.). First, individuals with SAD make negative predictions about what their social interactions will be like based on their assumptions about themselves and others in their social environment. This type of thinking is called *anticipatory processing* and usually causes individuals to believe they will perform poorly in social situations. Once in the social situation, socially anxious individuals become overly self-focused believing that if they focus enough attention on themselves, they can evaluate and alter how they perform in social situations in order to meet the high standards they have set for themselves. Unfortunately, this behavior, known as *self-focused attention*, often has the opposite effect and instead reinforces or even exaggerates the negative view socially anxious individuals have of themselves (D. A. Clark & A. T. Beck, 2012).

The third element of SAD consists of safety behaviors. *Safety behaviors* are actions individuals take to control or minimize their anxiety. Examples of safety behaviors include staying quiet in social situations, mentally rehearsing conversations, over-preparing for presentations and meetings, relying on alcohol or recreational drugs, avoiding eye contact, and constantly checking oneself for physical signs of anxiety. While these behaviors may reduce feelings of anxiety in the short-term, in the long-term they worsen social anxiety because they increase self-focused attention, prevent individuals from testing their fears, and lead to self-fulfilling prophesies. Use of safety behaviors over an extended period of time may also result in *anxiety-induced social skill deficits*, which is the fourth element of SAD. The final element of SAD is *post-event processing*, which is the process of reviewing what happened during an event after it is over in order to perform better in the future (D. A. Clark & A. T. Beck, 2012).

Broadly, there is a paucity of research examining SAD and its treatment among African Americans (Sibrava et al., 2013; Zerr et al., 2011). In the following section, I provide a review of the limited research on this topic, highlighting the role of racial discrimination and related cultural influences in the development of SAD among this population.

Social Anxiety in African Americans and the Role of Racial Discrimination

As stated, few studies explore the incidence and treatment of SAD among African Americans; however, a burgeoning body of research suggests that the experience of this disorder among this group of individuals is uniquely affected by encounters with race and racism (Buckner & Dean, 2017; Chou et al., 2012; Manning et al., 2017). A. B. Johnson (2006), for example, asserted that for African Americans, factors such as racism, stereotypes, and pressure to perform influence the social perceptions, biases, and experiences that shape the cognitions leading to social anxiety. Expounding on this assertion, A. B. Johnson (2006) explained that social anxiety is often correlated with social environments that do not support confident and independent behavior, which for African Americans is significant due to their social milieu of racial stigma and oppression. More specifically, the racially oppressed social status of African Americans has been associated with outcomes such as a general tendency toward self-focused attention and criticism, inhibited spontaneity, overly negative evaluations of social performance, exaggerated perceptions of disapproval, and beliefs that the expectations of others are too high to attain, all key features of social anxiety. Accordingly, the scrutiny, hostility, and/or disregard received from others due to racism, along with internalized racial stigma, all contribute to a clinical phenomenology in social anxiety with significant implications for assessment, conceptualization, and treatment among the African American population.

Unfortunately, racially hostile social situations that often lead to the development and maintenance of social anxiety may be worsened and become more dangerous when socially anxious behaviors and attitudes are exhibited. Of particular relevance given recent instances of police brutality in the African American community is the relationship between fears of negative evaluations and feelings of safety in the presence of police. According to Clevinger et al. (2018), heightened fears of negative evaluation are often associated with behavioral patterns such as a lowered gaze, avoidance of eye contact, fidgeting, and tensing of muscles, which are behaviors commonly believed to signal deception. Police officers who have been trained to interpret these behaviors as suspicious may misjudge and respond to individuals in ways that reinforce the perception of threat and socially anxious behavior among African Americans, creating a vicious cycle. In fact, one study of the relationship among racial group membership, fears of negative evaluation, and perceptions of safety in the presence of police officers found that the interaction between African American racial group membership and fears of negative evaluation does have an association with perceptions of safety in the presence of police, such that greater fears of negative evaluation lead to less feelings of safety in the presence of police (Clevinger et al., 2018). Although not mentioned by the study's authors, one implication for these results when working to empower African Americans to heal from racism concerns positive racial socialization and preparation for bias; that is, therapists may consider providing clients with psychoeducation on the way social anxiety may influence interactions with police in order to support surviving these interactions.

Beyond overt experiences with discrimination, cultural influences that may be conceptualized as traumatic responses to racism within the African American community (Menakem, 2022) have also been linked to SAD. One phenomenon known as *the acting White accusation*, for example, has been associated with social anxiety in multiple studies. According to Davis et al. (2018), "the acting White accusation (AWA) arises when a Black adolescent's ethnic/racial identity (ERI) is perceived as being not Black enough by another Black adolescent or group of adolescents" (p. 23). In their study of young Black women ages 10 to 18 years, these researchers found that in their sample of 31 participants, all had experienced the acting White accusation at least once in their life. Moreover, frequency and bother associated with the accusation were positively related to social anxiety, according to scores on the Acting White Experiences Questionnaire (Neal-Barnett et al., 2010) and the Multidimensional Anxiety Scale for Children-2nd edition (March, 2013). These results were replicated in another study of Black adolescents, which also found a predictive relationship between the acting White accusation and anxiety using the same measures, although only the total anxiety score was utilized in this research (Murray et al., 2012).

Findings from studies on the relationship between the acting White accusation and social anxiety suggest that negative feedback concerning one's racial identity may be internalized and lead to negative self-perceptions. Social anxiety as a result of negative feedback and self-perceptions may also be developed in response to stereotypes. *Stereotypes* are oversimplified generalizations about groups or categories of people. In Chapter 2, I discussed *stereotype threat*, which is defined as the fear of conforming to negative stereotypes about one's social group, leading to worsened task performance (C. M. Steele & Aronson, 1995; Stone et al., 2012). Another similar concept, *stereotype confirmation concerns*, has also been found to have a significant relationship to social anxiety more broadly. Stereotype confirmation concerns refer to the persistent worries people have about appearing to validate negative stereotypes concerning social groups to which they belong (Contrada et al., 2001). Recall that fear of negative evaluations from others is a key feature of SAD. According to research, stereotype confirmation concerns are predictive of fears of negative evaluations from others, such that greater concern predicts greater fear (S. B. Johnson & Anderson, 2014). Moreover, of particular relevance to the therapeutic process, stereotype confirmation concerns have also been found to predict attrition rates during therapy (S. Johnson et al., 2014).

Given the issues of marginalization and culture discussed above, researchers suggest that an individual's sociocultural background should be taken into consideration when evaluating their social behaviors and attitudes. A review of research on the cultural expression of SAD conducted by Hoffman and colleagues (2010), for example, found that for individuals who belong to collectivistic cultures, the significance of social behavior may be greater when compared to people from individualistic cultures, as deviations from cultural rules and guidelines may more readily lead to social sanctions. Moreover, individuals from collectivistic cultures may also possess self-construals that are more heavily dependent on interpersonal relationships and harmony with the group, such that individuals with dependent self-construals may more regularly adjust themselves to be in sync with the thoughts, feelings, and behaviors of important others. This has significant implications for the conceptualization of SAD among individuals from more collectivistic cultures, which as discussed in Chapter 3, broadly includes members of the African American community. Namely, interdependence may be positively correlated with embarrassability and fear of negative evaluations, which in turn may contribute to greater sensitivity and attention to social cues in social situations (Hofmann et al., 2010).

Based on the review of literature provided above, it is clear that racial discrimination may contribute to the etiology of SAD among African Americans. Conversely, positive racial socialization and relationships with family and community members may buffer against meeting criteria for SAD in this population. One study of African American and Black Caribbean adults, for example, found that emotional closeness and positive contact with family or friends were protective factors for SAD (Levine et al., 2015). Similarly, using structural equation modeling, a study of African American schoolchildren found that high ethnic pride was associated with high parental acceptance, which in turn, was associated with lower social anxiety among participants (Gray et al., 2011). As such, while therapists should be mindful of the negative relationship between racial oppression and social anxiety, acknowledgment of the beneficial aspects of race such as racial/ethnic pride and positive relationships with friends and family may highlight client strengths and culturally derived sources of coping.

Rapee-Heimberg Model

As mentioned in the introduction to this chapter, a number of cognitive models have been created to explain the development and maintenance of social anxiety. Some of these models include those developed by D. M. Clark and Wells (1995), Hofmann (2007), and Rapee and Heimberg (1997). Given the role of negative self-perceptions and self-focused attention in concerns that shape the structure of social anxiety among African Americans, particularly in anticipation of or when entering into a social situation, the Rapee-Heimberg (1997) model is highlighted in this chapter.

The Rapee-Heimberg (1997) cognitive behavioral model of social anxiety (see Figure 10.1) is based on two primary assumptions: (1) individuals with social anxiety believe people are inherently critical and likely to evaluate others negatively, and (2) individuals with social anxiety believe that being positively appraised by others is of fundamental importance. Accordingly, during social situations, individuals with social anxiety form mental representations of their external appearance and behavior, presumably as they believe they would been seen by others. Simultaneously, they focus their attention on this internal representation, as well as any perceived threats in the environment. These perceptions are informed by a variety of inputs, including internal proprioceptive and physical symptoms, as well as external feedback and indicators of negative evaluation from others. Once the negative internal or external cues are observed, the individual makes negative predictions about their ability to meet the audience's expectations, focusing on the negative observations of self and the audience's behavior and judging themselves inferior in the comparison, leading to the difficult behavioral, physical, and cognitive symptoms of social anxiety.

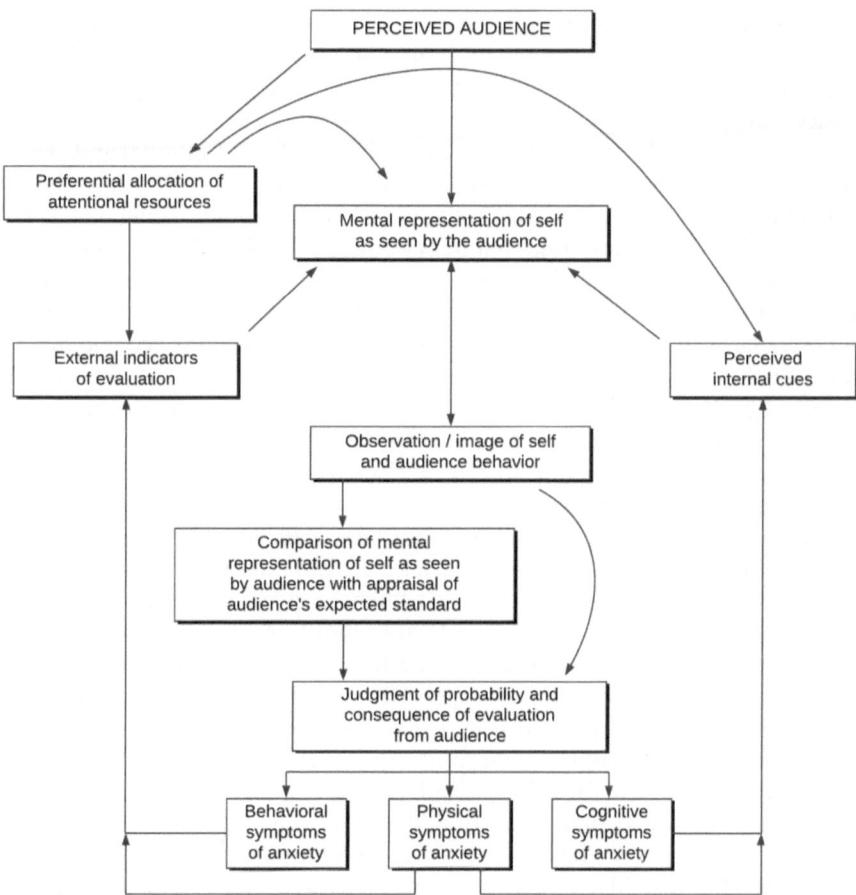

Figure 10.1 Rapee-Hiemberg Cognitive Model of Social Anxiety. Adapted from Heimberg, R. C., Brozovich, F. A., & Rapee, R. M. (2010). A cognitive behavioral model of social anxiety disorder: Update and extension. In S. G. Hofmann & P. M. DiBartolo (Eds.), *Social anxiety: Clinical, developmental, and social perspectives* (pp. 395–422). Elsevier Academic Press. https://doi.org/10.1016/B978-0-12-375096-9.00015-8

Consider Jordan, a young 17-year-old African American man recently diagnosed with SAD. Jordan was raised in a two-parent, upper-middle class family. During therapy, he admitted concerns about being perceived by others as weak or not masculine enough, which the therapist conceptualized as internalized gendered racial stereotypes (Harris, 1995). At his last session, Jordan discussed a situation in which he was in his family's hometown of Cleveland visiting for the summer break while on crutches recuperating from a torn Achilles tendon. One afternoon, he was invited by his cousin to go for a short walk in a popular shopping area of their community. In this situation,

Jordan imagined a perceived audience of his cousin and others in the community who might see his limited mobility and view him as vulnerable, which he defined as being an "easy target" to mock or cause physical harm.

According to the Rapee-Heimberg (1997) model, Jordan's mental representation was informed by his past experiences and a variety of internal and external cues. Specifically, Jordan was often teased for being "skinny" during school, and in the past, saw peers who did not appear "tough enough" being bullied by others. Jordan further reported that he is frequently told he should "stand up" for himself more, which he finds difficult due to his own nervousness and perception of himself as "corny." Additionally, when Jordan is in social situations he perceives as threatening, he notices that his voice and hands become shaky, which further contributes to his negative mental representation of himself. As theorized by Rapee and Heimberg (1997), Jordan's attentional resources during these situations are accordingly devoted to monitoring the salient aspects of his negative self-image and signs of external threats, which he described as "being on guard" in certain environments or when around "tough guys."

When considering the invitation to go on a walk in a popular shopping area, Jordan predicted that his injured leg and thin physique would lead others to view him as "weak," which would likely be evidenced by certain looks or even name calling from others and cause him to be embarrassed in front of his cousin. Initially, Jordan attempted to avoid the situation by claiming that he wanted to stay home to spend time with their grandmother. In response, the cousin explained they would not be gone for long and when Jordan refused the invitation a second time, the cousin accused Jordan of "being scarry." To save face, Jordan subsequently agreed to go on the walk. While there, he noted that much of his attention was devoted to constant scanning of the area while also trying to maintain an appearance of being unbothered because Black men are supposed to be tough. Despite his efforts, Jordan was unable to refute his negative predictions, perseverating on thoughts such as, "Something bad is probably going to happen" and "If I show any emotions, people will think I'm not strong," and experiencing physical reactions that included increased heart rate and hot flashes.

Assessment

Earlier in this chapter, I mentioned that differences may exist in the expression of social anxiety among individuals who belong to collectivistic cultures when compared to people with more individualistic worldviews (Hofmann et al., 2010). Specifically, individuals from collectivistic cultures may have self-construals that are more heavily dependent on interpersonal relationships and harmony with the group, which is correlated with embarrassability and fear of negative evaluations and may contribute to greater sensitivity to social cues in social situations. Asnaani et al. (2015), for example, described previous research which suggests individuals from collectivistic cultures may have greater fear of offending others, whereas those from individualistic cultures may experience greater fear of public performance due to a high regard for personal achievement. Among African Americans, studies have shown that these differences result in variability in the structure of social anxiety and feared social situations among this population when compared to their White counterparts. Results from a confirmatory factor analysis conducted by Melka et al. (2010), for example, showed that item loadings on the Fear of Negative Evaluation Scale (Watson & Friend, 1969) and the Social Avoidance and Distress Scale (Watson & Friend, 1969) were different across samples of African American and European American undergraduate students, with statistical tests suggesting that items on both measures be dropped for the African American sample. These findings, however, are contrasted with the results of a study that found a model of feared social situations that consisted of performance/public speaking, social interaction, and observational domains across Latinx, African American, and White populations (Asnaani et al., 2015).

Due to the potentially unique structure of SAD among African Americans, clinicians should select measures that have been found to be meaningful and accurate for use with this population when possible (Melka et al., 2010). The Positive and Negative Affect Scales of the Positive and Negative Affect Schedule–Expanded form (PANAS-X; Watson & L. A. Clark, 1994), for example, has been found to be reliable in predicting social anxiety in a sample of African American women (Petrie et al., 2013). This assessment consists of 60 items that measure positive and negative affect, as well as 11 items that measure other specific affects. Beyond the PANAS-X, there are several direct measures of social anxiety such as the Liebowitz Social Anxiety Scale (LSAS; Liebowitz, 1987) and the Social Phobia and Anxiety Inventory for Children (SPAI-C; Beidel et al. 1995), which are commonly used for the assessment of social anxiety. The LSAS (Liebowitz, 1987) consists of 24 social situations that are each rated for level of fear and avoidance and has been examined for use with African American populations (Beard et al., 2011). Likewise, the 26-item SPAI-C (Beidel et al. 1995) has also been examined for use with African Americans (Pina et al., 2014). However, given differences that may exist in the structure of social anxiety among African Americans, clinicians should exercise caution in their use of these assessments during diagnosis, being sure to utilize comprehensive assessment strategies that include interviews, behavioral assessments, and when working with youth, parent report (Ferrell et al., 2004). Moreover, clinicians should also be cognizant of other factors that may influence the assessment process, such as cultural mistrust and cultural differences in speech and communication (Turner & Mills, 2016).

Finally, several assessments are also available to measure specific cognitions and behaviors that may be useful for cognitive conceptualization and case formulation purposes in CBT according to D. M. Clark and Wells' (1995) model of social anxiety. The Social Cognitions Questionnaire (SCQ) assesses 22 of the most common social anxiety disorder–related negative automatic thoughts. The 29-item Social Behavior Questionnaire (SBQ) assesses client use of common social anxiety related safety behaviors. Last, the 50-item Social Attitudes Questionnaire (SAQ) assesses common core and intermediate beliefs that may increase vulnerability to social anxiety disorder. Each of these scales is available for clinician use at https://oxcadatresources.com/questionnaires/.

Culturally Adapted Cognitive Restructuring and Mindfulness

According to Cohen (2022), core elements of SAD include anxiety and shame. As previously discussed, anxiety during social situations develops as a result of fear of judgment from others, which might lead to embarrassment or feelings of rejection. Shame, on the other hand, occurs as a result of a sense of personal deficiency due to perfectionism. Effective social anxiety treatment, therefore, requires the integration of behavioral, cognitive, and mindfulness approaches to CBT to address the negative cognitions and avoidance behaviors associated with these elements of social anxiety, as well as the physiological symptoms and other internal cues that additionally contribute to elements of this condition.

Recall from the previous section, "Understanding Social Anxiety Disorder," that one of the maintaining factors of social anxiety, self-focused attention, while meant to prevent embarrassment and negative judgment from others, often has the opposite effect and instead reinforces or even exaggerates the negative view socially anxious individuals have of themselves (D. A. Clark & A. T. Beck, 2012). Within the Rapee-Heimberg (1997) model, this attention may be conceptualized as a preoccupation with the mental representation of self as seen by the audience and heightened awareness of internal proprioceptive and physical symptoms. Unfortunately, this ruminating behavior often inhibits spontaneity and contributes to deficits in social performance that may led to negative feedback from others, creating a vicious cycle (A. B. Johnson, 2006; Kelly-Turner & Radomsky, 2022; Meral & Vriends, 2021). Accordingly, mindfulness training is often implemented during CBT as a strategy to teach clients to become aware of their tendency to self-focus and to redirect their attentional processes (Bögels & Mansell, 2004; Bögels et al., 2006). More about the use of mindfulness-based interventions with African Americans is discussed in Chapter 11; however, it is important to note that due to cultural and religious beliefs, some African Americans may initially feel uncomfortable with use of such interventions. Therefore, therapists should be intentional in orienting clients to the use of these interventions, using neutral language that refers to mindfulness as non-judgmental attention to one's thoughts, emotions, and physical sensations, and encouraging clients to look to their own religious texts to learn what they say about mindfulness (Watson-Singleton et al., 2019). Additionally, consistent with research, therapists may want to emphasize external rather than internal mindfulness techniques in order to reinforce engagement with the here and now moment when working with socially anxious clients (Cohen, 2022).

Beyond mindfulness training, therapists should also utilize traditional cognitive restructuring techniques to address the negative automatic thoughts and underlying beliefs that lead to social anxiety. According to Cohen (2022), the most common hot thoughts in social anxiety concern appearance, performance, and judgment. This is consistent with the model of feared social situations that consists of performance/public speaking, social interaction, and observational domains identified by Asnaani et al. (2015). When considered within the context of healing from racism and issues such as stereotype confirmation concerns (Contrada et al., 2001) and the acting White accusation (Davis et al., 2018), examples of these thoughts may include, "I might look or sound too Black/White," "They won't think I'm good enough," and "They probably think I have an attitude." Cognitive restructuring strategies that may be used to address these thoughts and beliefs include thought records, analyzing anticipatory anxiety, recording social interactions, probing post-event rumination, reevaluating past experiences of social anxiety, assertive defense of the self, developing and strengthening new core beliefs, core belief continuums, and roleplays (D. A. Clark & A. T. Beck, 2012; Padesky, 1994, 1997).

Modified Exposure and Experiments

In addition to cognitive restructuring, exposure and behavioral experiments are also used during the treatment of social anxiety to address avoidance and test negative predictions in social situations (D. A. Clark & A. T. Beck, 2012). As discussed in Chapter 1, *exposure therapy* refers to interventions that help individuals take small, incremental steps toward engaging in feared situations. A benefit of these exercises is that they help clients increase their confidence in their ability to cope with threatening outcomes and reduce their sense of uncertainty in social situations. Generally, there are two types of exposure interventions: imaginal exposure and in-vivo exposure (Leahy et al., 2012). Imaginal exposure involves picturing oneself in a feared situation while implementing various coping and relaxation strategies, with the aim of becoming less distressed over time. Jordan, our previous clinical example, for instance, may have imagined himself in social settings he previously perceived as threatening, such as playing basketball or being in proximity to unfamiliar peers. In-vivo exposure, on the other hand, involves directly engaging in a feared situation, which allows clients to directly test the beliefs that lead to social anxiety. For Jordan, examples of in-vivo exposures may have included actually engaging in the basketball games or social situations with unfamiliar peers he envisioned during his imaginal exposures.

Among African Americans, one case study has found exposure therapy that includes racially relevant cues during imaginal and in-vivo exposures to be an effective treatment for social anxiety (Fink et al., 1996). In this research, the participant was a 39-year-old African American female physician who was often the only Black student in classes during residency. She endorsed particularly problematic fears during interactions with White male physicians and was accordingly provided with imaginal flooding scenes and in-vivo homework assignments that included racially salient content. Based on scores from pre- and post-administrations of several measures of social anxiety, this treatment, which was implemented within the context of group skills training and individual therapy, was effective in reducing social anxiety and associated distress. Moreover, her functioning was able to return to normal and she experienced improvement in impromptu speech and social interactions. Accordingly, this study demonstrates the increased value of exposure exercises that are modified to include racially salient material.

Combined with each other, imaginal and in-vivo exposures can be used to construct *exposure hierarchies*, which usually consist of 15 to 20 feared social situations ranked from least to most anxiety producing (Leahy et al., 2012). Information such as ratings of the expected level of anxiety or avoidance, as well as the anxious thoughts experienced in these situations, may also be included in the hierarchy (D. A. Clark & A. T. Beck, 2012). Implementation of an exposure hierarchy typically begins with situations that provoke a moderate level of anxiety, with the client successively engaging in increasingly distressing activities as they habituate to each situation. Roleplays may also be used during this process as a bridge between imaginal and in-vivo exposures (Leahy et al., 2012).

Finally, as mentioned, behavioral experiments are another intervention designed to assist clients with addressing avoidance behaviors and testing negative thoughts (J. S. Beck, 2020). More specifically, these experiments refer to social situations therapists and clients collaboratively devise to test hot thoughts, challenge negative predictions, and eliminate safety behaviors (Cohen, 2022). When constructing behavioral experiments, many therapists also teach clients to integrate external mindfulness into the process, which helps the client to be absorbed in the present moment and attuned to the cognitive and sensory information needed to test the validity of their thoughts. This includes defusing from distractions, focusing on the people one is with, and showing curious interest in the activities in which one is engaged without judgment (Cohen, 2022).

Because a primary goal of a behavioral experiment is to challenge maladaptive thinking, it is important that the therapist and client set up scenarios that are likely to succeed and engage in appropriate cognitive restructuring beforehand to decrease anticipatory anxiety and increase motivation and follow through (J. S. Beck, 2020; Cohen, 2022). Recall once more our clinical example, Jordan. One of the negative beliefs that increased Jordan's anxiety during social situations was, "Something bad is probably going to happen." To test this belief, Jordan agreed to attend one of his school's football games, which he typically avoided. Before the day of the game, Jordan completed a written arguments roleplay where he challenged negative thoughts and predictions associated with attending the event. Jordan also prepared for the game by practicing external mindfulness on a regular basis, focusing on the conversations and persons he interacts with rather than on self-focused thoughts and fears that his voice or hands might be shaking. Additionally, although there was low likelihood, Jordan and the therapist discussed possible negative outcomes, creating coping cards to address maladaptive thoughts that might occur in case something bad did happen (J. S. Beck, 2020).

Case Illustration: Shondra

Shondra is a 35-year-old African American woman who was referred to therapy by an executive career coach. Seven months prior to intake, Shondra was promoted to an Assistant Director position at a large and predominantly White non-profit organization. Before her promotion, Shondra was well-liked by most of her peers. However, since taking on additional leadership and management responsibilities, some of her colleagues have accused Shondra of being "difficult" and "unfriendly." Accordingly, Shondra, who was diagnosed with Social Phobia during college, reports an increase in worried and anxious thoughts, fearing embarrassment as a result of open hostility or insubordination from her juniors. In describing this concern further, Shondra reported that due to these fears, she typically avoids most staff meetings, often scheduling conflicting appointments outside of the office at the time of the meetings. When she does attend staff meetings, Shondra notices that she has poor concentration and is overly focused on her appearance and the tone of her voice. Shondra explained that her experiences at other places of employment were deeply affected by "the angry Black woman" stereotype, and that she was often accused of having an attitude for what Shondra called "just doing my job." Therefore, in her current interactions with others she attempts to communicate in ways she believes would be acceptable to her White colleagues, although Shondra admits that this strategy typically causes her to be withdrawn and restricted during her interactions rather than more accepted.

At intake, Shondra scored 39 and 28 on the Fear and Avoidance subscales of the LSAS, respectively (Liebowitz, 1987). Together, these two subscale scores resulted in a total score of 67, indicating a marked level of generalized social anxiety. Shondra also completed the Brief Fear of Negative Evaluation Scale (BFNE; Leary, 1983), a 12-item questionnaire that measures an individual's fears of being negatively evaluated. Her score was 47, which was clinically significant. During her diagnostic interview, Shondra additionally endorsed negative impacts to her functioning, noting impediments to her work performance, physiological complaints, and significant psychological distress as a result of her social anxiety, lasting more than six months. Given this data, Shondra's previous diagnosis of F40.11 Social Phobia, Generalized was confirmed. Her last course of therapy was 12 years prior, when she received her initial diagnosis during college.

Although Shondra's current course of therapy was precipitated by the difficulties at her place of employment, her social history revealed lifelong struggles with social anxiety. Shondra described herself as a naturally shy child, recalling crying every day for weeks at the start of each school year while in elementary school. Shondra, who was raised by her grandmother in a racially diverse community, stated that she was often ostracized by both Black and White peers, being mocked by Black peers for "talking White" and teased by White peers about aspects of her appearance such as her hair texture and for wearing Black hairstyles. Beyond her peers, Shondra also reported feeling overlooked by her teachers, the majority of whom were White. During her intake, Shondra, who always perceived herself as bright and capable, vividly recalled the embarrassment she felt during several interactions with her elementary school teachers. In one situation, Shondra was chastised by her teacher for using different phonetic spellings of her name on each assignment she submitted. In this situation, Shondra, who thought she would impress the teacher with her phonemic awareness, recalled thinking, "I must actually look dumb" and feeling embarrassed. In another situation, Shondra recalled having a similar thought and feeling when she asked her teacher if she would be in the academically talented program the next year. In this situation, Shondra interpreted the sheepish look on her teacher's face to mean that Shondra was foolish for asking. In her reflections on the incident in the years since it happened, Shondra has noted the clear distinction between how the White and African American students were treated during elementary school and the fact that there were no African American students in the academically talented program, leading to the belief, "African Americans are never really seen for who they are."

Case Formulation

Consistent with Spence and Rapee (2016) who suggest an etiology of SAD derived from a complex interplay of intraindividual and environmental inputs, several predisposing and contextual factors contributing to Shondra's social anxiety were identified throughout the course of her therapy. In terms of predisposing factors, what Shondra described as a "naturally shy temperament" appeared to be reflective of a larger pattern of behavioral inhibition evidenced since her childhood. Specifically, Shondra admitted to avoiding unfamiliar people and situations when she was a child and reported experiencing significant distress and arousal when forced to engage socially. She further admitted to avoidance and withdrawal symptoms during most interpersonal interactions at this time of her life, including difficulty making eye contact and staying quiet in most social settings. As a result, Shondra spent limited time engaged in social tasks, which created social skill deficits that led to negative feedback from peers and teachers, establishing a vicious cycle. Shondra also admitted to continued inhibited social behavior as an adult, for example, spending limited time at networking events, avoiding posting on social media, and experiencing sensitivity to criticism resulting in negative emotional states.

In terms of external factors, research suggests trauma and adverse life events increase the risk of developing SAD (Spence & Rapee, 2016). As emphasized throughout this text, racism and associated race-based social encounters are an ongoing source of trauma and adversity for many African Americans (Carter, 2007). The acting White accusations (Davis et al., 2018) Shondra received from Black peers and the racial "othering" experienced from White peers were particularly relevant to Shondra's difficulties with SAD, with Shondra experiencing constant worry about how aspects of her racial identity would cause her to appear to others. For example, Shondra frequently worried about sounding "too White" for Black people and "too Black" for White people. Although she had lighter skin, she also had concerns about having phenotypically Black features, wearing Black hairstyles, and being subjected to the "angry Black woman stereotype," which she believed automatically diminished her credibility and likeability in professional settings.

Due to the early childhood and sociocultural experiences described above, Shondra developed the core belief, "I don't fit in." Currently, this core belief is phrased, "African Americans are never really seen for who they are," and is strengthened by the interpersonal difficulties at her place of employment, as well as ongoing pressure to disconfirm negative stereotypes toward African Americans. In response to this core belief, Shondra has developed the attitude, "It's better to just avoid people." When she is unable to avoid social interaction, Shondra has the assumption, "If I think of all the ways I can look foolish or stereotypical, I can avoid them. If I don't, I won't be accepted." Her compensatory strategies include perfectionism, conforming to dominant cultural standards and code-switching, avoidance, self-focused attention, and anticipatory and post-event cognitive processing.

In Shondra's work environment, the above underlying cognitions are frequently evidenced in the negative automatic thoughts she has prior to staff meetings. Following Figure 10.1, the proceeding paragraphs illustrate Rapee and Heimberg's most recently updated model (Heimberg et al., 2010) for Shondra prior to her most recent staff meeting, an organizational year-end review.

As suggested by the Rapee-Heimberg model (Heimberg et al., 2010), prior to the meeting, Shondra imagined that a majority of her staff would be hostile due to their implicit bias toward Black women. Additionally, she believed that the organization's Director would be oblivious to the staff's hostility and through his silence, assent to their behavior. Shondra specifically recalled thinking, "Great, I get to be 'mad Black woman again,' and he's not going to do anything about it."

Shondra's expectations were informed by the personal history described previously, as well as experiences with her current work colleagues. An exchange with the organization's Events Coordinator discussed in Session 2 was especially distressing. During this situation, Shondra requested a calendar of events planned by the coordinator's department to meet the organization's six-month goal for increased community engagement. Initially, the Events Coordinator provided the calendar, but when Shondra asked for deliverables dates, the coordinator became upset and was overheard talking to another co-worker, accusing Shondra of being a "micromanager" and a "tyrant." While listening to the conversation, Shondra noticed that she began to feel hot and fearful that her face was turning red, decided not to address the issue.

As Shondra prepared to enter the year-end review, she recalled the situation with the Events Coordinator and again worried that her face would turn red during the meeting, causing her to be embarrassed. Shondra predicted that this outward sign of discomfort would further diminish the credibility she had with staff beyond the negative perceptions they held about her as a Black woman. Beliefs regarding her racial identity were particularly distressing for Shondra because rather than only interpreting her colleagues' perceptions as discriminatory stereotypes, she additionally attempted to prove that the stereotypes did not apply to her. Accordingly, as Shondra initiated the meeting, her attentional resources were devoted to monitoring the staff's body language, policing her own tone of voice and body gestures, and noticing any physiological signs of her anxiety, all while facilitating the meeting. As the meeting progressed, Shondra noticed that only a few of the staff members made eye contact with her during her presentation and generally appeared disengaged despite Shondra's use of several teambuilding and reflection exercises during her talk. This fed back into Shondra's mental representation of herself as seen by the audience and strengthened her belief, "I don't fit in." As a result, Shondra believed it was very likely that she would be evaluated negatively by her co-workers and that she would experience negative consequences due to these evaluations, including embarrassment or eventually being forced to quit. Her response was to avoid interaction with her co-workers by excusing herself from the room during breaks and focusing on her slide deck throughout the remainder of the presentation. Her thoughts during this time were, "None of these people like me," "They're going to think I have an attitude," and "This is a disaster."

Activity 10.1: Case Formulation in the Case of Shondra

Review the cognitive model presented as discussed in Shondra's case formulation and respond to the following questions:

- Which of Shondra's behaviors and cognitions might contribute to a vicious cycle of anxiety? How so?
- How are Shondra's behaviors and cognitions influenced by her sociocultural experience?

Treatment Plan

Recall that individuals with social anxiety believe that other people are inherently critical. Due to this assumption, people with social anxiety also believe that the probability they will be negatively judged by others is very high (Rapee & Heimberg, 1997). While the negative predictions associated with these beliefs may in some cases be distorted or exaggerated, the sad reality is that African Americans are often unfairly judged or criticized due to the color of their skin. Therefore, one of the therapist's overarching goals in developing a treatment plan in the case of Shondra was validating Shondra's experience and helping her to become more empowered, while also alerting Shondra to ways that biased attention, self-critical thoughts, social inhibition, and use of safety behaviors may worsen and maintain the sense of discomfort she feels in social situations (D. A. Clark & A. T. Beck, 2012). The specific treatment plan which includes Shondra's problem list and the treatment goals and interventions used to address these problems is presented in Table 10.1.

Problem List

Shondra reports an ongoing history with SAD. Accordingly, the issues identified in her problem list reflect the primary elements of social anxiety, including fear of negative evaluation, maladaptive thinking, and avoidance (D. A. Clark & A. T. Beck, 2012). Based on the discussion of these problems

Table 10.1 Shondra's Treatment Plan

Problem List
1. Fear of negative judgment from others and embarrassment
2. Perfectionism
3. Reluctant engagement/avoidance of social situations
4. Anxious thinking
5. Physical symptoms of anxiety including hot flashes and blushing

Treatment Goals:
1. Reduce fear of negative judgment from others
2. Eliminate safety behaviors
3. Eliminate avoidance
4. Restructure negative thoughts, highlighting negative self-appraisals and predictions developed in response to racism
5. Increase positive emotions
6. Reduce physical symptoms

Interventions
1. Modified exposure and behavioral experiments
2. Cognitive restructuring to modify distorted automatic thoughts, maladaptive assumptions, and dysfunctional schemas
3. Mindfulness, especially external mindfulness
4. Social skills training
5. Psychoeducation/bibliotherapy focused on stereotype confirmation concerns and other relevant sociocultural phenomena
6. Activities to facilitate positive emotions, such as joy and pride, especially racial pride

as precipitated by current events, the therapist anticipated that each problem would contain racially salient content. For example, Shondra's fear of negative judgments from others in her predominantly White work environment appeared to have been influenced by her experiences with stereotypes and fear of confirming stereotypes (Contrada et al., 2001; S. B. Johnson & Anderson, 2014; S. Johnson et al., 2014). Likewise, Shondra's therapist also hypothesized that Shondra's attempts to compensate through perfectionism might have reflected cultural phenomena within the African American community such as working twice as hard (DeSante, 2013; Palmer & Walker, 2020) or John Henryism (Kahsay & Mezuk, 2022). As such, efforts to address relevant racial and cultural factors are integrated into Shondra's treatment goals and interventions, which are discussed in the sections that follow.

Treatment Goals

To address the difficulties identified in her problem list, Shondra and the therapist collaborated to develop treatment goals that were evidenced-based and culturally responsive. Consistent with many evidenced-based approaches to social anxiety, the goals were designed to educate Shondra on social anxiety, increase insight into Shondra's personal social anxiety profile, teach coping skills, and expose Shondra to situations that would allow her to test her negative thoughts and practice new coping skills (Hope et al., 2019). To increase cultural sensitivity, Shondra's treatment goals additionally acknowledged the impact of racism on the thoughts targeted in the cognitive restructuring process.

Given that Shondra reported negative emotional states associated with her social anxiety, the therapist also suggested including a goal to increase positive emotions. Broadly, research suggests that individuals who are high on social anxiety tend to experience less positive emotion (Kashdan, 2007; Watson & L. A. Clark, 1994). More specifically, a study conducted by Cohen and Huppert (2018) found that when specific emotions such as pride and global positive affect were included in the same analysis, only pride was statistically associated with social anxiety. When multiple positive emotions (i.e., pride, love, joy, contentment, amusement, awe, and compassion) were in the same analysis, only pride and love were significantly related to social anxiety. Therefore, as the therapist considered the role of positive emotion in Shondra's treatment goals, she thought specifically about how pride, especially racial pride (Okeke-Adeyanju et al., 2014), could be utilized to enhance treatment outcomes as well.

Activity 10.2: Treatment Goals in the Case of Shondra

Given research which suggests that positive emotions such as pride and love are statistically associated with social anxiety (Cohen & Huppert, 2018), Shondra's therapist was intentional in considering the benefit drawing on racial pride might provide to Shondra's treatment. Based on your own clinical experience and/or ideas presented throughout this text, what other culturally relevant facets of positive emotion might be beneficial to Shondra's treatment?

Interventions

Consistent with findings from meta-analytic research, interventions identified in Shondra's treatment plan included exposure, cognitive restructuring, mindfulness, and social skills training (Gould et al., 1997; Liu et al., 2021). To enhance the development of critical consciousness and psychological empowerment, the therapist also utilized psychoeducation on relevant sociocultural phenomena such as stereotype confirmation concerns and other experiences connected to Shondra's marginalized social status (Graham et al., 2013). To support positive emotion, the therapist additionally incorporated activities designed to promote "radical self-care" into the treatment plan. According to Wyatt and Ampadu (2022),

> When practiced in Black communities, self-care is often executed as resistance to conditions of inequality, marginalization, and minoritization. Radical self-care also recognizes that the individual and the community have a reciprocal relationship. Such that, the individual that is embedded within the community is affected by the events of that community, and vice versa.
>
> (pp. 214–215)

Accordingly, self-care practices that increase a sense of liberation, interdependence, and wellness were emphasized, as well as strategies to overcome barriers to self-care.

Course of Treatment

As mentioned previously, there are several evidenced-based approaches to social anxiety treatment. Many of these treatments were developed for group counseling contexts (e.g., Heimberg & Becker, 2002). Shondra, however, elected to participate in individual therapy only. Accordingly, her therapist made cultural adaptations to the CBT treatment approach developed by Hope et al. (2019), which was developed primarily for use during individual counseling. As such, Shondra's therapy began with an overview of treatment, followed by psychoeducation, cognitive restructuring, and exposure.

To make appropriate cultural adaptations, Shondra's therapist followed recommendations made by Graham-LoPresti et al. (2017). In their work, these researchers presented case study data from a single participant of culturally adapted cognitive behavioral group therapy for social anxiety due to issues related to discrimination. The participant, a 22-year-old Mexican American woman, presented to therapy with fears that she would be perceived as incompetent and unintelligent in her predominantly White school and work environments. These fears were influenced by the participant's awareness and internalization of stereotypes pertaining to the participant's intersecting and marginalized racial and gender identities. As such, the recommended adaptations made to therapy included addressing issues of marginalization: (a) in the engagement session, (b) through cognitive restructuring, and (c) through exposures. Addressing issues of marginalization in the engagement session included initiating dialogue concerning the participant's experiences of marginalization and/or discrimination and how they contributed to her SAD. Adaptations made to cognitive restructuring included being careful to avoid implying that the participant's thoughts pertaining to discrimination were faulty or irrational, instead, focusing restructuring on the internalization of marginalized experiences. Last, addressing marginalization through exposures included developing scenarios that explicitly incorporated racially salient content (Graham-LoPresti et al., 2017).

The sections below describe a culturally adapted, evidenced-based course of treatment for SAD in the case of Shondra. Note the therapist's attention to the recommendations offered by Graham-LoPresti et al. (2017), as well as the therapist's inclusion of specific African-centered wellness principles such as liberation and interdependence (Wyatt & Ampadu, 2022). Additionally, before you read, revisit Chapters 2 and 3, and make note of any other cultural factors, interventions, or case formulation hypotheses that seem relevant to you for treatment with this client.

Beginning Phase of Treatment: Sessions 2 and 3

Shondra is a 35-year-old African American woman who presented to therapy with a previous diagnosis of SAD. Precipitating events at the time of her current course of therapy consisted of interpersonal difficulties at her place of employment after receiving a promotion. Specifically, Shondra reported experiencing fears of negative evaluation due to concerns that her colleagues now perceived her as "the angry Black woman" in her new leadership role. Other symptoms Shondra reported at the time of intake included avoidance, poor concentration, worsened work performance, self-focused attention, post-event processing, physiological complaints, and significant psychological distress as a result of her anxiety, lasting more than six months. Her scores on the Fear and Avoidance subscales of the LSAS (Liebowitz, 1987) at intake were 39 and 28, respectively. Together, these two subscale scores resulted in a total score of 67, indicating a marked level of generalized social anxiety. Her score on the BFNE (Leary, 1983) was 47, which was clinically significant.

When Shondra returned for Session 2, her score on the BFNE had increased slightly to 49. Shondra explained that the day prior to the session she facilitated a year-end review for her organization's staff, which she found distressing due to fears that her co-workers' perceptions of her as a Black woman would cause them to be hostile and diminish her credibility with the group. When Shondra finished explaining her increase in scores, the therapist validated Shondra's gendered racial experiences, stating, "Shondra, I am not African American, but I understand that many African American women experience hostility and discrimination based on stereotypes and that these experiences can be deeply painful." The therapist then probed the impact of racial discrimination further by asking, "Have there been other occasions where your experience as an African American woman have contributed to or worsened your social anxiety?" This honored Shondra's experiential reality and communicated a willingness to explore these issues throughout the remainder of therapy (Graham-LoPresti et al., 2017).

After reviewing prior events, Shondra and the therapist set the agenda for the session, which consisted of orienting Shondra to social anxiety treatment and exploring her view of the advantages and disadvantages of pursuing treatment. During this discussion, Shondra expressed that she was somewhat hopeless about experiencing change in her current situation due to the insidious nature of racism in the United States, stating, "No matter what I do, I'll never be a part of the club." She additionally expressed the belief that her anxiety helped to keep her alert and protected her from experiencing worse outcomes, especially in cross-racial settings. Specifically, Shondra had the assumption, "I have to make a good impression," and monitoring her behavior and "reading the room" was necessary "to keep others from thinking I'm incompetent." In response, the therapist again validated Shondra's concerns and acknowledged that hypervigilance may in fact have some protective value when confronted with racial bias or discrimination (Roberson & Carter, 2022). As such, Shondra and the therapist agreed to focus therapy on increasing her toolbox of positive coping strategies, as well as addressing any internalized racism that referenced her competence, intelligence, or self-worth (Graham et al., 2013). During the session, Shondra also identified personal values and strengths that could assist her in this process (Hope et al., 2019).

At Session 3, Shondra scored 47 on the BFNE. After reviewing updates and setting the session agenda, Shondra and the therapist continued psychoeducation on social anxiety and began completing Shondra's social anxiety profile. This included identifying the most common physical symptoms, thoughts, and behaviors Shondra experiences during anxiety provoking situations (Hope et al., 2019). Shondra reported that she often feels hot when anxious and that her face becomes flushed. This causes her to worry that others will notice and know that she is anxious. Shondra and the therapist then explored other thoughts Shondra typically had during anxiety provoking situations; however, to make this discussion more racially salient, the therapist utilized the technique applied on the Race-Based Traumatic Stress Symptom Scale and directed Shondra to think about three recent social or performance situations where race was a factor in her anxiety (Carter et al., 2013). In one of the situations, Shondra recalled thinking, "I can't give them any reason to doubt me" and "If I don't appear calm, they'll think I'm incompetent." In another situation, Shondra's thoughts were, "They're probably spending more time focused on my hair than what I'm saying" and "I'm so tired of having to fit in." In the final situation, Shondra thought, "My opinions mean nothing" and "It's better if the Director goes with me to explain things."

Using the Director's assistance as a safety behavior was typical, according to Shondra. Shondra viewed her director as an ally, and she tried her best to avoid giving staff new directives without his direct involvement. Other safety behaviors Shondra identified included avoiding eye contact, making efforts to get her words right, rehearsing what she is going to say, adhering to Eurocentric styles of dress and standards of beauty as much as possible, and staying on the periphery of groups, although Shondra reported that she tried to avoid groups as much as possible. For example, during breaks or downtime, Shondra would often escape opportunities to socialize with her co-workers, fleeing to her office or somewhere outside of the building. Additionally, Shondra reported that she also frequently avoided attending networking or conferences entirely, using her grandmother or other responsibilities as excuses. For homework, Shondra kept track of her thoughts, behaviors, and physiological responses and how they contributed to her cycle of social anxiety, recording them on a worksheet (Hope et al., 2019).

Middle Phase of Treatment: Sessions 4 through 7

In Sessions 4 and 5, Shondra scored 45 and 43 on the BFNE, respectively. During these sessions, Shondra and the therapist continued to examine to Shondra's unique experience with social anxiety by exploring aspects of her family environment and other important events that may have contributed to the development of her difficulties with SAD. Shondra shared that while she was growing up, her grandmother was very active politically, especially in the Black community. Accordingly, Shondra's grandmother was intentional in socializing Shondra into Black culture and preparing her to encounter bias from a very young age. Shondra recalled hearing her grandmother tell stories about racism she encountered while at work or in community settings, and teaching Shondra how she should respond when she encounters similar situations. Shondra reported that in response, she would worry about having her own experiences with racism in the future and feel uncertain that she would be able to handle them as well as her grandmother. About this, Shondra stated, "I guess I was right to worry, I'm a complete mess."

Shondra's therapist attempted to normalize her reaction to her grandmother's experiences with racism by sharing research which suggests that use of preparation for bias as socialization may actually have the opposite of its intended effect and contribute to internalizing behaviors in younger children (Liu & Lau, 2013; McKown & Weinstein, 2003). Osborne et al. (2021), for example, suggest that alerting children to racism before they have the vocabulary or abstract reasoning necessary to ask for help or process what was shared may increase feelings of pessimism, sadness, and anxiety rather than instill resilience. In response to the other experiences Shondra shared at intake and elaborated upon during these sessions, the therapist also provided Shondra with research on the acting White accusation (Davis et al., 2018; Neal-Barnett et al., 2010) and exposure to anti-Black attitudes

(Galán et al., 2022), which studies have shown may also contribute to poor mental health outcomes for Black youth. This information was validating for Shondra who stated, "It's helpful to know that there's not something inherently wrong with me. I think this way because of all of the experiences I've had."

With these experiences and recent situations in mind, Shondra and the therapist then worked on constructing a fear and avoidance hierarchy relevant to her therapy goals. To begin this process, Shondra started by first creating a list of eight to ten situations (Hope et al., 2019). To add context, Shondra then considered factors that made any of the situations more difficult. Shondra stated that she was especially fearful during cross-racial situations, expressing worries that the situation would somehow be influenced by stereotypes and bias. To conclude the exercise, Shondra rated each situation according to how much fear it evoked and how likely it was that she would avoid it. Fear was rated according to subjective units of discomfort (SUDS), which is a Likert-type scale that ranges from 0 to 100, where higher scores indicate greater anxiety/discomfort (Hope et al., 2019). Avoidance was also rated on a Likert-type scale ranging from 0 to 100. Shondra's final hierarchy ranked ordered by SUDS is presented in Table 10.2.

At Session 6, Shondra scored 44 on the BFNE. With the fear and avoidance hierarchy in place, she and the therapist began the process of cognitive restructuring, focusing on learning the cognitive model (J. S. Beck, 2020), how to identify negative automatic thoughts, and how to find thinking errors in automatic thoughts (Hope et al., 2019). This included psychoeducation on different types of cognitive distortions and guided practice in the use of a partial thought record. To complete the thought record, Shondra selected a recent situation representative of one of the situations listed on her hierarchy. Specifically, Shondra discussed a situation that occurred the day prior to Session 6 wherein she had to send an email to the Events Coordinator regarding his final plan for increased community engagement.

Table 10.2 Shondra's Fear and Avoidance Hierarchy

Situation	SUDS	Avoidance
1. Reprimanding a staff member	100	95
2. Giving a presentation/attending meetings	90	30
3. Conducting performance reviews	90	0
4. Socializing in the breakroom	70	100
5. Going to a conference	65	80
6. Receiving compliments	60	15
7. Sending interoffice emails	58	20
8. Sending emails/making phone calls to stakeholders	55	20
9. Posting something to social media	50	80

Shondra's primary thought before and while writing the email was, "How can I make sure I don't sound like I have an attitude?" Considering this question, Shondra peppered the email with praise and use of exclamation marks to soften her feedback. After sending the email, however, Shondra worried, "Maybe using exclamation marks makes me appear excessive and unprofessional." She also thought, "I'm so weak for worrying about what he thinks about me."

While discussing her thoughts, the therapist validated Shondra's concerns and acknowledged that gender bias is often a factor in computer-mediated communication. A study conducted by Waseleski (2006), for example, found that women used exclamation marks 73 percent more than men in professional settings. Although their analysis of the study's data suggested that women's most common use of exclamation marks was to convey friendliness and gratitude, exclamation points are traditionally viewed as "markers of excitability," that imply "instability and emotional randomness" due to gender bias (Waseleski, 2006, p. 1012). As such, Shondra's concerns that the Events Coordinator may have perceived the email as overly emotional or unprofessional were not completely irrational. These concerns were also unique to her racialized gender experience, as they additionally reflected her frequent fear of confirming the angry Black woman stereotype among her co-workers.

Another racialized gender concept the therapist acknowledged in relation to Shondra's thought record was the Strong Black Woman Schema. Recall from Chapter 2 that the *Strong Black Woman Schema* refers to a stereotype in which African American women are portrayed as capable of having and doing it all (Abrams et al., 2014). According to this stereotype, Black women are ascribed qualities such as unyielding strength, responsibility, and self-sacrifice, reflecting implicit obligations to: (a) "suppress fear and weakness, showcase strength, resist being vulnerable or dependent... and succeed despite limited resources," (b) "assume multiple roles such as financial providers and caregivers and possess the ability to independently support their families," and (c) "suffer quietly as they work to meet the expectations of their families, jobs, and larger society" (Abrams et al., 2014, pp. 503–504). While in some ways this phenomenon serves as a source of resilience, the Strong Black Woman Schema also contributes to psychological distress among African American women. In Shondra's case, the Strong Black Woman Schema, which was modeled in the relationship with her grandmother, appeared to contribute to her negative self-appraisals and poor coping ability. For homework, Shondra completed a partial thought record that included a column for identifying other societal influences on her cognitions.

In Session 7, Shondra scored 40 on the BFNE. At the start of the session, Shondra and the therapist reviewed the thought record she completed in between sessions, and Shondra remarked on her increased awareness of the extent to which racial factors influenced her difficulties with social anxiety. The therapist complimented Shondra on her insight and began exploration of strategies to replace her negative automatic thoughts. First, the therapist taught Shondra how to challenge her thoughts using various Socratic questioning strategies such as examining the evidence, devising alternative explanations, decatastrophizing and problem-solving, examining the utility, and gaining distance (J. S. Beck, 2020). Shondra and the therapist also explored other cognitive restructuring strategies. For example, Shondra and the therapist explored use of compassion to address negative self-appraisals that developed in response to her experiences with racism (Watson-Singleton et al., 2019). To reinforce use of compassion, the therapist provided Shondra with a self-compassion healing meditation script specific to one's experience with racism (J. M. Steele & Newton, 2023). Shondra agreed to integrate use of the script into her morning routine. To practice use of compassion to dispute specific negative automatic thoughts, the therapist taught Shondra how to use consensual roleplay (Cohen, 2022). This exercise involved engaging Shondra in a roleplay where she played two sides of herself: an emotional side and a compassionate side. Dialogue from Shondra's consensual roleplay is presented in the excerpt that follows.

Emotional Self: Shondra, you're so stupid and weak because of the way you've been struggling at work.

Compassionate Self: Shondra, the way you've been struggling doesn't make you stupid or weak at all. The way you feel is common for a lot of people, especially Black women who experience bias in the workplace.

Emotional Self: Yeah, but you struggle to do the simplest tasks, like send an email.

Compassionate Self: I have struggled to send emails in the past. The fact that I am able to do it anyway actually proves I'm not weak, I'm resilient.

Emotional Self: Well, you may be resilient, and you may be able to eventually get yourself to do your work, but you still feel bad and you're still anxious.

Compassionate Self: I am anxious some of the time, but even when I am, I'm still a success because I get through it. As I continue therapy, I'll learn more, and I'll get even better.

Final Phase of Treatment: Sessions 8 through 12

Shondra utilized the cognitive restructuring and compassion strategies she learned in Session 7, and by Session 8, her BFNE score dropped slightly to 35. During Session 8, the therapist shifted to the exposure component of treatment (Hope et al., 2019), using a graduated process. First, the therapist reviewed the psychoeducation on SAD and its behavioral and avoidance elements discussed at the start of therapy. Then, the therapist provided additional psychoeducation on exposure and its benefits in relation to the behavioral and avoidance aspects of SAD. This included teaching Shondra about the different types of exposure (i.e., imaginal, roleplay, and in-vivo exposures) and various elements related to the process such as distress tolerance, safety behaviors, and external mindfulness (Leahy et al., 2012). The therapist was especially intentional in highlighting benefits, which included: (a) the ability to practice use of appropriate social and distress tolerance skills, (b) identification of negative automatic thoughts, and (c) testing the accuracy of negative automatic thoughts (Hope et al., 2019).

After the psychoeducation, Shondra and the therapist completed steps to design her first exposure activity (see Table 10.3). To begin, Shondra selected

Table 10.3 Shondra's Exposure Exercise

Situation: Make a post about an upcoming charity event on my LinkedIn page

Negative Automatic Thoughts:
• I hate my picture
• If I draw attention to myself, people might find something to criticize
• People might not be interested in the event if they see that I am Black

Alternative Thoughts:
• I don't have to like my picture, I can accept it and focus on the information I need to communicate in the post instead
• It's normal for people to have opinions, if someone has useful feedback, I can accept it and if not I can let it go
• It's true that some people might not pay attention to my post or be less interested in the event because of their unconscious bias, but this thought isn't helpful in this moment and not making the post would perpetuate racism by keeping me from doing my job to the best of my ability

Safety Behaviors to Eliminate:
• Reposting another staff member's post
• Posting a flyer for the event with no message
• Avoiding attention

Coping Strategies to Implement:
• Compassion
• Acceptance
• Mindfulness of breath
• Helpful thinking

Behavioral Goals:
• Use a staff photo that includes a picture of myself in the post
• Make the post myself rather than reposting someone else's original post
• Include a personally written message about the event in the post

---

Situation 9 from her fear and avoidance hierarchy to be the target of her exposure exercise, stating that she wanted to make a post about an upcoming charity event on her LinkedIn page. With this in mind, the therapist guided Shondra in writing behavioral goals describing specific observable behaviors that would let Shondra know the exposure was a success (Hope et al., 2019). Shondra stated that she would know the exposure was a success if she used a staff photo that included a picture of herself in the post, made the post herself rather than sharing a post about the event originally made by another staff person, and if she included a personally written message about the event in the post. Once the exposure activity and behavioral goals were set, Shondra finished planning for the exposure by identifying typical anxious thoughts to modify, corrected alternative thoughts, maladaptive safety behaviors to eliminate, and coping strategies to implement (D. A. Clark & A. T. Beck, 2012).

To further assist Shondra with implementing the exposure activity, the therapist guided her in an imaginal exercise where Shondra imagined herself sitting at her office desk, writing the post. Shondra engaged in three trials of the imaginal exposure during the session, rating her distress before, during, and after each repetition and practicing use of her coping strategies. After the third trial, Shondra stated that she felt confident she would be able to make the post the next day at work, emphasizing that not making the post would be to reinforce racist beliefs about her ability to do her job competently and contribute to internalized racism as well (Bivens, 1995). This was consistent with Graham-LoPresti et al. (2017), who suggested that culturally adapted exposure activities should be modified to explicitly address experiences with marginalization.

In Sessions 9 and 10, Shondra's scores on the BFNE continued to decrease, with Shondra scoring 33 and 29 at each session, respectively. During Session 9, Shondra confirmed that she completed her exposure activity, making the LinkedIn post and using her coping strategies to manage anxiety and challenge negative thoughts while doing so. In Session 9, Shondra and the therapist also debriefed the exposure activity, discussing what she feared would happen as a result of making the post, what actually happened, and what she learned from the exercise (Hope et al., 2019). Shondra stated that her most distressing fear was that drawing attention to herself would attract criticism from others. She acknowledged that while no one had directly expressed any criticisms, she believed that it was highly likely that people held negative opinions about the post that simply had not been expressed to her.

Based on Shondra's comments and her history of painful self-critical cognitive patterns, particularly within the context of racism (e.g., "I must look dumb," "I don't fit," and "I'm a complete mess"), the therapist hypothesized that Shondra's fear was rooted in shame derived from internalized beliefs about being defective or lesser than. According to a systematic review of literature on the relationship between shame and social anxiety conducted by Swee et al. (2021), shame may be related to the development and maintenance of social anxiety through a number of central features. Specifically, within the context of the Rapee-Heimberg model, these authors suggest that shame results from environmental experiences that predispose individuals to preferentially allocate attentional resources toward detecting threat in the environment. Second, shame may have a bidirectional influence on how individuals imagine themselves and the cognitive processes that lead to perceived negative evaluation from others. As such, shame manifests itself in post-event cognitive processes that perpetuate social anxiety, as well as the behavioral manifestations that perpetuate the condition.

Of particular relevance to Shondra's experience of gendered racial marginalization, Swee et al. (2021) specified that shame is inextricably linked to perceptions of low social rank and inferior social status. Although the mechanisms that foster and maintain this relationship are unclear, this finding is consistent with literature on the association between shame and racism among African Americans. According to A. J. Johnson (2020), negative racial and gender expectations provide the foundation and reinforcement of negative African American stereotypes, which in turn prompt social rejection and unacceptance through stigmatized social interactions. Exploring this idea in greater depth, Watts-Jones (2002) argued that racism, specifically internalized racism, involves two levels of shame: (1) internalized anti-Black attitudes, and (2) the shame of being ashamed. According to Watts-Jones (2002), the first shame is related to the trauma of slavery and oppression, while the second shame is about being victimized. In the United States, and among the African American community more specifically, stigma is often attached to being vulnerable or hurt by others due to the implication that the victim is passive or deficient (Watts-Jones, 2002). Accordingly, many African Americans have difficulty acknowledging the pain associated with the vulnerability of belonging to a marginalized racial group, focusing instead on projecting their strength and resilience. When discussed during therapy, this idea resonated with Shondra who acknowledged that many of her compensatory strategies, especially perfectionism, represented efforts to reduce the sense of defenselessness she feels in social situations, particularly during cross-racial interactions. As such, Shondra and the therapist agreed that it would be beneficial to explore her perfectionistic beliefs and engage in core belief work in future sessions. To address internalized anti-Black attitudes, Shondra also created a list of activities to cultivate racial pride, which included reflecting on achievements made by family members and significant Black historical figures, as well as reconnecting with various community and cultural institutions focused on uplifting the Black community (J. M. Steele & Newton, 2023).

In Session 10, Shondra and the therapist did another in-session exposure and also began exploring the underlying cognitions contributing to Shondra's anxiety in social situations. For the exposure exercise, Shondra brought her phone to session and used it to compose and send an email to her colleagues (Situation 7 on her fear and avoidance hierarchy). During this activity, the therapist used discussion of Shondra's negative automatic thoughts as a segue to explore her perfectionistic beliefs. In this process, use of the downward arrow technique uncovered important intermediate and core beliefs. Shondra had the attitude, "It's embarrassing to confirm a stereotype" and the assumption, "If I make mistakes, people will think I'm just another stereotype." Implicit in this discussion was the rule, "Don't make mistakes." The attitude, assumption, and rule all stemmed from the core belief, "I don't fit in." The dialogue that follows is an excerpt of the therapist's use of the downward arrow technique to discover these beliefs (J. S. Beck, 2020).

Therapist: Shondra, you stated that one of the things that upsets you when you write emails is that no matter how many times you proofread it, you often have typos or later think of ways you could have said things better, is that correct?

Shondra: Yes.

Therapist: What's the worst part about having typos in your email or not saying things in a certain way?

Shondra: Well, you know there's a stereotype that African Americans don't write or speak well.

Therapist: Yes, it's unfair, but that stereotype does exist. What's does that mean for you in this situation?

Shondra: It means that if I make mistakes, people will think I'm just another stereotype.

Therapist: Shondra, I hear that's something you're trying to avoid. What would be so bad about people thinking you're just another stereotype?

Shondra: It would be embarrassing.

Therapist: I see. And what would it mean *about you* if people thought you were just another stereotype?

Shondra: It's proof that I don't fit in.

In Session 11, Shondra scored 29 on the BFNE again. During the session, Shondra and the therapist did an exposure focused on Situation 4 from her fear and avoidance hierarchy, socializing in the breakroom. First, Shondra and the therapist reviewed social skills such as starting and maintaining conversations and paying and accepting compliments (Olivares-Olivares et al., 2019). They then did roleplays of the situation twice, each time emphasizing the use of external mindfulness; that is, being absorbed in the present moment and attuned to the cognitive and sensory information needed to test the validity of their thoughts. This included defusing from distractions, focusing on the people one is with, and showing curious interest in the activities in which one is engaged without judgment (Cohen, 2022). Shondra observed that by redirecting her attentional resources to listening and being interested, she had more to say and felt less anxious. She also noted that she accomplished her behavioral goals, which were to learn three things about the other person, ask one follow-up question, and share one thing about herself (Hope et al., 2019).

Based on what she learned from the exposure, the therapist worked with Shondra to develop a new core belief. Shondra stated that she wanted to focus the new belief on her inherent worth rather than her ability to live up to the expectations of others, whether these expectations were real or imagined. The therapist supported Shondra in her reasoning and encouraged her to consider cultural or religious values that might help inform her new belief. Accordingly, Shondra identified the new more adaptive belief, "I bring value to relationships." Explaining her decision, Shondra stated that according to her faith and community values, each person has a purpose and role in helping to build and support others. Through the therapeutic process, she realized that her ability to be promoted and excel in leadership roles despite her anxiety was evidence of this. With this in mind, the therapist guided Shondra in the use of a positive data log to strengthen this belief as she became more attuned to schema-contradictory evidence (Padesky, 1994). For homework, Shondra did an in-vivo exposure, socializing in the breakroom.

At Session 12, Shondra scored a 23 on the BFNE. She reported completing her in-vivo exposure and recording observations from the activity in her positive data log. Overall, Shondra reported having a positive experience in therapy and being hopeful about continued reductions in her SAD symptoms. To strengthen Shondra's therapeutic gains, she and the therapist engaged in another in-session exposure, roleplaying Situation 2 from the fear and avoidance hierarchy, giving a presentation/attending meetings. To conduct the roleplay, Shondra used her phone to video record the presentation, and the therapist guided Shondra in the use of video feedback to predict what she believed she would see in the video and how she came across (Hope et al., 2019). Then, Shondra watched the video as if she were watching a stranger, giving new ratings to her performance and anxiety. Shondra stated that overall, her anxiety was less apparent than she thought it would be. She also communicated the material better than she thought she would. Most importantly, Shondra stated that the African American speech and communications patterns observed during the presentation were not embarrassing, but a reflection of her unique cultural experiences and something that actually connected her to the population her organization serves.

At the conclusion of Session 12, Shondra and the therapist agreed to taper sessions and plan for termination of therapy. As such, sessions were reduced to bi-weekly appointments where Shondra and the therapist continued exposure and cognitive restructuring exercises, emphasizing her experiences of marginalization and their contribution to her social anxiety. In their final session, Shondra and the therapist discussed how to continue making progress, what to anticipate with new challenges, and goals for after treatment ends (Hope et al., 2019). Shondra ended individual therapy with new coping skills and a greater ability to challenge the negative thoughts, feelings, and behaviors developed as a result of her lived experience as an African American woman.

References

Abrams, J. A., Maxwell, M., Pope, M., & Belgrave, F. Z. (2014). Carrying the world with the grace of a lady and the grit of a warrior: Deepening our understanding of the "Strong Black Woman" Schema. *Psychology of Women Quarterly, 38*(4), 503–518. https://doi.org/10.1177/0361684314541418

Alvarez, K., Fillbrunn, M., Green, J. G., Jackson, J. S., Kessler, R. C., McLaughlin, K. A., Sadikova, E., Sampson, N. A., & Alegría, M. (2019). Race/ethnicity, nativity, and lifetime risk of mental disorders in US adults. *Social Psychiatry and Psychiatric Epidemiology, 54*(5), 553–565. https://doi.org/10.1007/s00127-018-1644-5

American Psychiatric Association. (2013). *Diagnostic and statistical manual of mental disorders* (5th ed.). American Psychiatric Association. https://doi.org/10.1176/appi.books.9780890425596

Asnaani, A., Aderka, I. M., Marques, L., Simon, N., Robinaugh, D. J., & Hofmann, S. G. (2015). The structure of feared social situations among race-ethnic minorities and Whites with social anxiety disorder in the United States. *Transcultural Psychiatry, 52*(6), 791–807. https://doi.org/10.1177/1363461515576823

Bandelow, B., & Michaelis, S. (2015). Epidemiology of anxiety disorders in the 21st century. *Dialogues in Clinical Neuroscience, 17*(3), 327–335. https://doi.org/10.31887/DCNS.2015.17.3/bbandelow

Beard, C., Rodriguez, B. F., Moitra, E., Sibrava, N. J., Bjornsson, A., Weisberg, R. B., & Keller, M. B. (2011). Psychometric properties of the Liebowitz Social Anxiety Scale (LSAS) in a longitudinal study of African Americans with anxiety disorders. *Journal of Anxiety Disorders, 25*(5), 722–726. https://doi.org/10.1016/j.janxdis.2011.03.009

Beck, J. S. (2020). *Cognitive behavior therapy: Basics and beyond* (3rd ed.). Guilford Press.

Beck Institute. (n.d.). CBT for anxiety disorders: Online course. https://beckinstitute.org/training/online-training

Beidel, D. C., Turner, S. M., & Morris, T. L. (1995). A new inventory to assess childhood social anxiety and phobia: The Social Phobia and Anxiety Inventory for Children. *Psychological Assessment, 7*(1), 73–79. https://doi.org/10.1037/1040-3590.7.1.73

Bivens, D. (1995). *Internalized racism: A definition*. https://www.racialequitytools.org/resourcefiles/bivens.pdf

Bögels, S. M., & Mansell, W. (2004). Attention processes in the maintenance and treatment of social phobia: Hypervigilance, avoidance and self-focused attention. *Clinical Psychology Review*, *24*(7), 827–856. https://doi.org/10.1016/j.cpr.2004.06.005

Bögels, S. M., Sijbers, G. F. V. M., & Voncken, M. (2006). Mindfulness and task concentration training for social phobia: A pilot study. *Journal of Cognitive Psychotherapy*, *20*(1), 33–44. https://doi.org/10.1891/jcop.20.1.33

Buckner, J. D., & Dean, K. E. (2017). Social anxiety and post-event processing among African-American individuals. *Anxiety, Stress, and Coping*, *30*(2), 219–227. https://doi.org/10.1080/10615806.2016.1220549

Carter, R. T. (2007). Racism and psychological and emotional injury: Recognizing and assessing race-based traumatic stress. *The Counseling Psychologist*, *35*(1), 13–105. https://doi.org/10.1177/0011000006292033

Carter, R. T., Mazzula, S., Victoria, R., Vazquez, R., Hall, S., Smith, S., Sant-Barket, S., Forsyth, J., Bazelais, K., & Williams, B. (2013). Initial development of the Race-Based Traumatic Stress Symptom Scale: Assessing the emotional impact of racism. *Psychological Trauma: Theory, Research, Practice, and Policy*, *5*(1), 1–9. https://doi.org/10.1037/a0025911

Chou, T., Asnaani, A., & Hofmann, S. G. (2012). Perception of racial discrimination and psychopathology across three U.S. ethnic minority groups. *Cultural Diversity & Ethnic Minority Psychology*, *18*(1), 74–81. https://doi.org/10.1037/a0025432

Clark, D. A., & Beck, A. T. (2011). *Cognitive therapy of anxiety disorders: Science and practice*. Guilford Press.

Clark, D. A., & Beck, A. T. (2012). *The anxiety & worry workbook: The cognitive behavioral solution*. Guilford Press.

Clark, D. M., & Wells, A. (1995). A cognitive model of social phobia. In R. G. Heimberg, M. R. Liebowitz, D. A. Hope, & F. R. Schneier (Eds.), *Social phobia: Diagnosis, assessment, and treatment* (pp. 69–93). Guilford Press.

Clevinger, A. M., Kleider-Offutt, H. M., & Tone, E. B. (2018). In the eyes of the law: Associations among fear of negative evaluation, race, and feelings of safety in the presence of police officers. *Personality and Individual Differences*, *135*, 201–206. https://doi.org/10.1016/j.paid.2018.06.041

Cohen, L. (2022). Social anxiety disorder comprehensive training course: Evidence-based CBT strategies to overcome fear, shame, and avoidance. *Psychotherapy Networker*. https://catalog.psychotherapynetworker.org/sales/pn_c_001659_social anxietydisorder_organic-496846

Cohen, L., & Huppert, J. D. (2018). Positive emotions and social anxiety: The unique role of pride. *Cognitive Therapy and Research*, *42*(4), 524–538. https://doi.org/10.1007/s10608-018-9900-2

Contrada, R. J., Ashmore, R. D., Gary, M. L., Coups, E., Egeth, J. D., Sewell, A., Ewell, K., Goyal, T. M., & Chasse, V. (2001). Measures of ethnicity-related stress: Psychometric properties, ethnic group differences, and associations with well-being. *Journal of Applied Social Psychology*, *31*(9), 1775–1820. https://doi.org/10.1111/j.1559-1816.2001.tb00205.x

Davis, M., Stadulis, R., & Neal-Barnett, A. (2018). Assessing the effects of the acting White accusation among Black girls: Social anxiety and bullying victimization. *Journal of the National Medical Association*, *110*(1), 23–28. https://doi.org/10.1016/j.jnma.2017.06.016

DeSante, C. D. (2013). Working twice as hard to get half as far: Race, work ethic, and America's deserving poor. *American Journal of Political Science, 57*(2), 342–356. https://doi.org/10.1111/ajps.12006

Ferrell, C. B., Beidel, D. C., & Turner, S. M. (2004). Assessment and treatment of socially phobic children: A cross cultural comparison. *Journal of Clinical Child and Adolescent Psychology, 33*(2), 260–268. https://doi.org/10.1207/s15374424jc cp3302_6

Fink, C. M., Turner, S. M., & Beidel, D. C. (1996). Culturally relevant factors in the behavioral treatment of social phobia: A case study. *Journal of Anxiety Disorders, 10*(3), 201–209. https://doi.org/10.1016/0887-6185(96)00005-9

Galán, C. A., Auguste, E. E., Smith, N. A., & Meza, J. I. (2022). An intersectional-contextual approach to racial trauma exposure risk and coping among Black youth. *Journal of Research on Adolescence, 32*(2), 583–595. https://doi.org/10.1111/jora.12757

Gould, R. A., Buckminster, S., Pollack, M. H., Otto, M. W., & Yap, L. (1997). Cognitive-behavioral and pharmacological treatment for social phobia: A meta-analysis. *Clinical Psychology: Science and Practice, 4*(4), 291–306. https://doi.org/10.1111/j.1468-2850.1997.tb00123.x

Graham, J. R., Sorenson, S., & Hayes-Skelton, S. A. (2013). Enhancing the cultural sensitivity of cognitive behavioral interventions for anxiety in diverse populations. *The Behavior Therapist, 36*(5), 101–108.

Graham-LoPresti, J. R., Gautier, S. W., Sorenson, S., & Hayes-Skelton, S. A. (2017). Culturally sensitive adaptations to evidence-based cognitive behavioral treatment for social anxiety disorder: A case paper. *Cognitive and Behavioral Practice, 24*(4), 459–471. https://doi.org/10.1016/j.cbpra.2016.12.003

Gray, C. M. K., Carter, R., & Silverman, W. K. (2011). Anxiety symptoms in African American children: Relations with ethnic pride, anxiety sensitivity, and parenting. *Journal of Child and Family Studies, 20*(2), 205–213. https://doi.org/10.1007/s10826-010-9422-3

Harris, S. M. (1995). Psychosocial development and Black male masculinity: Implications for counseling economically disadvantaged African American male adolescents. *Journal of Counseling & Development, 73*(3), 279–287. https://doi.org/10.1002/j.1556-6676.1995.tb01749.x

Heimberg, R. G., & Becker, R. E. (2002). *Cognitive-behavioral group therapy for social phobia: Basic mechanisms and clinical strategies*. Guilford Press.

Heimberg, R. G., Brozovich, F. A., & Rapee, R. M. (2010). A cognitive behavioral model of social anxiety disorder: Update and extension. In S. G. Hofmann & P. M. DiBartolo (Eds.), *Social anxiety: Clinical, developmental, and social perspectives* (pp. 395–422). Elsevier Academic Press. https://doi.org/10.1016/B978-0-12-375096-9.00015-8

Hofmann, S. G. (2007). Cognitive factors that maintain social anxiety disorder: A comprehensive model and its treatment implications. *Cognitive Behaviour Therapy, 36*(4), 193–209. https://doi.org/10.1080/16506070701421313

Hofmann, S. G., Anu Asnaani, M. A., & Hinton, D. E. (2010). Cultural aspects in social anxiety and social anxiety disorder. *Depression and Anxiety, 27*(12), 1117–1127. https://doi.org/10.1002/da.20759

Hope, D. A., Heimberg, R. G., & Turk, C. L. (2019). *Managing social anxiety: A cognitive–behavioral therapy approach: Therapist guide* (3rd ed.). Oxford University Press. https://doi.org/10.1093/med-psych/9780190247591.001.0001

Johnson, A. B. (2006). Performance anxiety among African-American college students: Racial bias as a factor in social phobia. *Journal of College Student Psychotherapy, 20*(4), 31–38. https://doi.org/10.1300/J035v20n04_04

Johnson, A. J. (2020). Examining associations between racism, internalized shame, and self-esteem among African Americans. *Cogent Psychology, 7*(1), Article 1757857. https://doi.org/10.1080/23311908.2020.1757857

Johnson, S., Price, M., Mehta, N., & Anderson, P. L. (2014). Stereotype confirmation concerns predict dropout from cognitive behavioral therapy for social anxiety disorder. *BMC Psychiatry, 14*, 233. https://doi.org/10.1186/s12888-014-0233-8

Johnson, S. B., & Anderson, P. L. (2014). Stereotype confirmation concern and fear of negative evaluation among African Americans and Caucasians with social anxiety disorder. *Journal of Anxiety Disorders, 28*(4), 390–393. https://doi.org/10.1016/j.janxdis.2014.03.003

Kahsay, E., & Mezuk, B. (2022). The association between John Henryism and depression and suicidal ideation among African-American and Caribbean Black adolescents in the United States. *Journal of Adolescent Health, 71*(6), 721–728. https://doi.org/10.1016/j.jadohealth.2022.07.006

Kashdan, T. B. (2007). Social anxiety spectrum and diminished positive experiences: Theoretical synthesis and meta-analysis. *Clinical Psychology Review, 27*(3), 348–365. https://doi.org/10.1016/j.cpr.2006.12.003

Kelly-Turner, K., & Radomsky, A. S. (2022). Always saying the wrong thing: Negative beliefs about losing control cause symptoms of social anxiety. *Cognitive Therapy and Research, 46*(6), 1137–1149. https://doi.org/10.1007/s10608-022-10325-w

Leahy, R., Holland, S. J. F., & McGinn, L. K. (2012). *Treatment plans and interventions for depression and anxiety disorders*. Guilford Press.

Leary, M. R. (1983). A brief version of the Fear of Negative Evaluation Scale. *Personality and Social Psychology Bulletin, 9*(3), 371–375. https://doi.org/10.1177/0146167283093007

Levine, D. S., Taylor, R. J., Nguyen, A. W., Chatters, L. M., & Himle, J. A. (2015). Family and friendship informal support networks and social anxiety disorder among African Americans and Black Caribbeans. *Social Psychiatry and Psychiatric Epidemiology, 50*(7), 1121–1133. https://doi.org/10.1007/s00127-015-1023-4

Liebowitz, M. R. (1987). Social phobia. *Modern Problems of Pharmacopsychiatry, 22*, 141–173. https://doi.org/10.1159/000414022

Liu, L. L., & Lau, A. S. (2013). Teaching about race/ethnicity and racism matters: An examination of how perceived ethnic racial socialization processes are associated with depression symptoms. *Cultural Diversity & Ethnic Minority Psychology, 19*(4), 383–394. https://doi.org/10.1037/a0033447

Liu, X., Yi, P., Ma, L., Liu, W., Deng, W., Yang, X., Liang, M., Luo, J., Li, N., & Li, X. (2021). Mindfulness-based interventions for social anxiety disorder: A systematic review and meta-analysis. *Psychiatry Research, 300*, 113935. https://doi.org/10.1016/j.psychres.2021.113935

Manning, K., Bakhshaie, J., Mcleish, A. C., Luberto, C., Walker, R. L., & Zvolensky, M. J. (2017). Emotional nonacceptance and anxiety sensitivity in relation to anxious arousal, social anxiety, and depressive symptoms among African American young adults. *Journal of Black Psychology*, *43*(7), 669–687. https://doi.org/10. 1177/0095798416670780

March, J. S. (2013). *Multidimensional Anxiety Scale for Children–2nd edition: Technical manual*. Multi-Health Systems.

McKown, C., & Weinstein, R. S. (2003). The development and consequences of stereotype consciousness in middle childhood. *Child Development*, *74*(2), 498–515. https://doi.org/10.1111/1467-8624.7402012

Melka, S. E., Lancaster, S. L., Adams, L. J., Howarth, E. A., & Rodriguez, B. F. (2010). Social anxiety across ethnicity: A confirmatory factor analysis of the FNE and SAD. *Journal of Anxiety Disorders*, *24*(7), 680–685. https://doi.org/10.1016/j. janxdis.2010.04.011

Menakem, R. (2022). *The quaking of America: An embodied guide to navigating our nation's upheaval and racial reckoning*. Central Recovery Press.

Meral, Y., & Vriends, N. (2021). Self-image and self-focused attention in a social interaction situation: What is relevant for social anxiety? *Behavioural and Cognitive Psychotherapy*, 1–11. Advance online publication. https://doi.org/10.1017/S13524 65821000424

Murray, M. S., Neal-Barnett, A., Demmings, J. L., & Stadulis, R. E. (2012). The acting White accusation, racial identity, and anxiety in African American adolescents. *Journal of Anxiety Disorders*, *26*(4), 526–531. https://doi.org/10.1016/j.janxdis.2012.02.006

Neal-Barnett, A., Stadulis, R., Singer, N., Murray, M., & Demmings, J. (2010). Assessing the effects of experiencing the acting White accusation. *The Urban Review*, *42*(2), 102–122. https://doi.org/10.1007/s11256-009-0130-5

Okeke-Adeyanju, N., Taylor, L. C., Craig, A. B., Smith, R. E., Thomas, A., Boyle, A. E., & DeRosier, M. E. (2014). Celebrating the strengths of Black youth: Increasing self-esteem and implications for prevention. *The Journal of Primary Prevention*, *35*(5), 357–369. https://doi.org/10.1007/s10935-014-0356-1

Olivares-Olivares, P. J., Ortiz-González, P. F., & Olivares, J. (2019). Role of social skills training in adolescents with social anxiety disorder. *International Journal of Clinical and Health Psychology*, *19*(1), 41–48. https://doi.org/10.1016/j.ijchp.2018. 11.002

Osborne, K. R., Caughy, M. O., Oshri, A., Smith, E. P., & Owen, M. T. (2021). Racism and preparation for bias within African American families. *Cultural Diversity and Ethnic Minority Psychology*, *27*(2), 269–279. https://doi.org/10.1037/cdp0000339

Padesky, C. A. (1994). Schema change processes in cognitive therapy. *Clinical Psychology and Psychotherapy*, *1*(5), 267–278. https://doi.org/10.1002/cpp.5640010502

Padesky, C. A. (1997). A more effective treatment focus for social phobia? *International Cognitive Therapy Newsletter*, *11*(1), 1–3.

Palmer, R. T., & Walker, L. J. (2020, July 6). Proposing a concept of the Black tax to understand the experiences of Blacks in America. *Diverse Issues in Higher Education*. https://diverseeducation.com/article/182837/

Petrie, J. M., Chapman, L. K., & Vines, L. M. (2013). Utility of the PANAS-X in predicting social phobia in African American females. *Journal of Black Psychology*, *39*(2), 131–155. https://doi.org/10.1177/0095798412454677

Pina, A. A., Little, M., Wynne, H., & Beidel, D. C. (2014). Assessing social anxiety in African American youth using the social phobia and anxiety inventory for children. *Journal of Abnormal Child Psychology*, *42*(2), 311–320. https://doi.org/10.1007/s10802-013-9775-3

Rapee, R. M., & Heimberg, R. G. (1997). A cognitive-behavioral model of anxiety in social phobia. *Behaviour Research and Therapy*, *35*(8), 741–756. https://doi.org/10.1016/s0005-7967(97)00022-3

Roberson, K., & Carter, R. T. (2022). The relationship between race-based traumatic stress and the Trauma Symptom Checklist: Does racial trauma differ in symptom presentation? *Traumatology*, *28*(1), 120–128. https://doi.org/10.1037/trm0000306

Sibrava, N. J., Beard, C., Bjornsson, A. S., Moitra, E., Weisberg, R. B., & Keller, M. B. (2013). Two-year course of generalized anxiety disorder, social anxiety disorder, and panic disorder in a longitudinal sample of African American adults. *Journal of Consulting and Clinical Psychology*, *81*(6), 1052–1062. https://doi.org/10.1037/a0034382

Spence, S. H., & Rapee, R. M. (2016). The etiology of social anxiety disorder: An evidence-based model. *Behaviour Research and Therapy*, *86*, 50–67. https://doi.org/10.1016/j.brat.2016.06.007

Steele, C. M., & Aronson, J. (1995). Stereotype threat and the intellectual test performance of African-Americans. *Journal of Personality and Social Psychology*, *69*(5), 797–811. https://doi.org/10.1037/0022-3514.69.5.797

Steele, J. M., & Newton, C. S. (2023). *Black lives are beautiful: 50 tools to heal from trauma and promote positive racial identity*. Routledge.

Stone, J., Harrison, C., & Mottley, J. (2012). "Don't call me a student-athlete": The effect of identity priming on stereotype threat for academically engaged African American college athletes. *Basic and Applied Social Psychology*, *34*(2), 99–106. https://doi.org/10.1080/01973533.2012.655624

Swee, M. B., Hudson, C. C., & Heimberg, R. G. (2021). Examining the relationship between shame and social anxiety disorder: A systematic review. *Clinical Psychology Review*, *90*, 102088. https://doi.org/10.1016/j.cpr.2021.102088

Turner, E. A., & Mills, C. J. (2016). Culturally relevant diagnosis and assessment of mental illness. In A. Breland-Noble, C. S. Al-Mateen, & N. N. Singh (Eds.), *Handbook of mental health in African American youth* (pp. 21–35). Springer International Publishing/Springer Nature. https://doi.org/10.1007/978-3-319-25501-9_2

Waseleski, C. (2006). Gender and the use of exclamation points in computer-mediated communication: An analysis of exclamations posted to two electronic discussion lists. *Journal of Computer-Mediated Communication*, *11*(4), 1012–1024. https://doi.org/10.1111/j.1083-6101.2006.00305.x

Watson, D., & Clark, L. A. (1994). *The PANAS-X: Manual for the Positive and Negative Affect Schedule-Expanded Form*. University of Iowa.

Watson, D., & Friend, R. (1969). Measurement of social-evaluative anxiety. *Journal of Consulting and Clinical Psychology*, *33*(4), 448–457. https://doi.org/10.1037/h0027806

Watson-Singleton, N. N., Black, A. R., & Spivey, B. N. (2019). Recommendations for a culturally-responsive mindfulness-based intervention for African Americans. *Complementary Therapy in Clinical Practice*, *34*, 132–138. https://doi.org/10.1016/j.ctcp.2018.11.013

Watts-Jones, D. (2002). Healing internalized racism: The role of a within-group sanctuary among people of African descent. *Family Process, 41*(4), 591–601. https://doi.org/10.1111/j.1545-5300.2002.00591.x

Wyatt, J. P., & Ampadu, G. G. (2022). Reclaiming self-care: Self-care as a social justice tool for Black wellness. *Community Mental Health Journal, 58*(2), 213–221. https://doi.org/10.1007/s10597-021-00884-9

Zerr, A. A., Holly, L. E., & Pina, A. A. (2011). Cultural influences on social anxiety in African American, Asian American, Hispanic and Latino, and Native American adolescents and young adults. In C. A. Alfano & D. C. Beidel (Eds.), *Social anxiety in adolescents and young adults: Translating developmental science into practice* (pp. 203–222). American Psychological Association. https://doi.org/10.1037/12315-011

Chapter 11

Putting It All Together

Posttraumatic Stress Disorder

Due to the historical legacy of slavery and ongoing systems of racial oppression in the United States, trauma is an experience woven into the lives of many African Americans. According to Carter (2007), *trauma* refers to severe stress reactions to "emotionally painful events that are sudden, negative, and out of one's control and that result in primary symptom clusters that include avoidance, arousal, and intrusion" (p. 18). When these reactions happen within the context of racism, they are referred to as *racial trauma*. More specifically defined, racial trauma may be conceptualized as "a traumatic response to race-related experiences that are collectively characterized as racism, including acts of prejudice, discrimination, or violence against a subordinate racial group based on attitudes of superiority held by the dominant group" (M. T. Williams et al., 2018, p. 181). Other terms for racial trauma include *racialized trauma*, *race-based stress*, and *race-based traumatic stress*. Diagnostically, racial trauma and other formally recognized trauma disorders such as Posttraumatic Stress Disorder (PTSD) share a similar constellation of symptoms. Accordingly, this chapter focuses on using CBT to empower healing from PTSD within the context of racism, while also drawing from studies on racial trauma and other related topics.

Current research suggests that most therapists will work with clients who report racial trauma at some point in their careers. Prior to the COVID-19 pandemic and the highly publicized murders of individuals such as George Floyd, Ahmaud Arbery, and Breonna Taylor, one study found that a majority, 70.8 percent, of counselors had worked with clients who reported experiences with race-based trauma (Hemmings & Evans, 2018). Since that time, this percentage has increased, with 96.5 percent of counselors indicating they hear at least one report of discrimination from clients of color at least occasionally during therapy (Giordano et al., 2021). Unfortunately, despite the high percentages of therapists who see clients with racial trauma, many have not received training in identifying and treating race-based trauma among people of color (Hemmings & Evans, 2018). Beyond formal training,

DOI: 10.4324/9781003196303-11

there is also a dearth of theory-based literature to guide therapists in addressing the various aspects of racial trauma (Banks et al., 2021).

In this chapter, I discuss how culturally adapted CBT that emphasizes various third wave CBT mindfulness-based techniques may be utilized to help clients address maladaptive cognitions and heightened stress responses that develop as a result of trauma within the context of racial oppression. First, I discuss PTSD and the African American experience of PTSD due to encounters with racism. I then describe models of PTSD and race-based traumatic stress and discuss assessment and treatment approaches for these conditions. I conclude the chapter with the presentation of a case example and illustration of cognitive conceptualization and treatment planning using the case example. Please note that the case describes the course of treatment for an African American woman with birth trauma, which some readers may find triggering.

Understanding Posttraumatic Stress Disorder

Posttraumatic Stress Disorder is a mental health condition that develops following exposure to a traumatic event. While the clinical presentation of PTSD symptoms varies across individuals, the disorder is characterized by five primary criteria: (A) exposure to actual or threatened death, serious injury, or sexual violence; (B) intrusion associated with the traumatic event; (C) persistent avoidance of stimuli associated with the traumatic event; (D) negative alterations in cognition and mood; and (E) alterations in arousal and reactivity (American Psychiatric Association, 2013). Intrusion, persistent avoidance of stimuli, negative alterations in cognition and mood, and alterations in arousal and reactivity (Criteria B through E) must occur for more than one month.

Changes to Criterion A reflected in the most recent edition of the *DSM* clarify what constitutes a traumatic event (American Psychiatric Association, 2013). As previously indicated, a traumatic event is defined in the *DSM-5* as exposure to actual or threatened death, serious injury, or sexual violence (American Psychiatric Association, 2013). These exposures are limited to: (1) directly experiencing the event, (2) witnessing the event in person, (3) learning that the event happened to a close family member or friend, and (4) experiencing extreme or repeated exposure to aversive details of the event. Of relevance to the experience of PTSD among African Americans, Criterion A4 excludes exposure to aversive details through electronic media, television, movies, or pictures, unless the exposure is work-related. This means that symptoms precipitated by traumatic events commonly experienced within the African American population such as vicarious exposures to police brutality via the news or social media, or the collective pain felt with the murders of Trayvon Martin and Tamir Rice in light of the historical murders of Emmett Till and countless other young Black boys and girls would not meet the criteria for PTSD.

Due to the gap between the lived experiences of people of color and current *DSM-5* criteria, scholars have called for the inclusion of exposure to racism and other forms of oppression as traumatic events in the diagnosis of PTSD (M. T. Williams et al., 2018). Among African Americans, extant research suggests PTSD is associated with a variety of concerns not limited to alcohol-related problems (Fischer et al., 2022), dysfunctional emotional regulation strategies (Sun et al., 2020), problematic parenting and parental distress (Cross et al., 2018), and comorbidities with Major Depressive Episodes and Substance Use Disorder (Pahl et al., 2020), underscoring the significance of accurate diagnosis and treatment within this population. Without inclusion of racism as a precipitant to PTSD, accurate diagnosis and treatment becomes difficult.

Posttraumatic Stress Disorder in African Americans and the Role of Racial Oppression

Broadly, African Americans experience more PTSD symptomatology and greater lifetime prevalence when compared to other racial groups (Mekawi et al., 2021). In Chapter 2, I discussed social determinants of mental health derived from the historical legacy of slavery, including disparate incarceration and poverty statistics. Violence associated with these determinants when conceptualized as encounters with law enforcement and crime in racially segregated low SES neighborhoods has been found to be correlated with the incidence of PTSD in the African American population. A synthesis of research provided by Isen (2022), for example, found that one sample of 38,993 Black Americans experienced an increase in poor mental health days after the police killing of an unarmed Black man in their state, according to interviews conducted zero to three months later (see Bor et al., 2018). In another example, research presented by Tynes et al. (2019) found that among Black, Latinx, and Hispanic adolescents, frequency of viewing traumatic events such as videos of someone from their ethnic group being beaten, arrested, or detained, or a viral video of a Black American being shot by a police officer online resulted in an increase of PTSD-specific symptoms. Furthermore, as it relates to neighborhood crime, a substantial body of evidence shows that pervasive exposure to violence in poor and predominantly African American communities also has a strong correlation to PTSD among this population. A study conducted by Goldmann et al. (2011), for example, found that among 1,306 randomly selected African American residents of Detroit, lifetime prevalence of exposure to at least one traumatic event was 87 percent, with assault representing 51 percent of these events. Moreover, approximately 17 percent of those who experienced a traumatic event also met criteria for probable lifetime PTSD, highlighting the ongoing deleterious effect of socially determined mental health conditions such as PTSD in the African American population.

As stated, to meet *DSM-5* criteria for PTSD, an individual must experience or witness an event that leads to actual or threatened death, serious injury, or sexual violence (American Psychiatric Association, 2013). Recall from Chapter 6 that in some cases the traumatic events associated with racial discrimination and harassment meet this criterion. These events include overt racially motivated threats of violence, physical assaults or threats from law enforcement, racially motivated threats of violence in the workplace, community violence, medical mistreatment, physical or sexual assault while in prison, and deportation (M. T. Williams et al., 2018). Other types of race-related experiences such as repeated microaggressions, being denied access or services, being stereotyped, being ignored, verbal assaults, or being profiled, however, do not qualify as traumatic events as defined by the *DSM-5*. Nevertheless, these events when varied, chronic, pervasive, uncontrollable, and stressful in nature frequently lead to the full clinical syndrome of PTSD symptoms (Abdullah et al., 2021; Kirkinis et al., 2021).

Understanding the types of trauma reactions that may occur across various experiences with racism can help improve treatment and the therapist's ability to assist African American clients in processing their trauma. According to research conducted by Carter and Forsyth (2010), individuals who have direct experiences with discrimination have stronger trauma reactions than those whose experiences are vicarious. In their research, trauma reactions were measured according to the Emotions and Coping Checklist (Harrell, 1997) and consisted of intrusion, hypervigilance, avoidance/numbing, depression, anxiety, anger, low self-esteem, positive/vigor, and guilt/shame. When examining differences in these symptoms according to the experiences of racial discrimination versus racial harassment, their research additionally found that individuals whose symptoms were precipitated by racial harassment experienced more anxiety and hypervigilance when compared to individuals who identified their symptoms as resulting from racial discrimination. Accordingly, when treating PTSD, therapists should pay careful attention to whether the trauma was experienced directly and if it was experienced as harassment, as these factors may contribute to more distressing symptoms.

Other, more recent research conducted by Roberson and Carter (2022) further elucidates the unique experience of trauma within the African American community. In their study of Black Americans, Roberson and Carter (2022) explored differences in the presentation of race-based traumatic stress symptoms and traditional trauma symptoms and found that among those who experienced racial stress, depression, intrusion, anger, and low self-esteem primarily drove the relationship between race-based traumatic stress symptoms and trauma reactions; however, hypervigilance, a common trauma symptom, was not predictive of trauma reactions within this group. These findings are contrary to the results of other studies that suggest hypervigilance is the most common symptom of trauma for African Americans and warrant further exploration (Smith & Patton, 2016). Nonetheless, based on these findings, Roberson and Carter (2022) suggest that when assessing and treatment planning for racial trauma, caution should be taken, as hypervigilance may not be as prevalent and low self-esteem may need to be emphasized instead. The researchers further suggest that for Black Americans, increased arousal may be an adaptive coping strategy used to navigate racially charged situations and increase safety. Therapists, therefore, should be cognizant of this potentially distinguishing feature of racial trauma, especially within the context of the current sociopolitical environment.

Finally, while definitions of PTSD tend to emphasize their emotional, cognitive, physical, and relational components, findings made possible by recent advances in neuroscience implicate several brain structures in the makeup of trauma, including racial trauma (U. S. Clark et al., 2018; Fani et al., 2021; Harnett, 2020; van der Kolk, 2002). An in-depth review of trauma neuroscience is beyond the scope of this chapter; however, decades of neuroscience research prove there is a reciprocal relationship between trauma and the brain (van der Kolk, 2014). Traditionally, the human brain is conceptualized as a complex structure that can be divided into three primary layers—the *brain stem*, the *subcortical region*, and the *cortex* (MacLean, 1990). The cortex, also known as the *primate* or *human brain*, is the largest and most sophisticated layer of the brain. It is responsible for higher mental functions such as complex reasoning, abstract thoughts, imagination, language, empathy, and regulation of attention, feelings, and desires. The subcortical region, known as the *mammalian brain*, on the other hand, is responsible for functions that include motivation, satisfaction, emotions, learning, and memory. Finally, the brain stem and cerebellum, known as the *reptilian brain*, is responsible for survival and maintenance. Its functions include regulation of heartrate, breathing, and other vital organs. Evolutionarily, the subcortical and stem regions of the brain are more primitive and not under conscious control (van der Kolk, 2002). These areas of the brain manage the body's detection of threat or danger and consequently are responsible for its protection response, frequently referred to as the *fight-flight-freeze response*.

When people encounter a situation perceived as dangerous, the reptilian brain overrides the part of the brain where humans think and reason, the cortex, and initiates the fight-flight-freeze response (van der Kolk, 2002). Structurally, this involves the secretion of hormones that regulate arousal and attention, namely, cortisol and norepinephrine. *Cortisol* helps an individual mobilize to encounter danger by increasing vigilance behaviors critical for coping with acute threat, while *norepinephrine* increases heartrate and provides the body the energy it needs to fight or flee (Bremner, 2006; Pan et al., 2018). For people with PTSD, these stress responses result in physiological reactions such as hypervigilance, panic attacks, exaggerated startle response, and muscular tension, which occur in response to specific reminders of the trauma or in response to intense but neutral stimuli, such as loud noises (van der Kolk, 2002). Additionally, because these stress responses also have an effect on the parts of the brain involved in emotion and memory, that is, the amygdala and the hippocampus, individuals with PTSD may moreover experience conditioned fear responses when confronted with stimuli that invoke emotionally intense memories, including emotional numbing, avoidance, flashbacks, and nightmares.

The fight-flight-freeze response is reflexive in nature and occurs in a fraction of a second (Menakem, 2017). As mentioned, individuals who suffer distress due to trauma often become triggered when encountering stimuli that remind them of the original trauma. Among individuals with PTSD, or among those with what might be informally categorized as racial trauma when not meeting criteria for PTSD, research suggests that over time, racist encounters become stimuli that sensitize threat response systems, whereby more frequent exposure to these encounters produces chronically heightened vigilance for potential threat (U. S. Clark et al., 2018; Fani et al., 2021; Harnett 2020). Fani et al. (2021), for example, used functional MRI (fMRI) data to examine associations between discriminatory experiences and brainwide response to threat-relevant cues in Black women and found that greater racial discrimination experiences were significantly associated with increased responses in the visual attention, emotion regulation, and fear inhibition regions of the brain when participants were exposed to trauma-relevant distractors vs neutral distractors during attentional control tasks. Essentially, the results of their study indicate that experiences with racism are associated with greater vigilance for potential threat and heightened efforts to suppress threat responses, which can exacerbate the development and expression of PTSD symptoms over time. These results are similar to another fMRI study wherein racial discrimination was found to be associated with greater spontaneous activity in the amygdala, which has been related to mental health outcomes such as higher levels of stress, physiological arousal, and vigilance (U. S. Clark et al., 2018).

Ultimately, the body of research derived from recent advances in neuropsychology indicate that PTSD and racial trauma begin in the brain and live in the body through symptoms such as increased somatic complaints, physical arousal, dissociation, and vigilance. Given this indication, therapists must be equipped to address the cognitive and emotional aspects of trauma, as well as physiological symptoms prompted by the threat response systems of the brain. Moreover, given literature which also describes the importance of psychological liberation in healing from racial trauma in particular, therapists must additionally be equipped to promote empowerment and resilience in the face of systemic oppression (Bryant-Davis et al., 2021; Chavez-Dueñas et al., 2019). Accordingly, the case illustration included later in this chapter emphasizes the integration of cognitive restructuring with liberation frameworks and third wave CBT techniques that address somatic and arousal symptoms characteristic of PTSD.

Ehlers and Clark's Cognitive Model of Posttraumatic Stress Disorder

Cognitive therapy (CT) for PTSD (Ehlers & D. M. Clark, 2000) is a highly effective and empirically validated trauma approach (Ehlers et al., 2005). Another approach, cognitive processing therapy (CPT, Resick et al., 2017), has also been found to be highly effective; however, CPT is a manualized treatment consisting of 12 sessions, whereas CT-PTSD has been found to be effective in a shorter self-study format consisting of six sessions and six self-study modules in between sessions (Grey et al., 2009; Wild & Ehlers, 2010). Given barriers to treatment discussed in Chapter 1 including limited time to access services, CT-PTSD was therefore selected as the theoretical framework for the purpose of this chapter (the reader is referred to Resick et al. (2017) for a review of CPT). The model upon which CT-PTSD is grounded, Ehlers and D. M. Clark's (2000) cognitive model of PTSD, is based on the premise that individuals develop PTSD when trauma is processed in ways that lead to a sense of serious, current threat. This processing includes: (1) negative appraisals of the trauma and its sequelae and (2) a disturbance of memory characterized by poor elaboration, strong associative memory, and strong perceptual priming. *Negative appraisals* refer to the personal meanings ascribed to the trauma. They are idiosyncratic in nature but signal (a) perceived external threat due to impending danger (e.g., "Black people are never safe") or the unfairness of the trauma (e.g., "The world is unfair to people like me"), and (b) perceived internal threat, which typically relates to beliefs about one's reactions, emotions, or behavior during the trauma (e.g., "I should be stronger" or "I'm not as good as others") (Ehlers & Wild, 2020).

The second processing difficulty in Ehlers and D. M. Clark's (2000) model, *disturbance of memory*, refers to disjointed, decontextualized recollections that induce a sense of threat similar to the threat experienced in the initial trauma (Ehlers & Wild, 2020). Recall earlier in this chapter where it was noted that neuropsychologically, stress responses originating in the amygdala and the hippocampus have a significant effect on memory during a traumatic event. Specifically, when the amygdala senses a threat, it signals the hypothalamus, which activates the sympathetic nervous system and releases stress hormones including cortisol and norepinephrine (Wolkin, 2016). Cortisol affects the strength of the memories associated with traumatic events, and norepinephrine increases heartrate and controls the fight-flight-freeze response. As these chemicals are released, the brain shifts the body into survival mode, shutting down all non-essential body and mind processes. At the same time, the hippocampus, which is in charge of memories, also interacts with the amygdala by producing fragmented memories and flashbacks that further trigger the amygdala's fight-flight-freeze response. Normally, the hippocampus connects and organizes memories within their proper time, place, and context. However, when trauma has occurred, the hippocampus has difficulty discriminating past from present and memory from factual knowledge.

Cognitively, these processes are problematic because they prevent people with PTSD from accessing information needed to correct negative predictions made at the time of the traumatic event (Ehlers & Wild, 2020). For example, Tanesha was an African American woman who along with her husband, Malakai, was pulled over by the police for what should have been a routine traffic stop. During the interaction, Malakai was asked to step out of the car where an unprovoked physical altercation took place. As Tanesha watched police assault her husband, she thought to herself, "He is going to die, and I am going to be alone." When subsequently recalling this moment, Tanesha had difficulty integrating the fact that her husband did not die into her memory of the event. As a result, Tanesha's memories of the interaction with police had the effect of inducing an ongoing sense of threat similar to the threat she felt on that day, including a reexperiencing of the same high emotions and arousal (Ehlers & Wild, 2020). Moreover, consistent with Ehlers and D. M. Clark's (2000) model, these memories were easily triggered by sensory cues that overlapped with sensory features of the initial trauma, such that whenever Tanesha heard sirens or loud voices, saw police in her community, or even saw uniformed police on the television she experienced significant distress, including flashbacks and panic. Essentially, through associative learning, Tanesha had come to associate these sights and sounds with a prediction of severe danger (Ehlers & D. M. Clark, 2000). Additionally, due to strong perceptual priming, these stimuli were triggering even in situations that were different from the original trauma, for example, when hearing loud voices at a family gathering.

According to Ehlers and D. M. Clark (2000), PTSD symptoms like those described in the case of Tanesha are maintained by maladaptive behavioral and cognitive strategies. Examples of these strategies include trying to stop the thought, selective attention to threat cues, rumination, avoidance of reminders, dissociation, substance use, and use of safety behaviors to prevent or minimize future occurrences of the event (Ehlers & D. M. Clark, 2000; Ehlers & Wild, 2020). While meant to control the sense of threat, these strategies actually worsen PTSD symptoms because they directly produce PTSD symptoms, prevent change in negative appraisals, or prevent change in the trauma memory. In Tanesha's case, efforts to avoid reminders of her trauma such as limiting driving, staying at home, and being overprotective of her husband prevented her from challenging appraisals such as "Nowhere is safe" and "If we don't stay hidden, we will be targeted again." Constant scanning of her environment when she did go outside also increased her awareness of police presence, even when faraway, which additionally brought on arousal and trauma-related emotions.

To address the appraisals, memory difficulties, and behavioral and cognitive strategies that maintain a sense of current threat and PTSD symptoms, Ehlers and D. M. Clark (2000) suggest three treatment goals: (1) modification of problematic appraisals, (2) elaboration of the trauma memory to include prior and subsequent experience and enhanced trigger discrimination in order to reduce reexperiencing of the trauma, and (3) reduction in the use of dysfunctional behavioral and cognitive strategies. Clinical guidelines in this process include developing a therapeutic relationship characterized by trust and collaborative empiricism, regular monitoring of client symptomatology, psychoeducation, and individualized case formulation. Specific interventions in CT-PTSD include reclaiming/rebuilding your life assignments, the updating trauma memories procedure, narrative writing, imagery, and developing a blueprint (Ehlers & Wild, 2020). Other broad categories of PTSD interventions include relaxation, systematic desensitization, stress inoculation training, prolonged exposure, and cognitive restructuring (Leahy et al., 2012).

Research on the treatment of PTSD using CBT in the African American population is scant, with virtually no studies examining CBT as a treatment to PTSD developed in response to racism. Instead, much of the extant literature focuses on the use of CBT and trauma-focused CBT broadly among African American youth. For example, Scheeringa et al. (2011) found that TF-CBT was effective for treating PTSD in a majority Black sample of three- through six-year-old children exposed to heterogeneous types of traumas. In this study, treatment included psychoeducation about PTSD, recognition of feelings, trainings in coping skills, graduated exposures to trauma-related reminders with three modalities (drawings, imaginal, and in vivo), and safety planning. Studies among African American adults, conversely, have primarily focused on veteran (e.g., Trahan et al., 2016) and sexual assault populations (e.g., Holliday et al., 2017). While still not specific to experiences with racism, these studies also show CBT to be effective in the treatment of PTSD among African Americans.

Carter's Race-Based Traumatic Stress Injury Model

In Chapter 2, I briefly introduced Carter's (2007) race-based traumatic stress injury model. Recall that according to this model, racial trauma is the result of mental and emotional injury caused by encounters with racism (Carter, 2007). Racism, as conceptualized by Carter (2007), can be categorized into three types: (1) racial harassment, (2) racial discrimination, or (3) discriminatory harassment. *Racial harassment* refers to physical, interpersonal, and verbal assaults, treatment as stereotype, and assumptions of criminality or dangerousness. *Racial discrimination* refers to behaviors such as barring access, exclusion, withholding information, and use of deception on the basis of race. *Discriminatory harassment* refers to aversive behaviors such as "White flight," isolation at work, denial of promotions, and questioning of qualifications. According to the race-based traumatic stress injury model, when individuals experience their encounters with any of these three types of racism as negative, memorable, sudden, and uncontrollable they develop trauma reactions; that is, reactions characterized by intrusion, avoidance, and arousal. These reactions, in turn, produce significant psychological distress and negative impacts to the individual's functioning (Carter et al., 2017). A diagram of the race-based traumatic stress injury model applied to the case of Tanesha is shown in Figure 11.1.

Research using Carter's (2007) model as an organizing framework offers insight into the ways racism elicits a trauma response comparable to PTSD. Polanco-Roman et al. (2016), for example, found that racial discrimination was positively associated with dissociation, which as discussed previously, is a common reaction to trauma initiated by the brain's response to perceived threat. According to Polanco-Roman et al. (2016), *dissociation* may be more

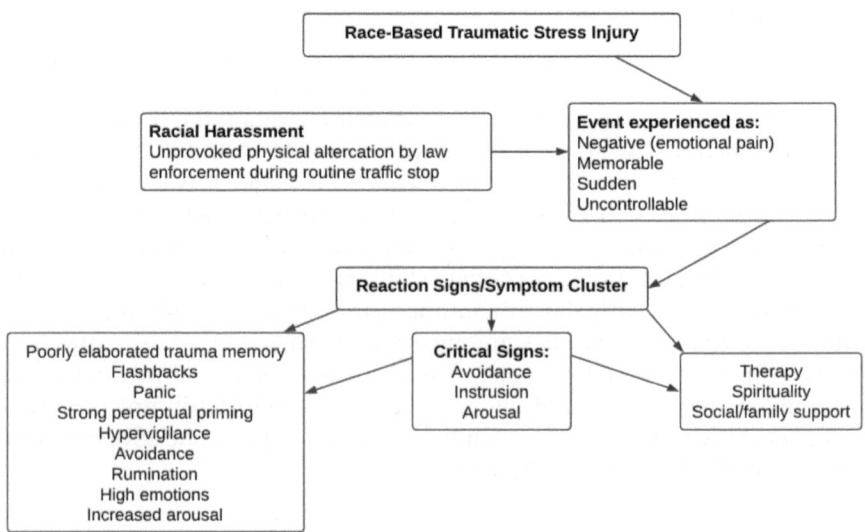

Figure 11.1 Race-Based Traumatic Stress Injury Model in the Case of Tanesha. Adapted from Carter, R. T. (2007). Racism and psychological and emotional injury: Recognizing and assessing race-based traumatic stress. *The Counseling Psychologist, 35*(1), 13–105. https://doi.org/10.1177/0011000006292033

specifically defined as "an experienced loss of control over mental processes that result in alterations in conscious awareness and self-attribution" (p. 610). When considered within the race-based traumatic stress injury model, dissociation in the study reflected one type of a critical reaction (i.e., intrusion, avoidance, and arousal) developed in response to racial discrimination that was experienced as negative, memorable, sudden, and out of one's control. As hypothesized according to the premise of the model, racial discrimination as measured by the Experiences of Discrimination Scale (Krieger et al., 2005) had a significant relationship with dissociative symptoms that was not explained by exposure to other traumatic life events as measured by the Life Events Checklist (Gray et al., 2004), lending empirical support to the assertion that racial discrimination produces symptoms similar to PTSD.

Assessment

PTSD assessment should incorporate use of both tests and clinical interviews (Leahy et al., 2012). One of the most commonly utilized quantitative tests of PTSD symptoms is the PTSD Checklist (PCL-5; Blevins et al., 2015). This measure is a 20-item questionnaire that assesses PTSD symptoms according to the *DSM-5*. For each symptom, respondents rate how much they were bothered in the past month on a Likert-type scale ranging from 0 (*not at all*) to 4 (*extremely*). A total symptom severity score, which ranges from 0 to 80, can be obtained by summing the responses for each item. Scores corresponding to *DSM-5* PTSD criteria can be obtained by summing the scores for the items within a given criterion. For more information on the PCL-5, the reader is referred to Table 6.1 in Chapter 6. A structured clinical interview known as the Clinician-Administered PTSD Scale (CAPS-5; Weathers et al., 2013, 2018) is also available. The Posttraumatic Cognitions Inventory (PTCI; Foa et al., 1999), on the other hand, is a 33-item self-report measure of negative posttraumatic appraisals that is rated on a Likert-type scale that ranges from 1 (*totally disagree*) to 7 (*totally agree*). Scores on the measure are obtained for three subscales: (1) Negative Cognitions About Self (21 items), (2) Negative Cognitions About the World (7 items), and (3) Self-Blame (5 items). Subscale scores are computed as the mean item response for each subscale. A total score is calculated by summing responses across all items.

In terms of the clinical interview, Ehlers and D. M. Clark (2000) note that a primary goal should be articulation of the client's idiosyncratic experience of the three aspects of PTSD according to their model: (1) negative appraisals, (2) trauma memories, and (3) problematic behavioral and cognitive strategies. To examine negative appraisals, the researchers recommend asking clients about what has been most distressing since the event and exploring the client's corresponding beliefs about their symptoms, their future, and the behavior of others. This would include identifying experiences that evoked particularly strong distress, known as "hotspots." Concerning trauma memory, emphasis is placed on gathering information on where there are gaps in memory, and the extent to which memories and intrusions have a "here and now" quality and strong sensory components. Behavioral and cognitive strategies are examined by asking clients about various methods of coping with their trauma (Ehlers & D. M. Clark, 2000).

Given the differential nature of PTSD and racial trauma, assessment of race-based stress is generally acknowledged as an additional first step in the treatment of trauma due to experiences with racism (Bryant-Davis & Ocampo, 2006; Malcoun et al., 2015). It includes: (1) attention to the counseling relationship, (2) use of quantitative assessment, and (3) use of clinical interview (Carter & Pieterse, 2020). In terms of the counseling relationship, the importance of building rapport with clients is emphasized from the first point of contact. Due to the sensitive nature of race and racial trauma, therapists should be particularly intentional in establishing safety and building a strong therapeutic alliance at this stage of therapy (Markin & Coleman, 2021). As discussed in Chapter 5, traditionally, the therapeutic alliance is conceptualized as consisting of three interrelated components: (1) client/therapist agreement on treatment goals, (2) client/therapist agreement on the tasks that will be used to achieve those goals, and (3) a bond between the client/therapist that is experienced as secure, warm, and friendly (Boswell & Constantino, 2022, pp. 113–114). More recently, scholars have also recognized the significance of cultural humility in the establishment of a strong therapeutic alliance, especially during counseling with people of color (Davis et al., 2018). Recall that *cultural humility* is defined as "the ability to maintain an interpersonal stance that is other-oriented (or open to the other) in relation to aspects of cultural identity that are most important to the client" (Hook et al., 2013, p. 354). Accordingly, use of basic counseling techniques such as warmth, empathy, and validation should be emphasized to facilitate aspects of the therapeutic alliance such as trust and safety; however, when additionally conceptualizing cultural humility as a primary aspect of the therapeutic alliance, therapists should also be skilled in use of advanced counseling techniques such as broaching during the assessment phase of counseling and continue use of these skills across sessions (Day-Vines et al., 2018, 2020; Malott & Schaefle, 2015; Steele & Newton, 2022). During initial assessments with clients who directly report stress or trauma due to racism, this may be demonstrated with an intracounseling dynamics focused broaching statement such as, "Although we are both women and share some similarities, we also share some differences based on race. How do you think these differences might impact our relationship?" "Would you be willing to tell me if I do or say something that doesn't sit well with you during our work together?" Among clients who do not initially report racial trauma, broaching may be more inter-racially focused with a statement such as, "In what ways, if any, does race/racism influence your current problems?" (American Psychiatric Association, 2013; Day-Vines et al., 2021; King, 2021).

Beyond attention to the therapeutic relationship, assessment with clients who have experienced racial trauma is enhanced with use of standardized quantitative measures of the construct (Carter & Pieterse, 2020; M. T. Williams et al., 2022b). A review of these measures is provided in Chapter 6 (see Table 6.2). In addition to quantitative assessment of the client's symptomatology, a thorough assessment of racial trauma also incorporates taking the client's complete history to learn more about their racial background, including when the client became aware of race and how they came to think of themselves as a racial being, as well as their coping strategies, strengths, psychological history, and explanatory models about the trauma (Bryant-Davis & Ocampo, 2006; Carter & Pieterse, 2020). In a more structured approach, Carter and Pieterse (2020) developed a clinical interview protocol which mimics the RBTSSS in its exploration of race-based stress. These authors note, however, that the interview protocol should be used to explore one specific incident of race-based stress, thereby, complimenting rather than replacing exploration of the client's personal history.

Embodied Healing

Given neuropsychological research which indicates racial trauma, in part, represents the body's protective response to race-based events, the initial assessment stage of treatment typically yields information about physiological symptoms resulting from the trauma (Carter et al., 2013). Consistent with a CBT approach, addressing these symptoms should begin with psychoeducation that highlights the physiological aspects of trauma and emphasizes the importance of healing through the body. A second step involves teaching the client somatic-based exercises to increase awareness of their body's trauma responses, when and where they activate, the emotions they give rise to, and how to settle these emotions and physiological responses (Gutiérrez, 2022; Menakem, 2017). With increased frequency, this approach to trauma is becoming known as *embodied healing* (Menakem, 2022). As discussed in Chapter 6, Menakem (2017) conceptualized embodied healing from racial trauma as a five-part process that consists of:

(1) soothing yourself to quiet your mind, calm your heart, and settle your body, (2) noticing the sensations and emotions in your body, (3) accepting any discomfort you are experiencing rather than attempting to flee from it, (4) staying present in your body as your pain unfolds and responding to it from the best parts of yourself, and (5) safely discharging any remaining energy.

(p. 168)

Various interventions that facilitate this healing are collectively known as *mindfulness-based* or *mind-body* interventions (Hinton et al., 2011; Watson-Singleton et al., 2019; Woods-Giscombé & Black, 2010). Specific examples of these interventions include meditation, grounding, breathing, and relaxation exercises. Their use in the treatment of racial trauma is discussed in the paragraphs below.

Meditation

Meditation refers to nonjudgmental attention focused on a particular object, thought, or activity (Kabat-Zinn, 2013). As an intervention in the treatment of racial trauma, meditation can be beneficial by helping clients become more aware of the distressing thoughts, emotions, or physical sensations they experience in their bodies, while simultaneously providing a pathway to increase calm and restore health (Watson-Singleton et al., 2019; Woods-Giscombé & Black, 2010). Among African American women, Woods-Giscombé and Black (2010) found that meditation focused on loving-kindness results in a reduction of debilitating emotions, greater self-forgiveness, improved self-care, and greater capacity for more healthy relationships. Similarly, Hinton et al. (2013) found loving-kindness meditations are therapeutic for refugees and racial minority populations because of their potential for increasing emotional flexibility, decreasing rumination, and serving as emotional regulation techniques. In my clinical work, I have found that for people who have experienced racial trauma, meditation focused on self-compassion may also be especially beneficial. Individuals with racial trauma often experience feelings of helplessness, hopelessness, shame, and humiliation. Self-compassion teaches clients to acknowledge this pain without judging themselves for having it (Gutiérrez, 2022). As a result, clients with greater self-compassion tend to experience decreased shame, humiliation, self-criticism, and resulting somatic complaints (M. T. Williams et al., 2022a). Questions to help clients achieve these goals and process self-compassion or other meditative practices include: "How can self-compassion (acceptance, loving-kindness, etc.) help you deal with racial trauma?" "What else do you need to say to express compassion (acceptance, loving-kindness, etc.) toward yourself?" and "What goal-directed behavior can you engage in now? For example, what can you do to feel accomplished or to help someone else?" (Steele & Newton, 2023).

Grounding

As previously discussed, racial trauma often leads to PTSD symptoms such as dissociation and panic (Carter et al., 2020; Polanco-Roman et al., 2016). *Grounding* is a term used to describe techniques that help clients interrupt these physiological responses and reconnect to the present moment. One example of a grounding technique known as the *five senses grounding technique* or the *5-4-3-2-1 method* involves identifying five things you can see, four things you can touch, three things you can hear, two things you can smell, and one thing you can taste. This process helps deal directly with the problem of dissociation, which refers to momentary lapses with reality, by drawing attention to the external environment and providing opportunities for more active coping (Polanco-Roman et al., 2016; Punkanen & Buckley, 2021). With clients who feel strongly connected to their culture or ancestors, or for those who want to increase access to ancestral wisdom and support, this method can be adapted by encouraging clients to identify something connected to their cultural identity that grounds them or makes them feel relaxed and at ease (Gutiérrez, 2022). Focusing on each of the five senses, examples of this recommended by my colleague, Dr. Charmeka Newton, might include, looking at a picture of their grandmother, listening to gospel music, getting a hug from someone who validates and understands their trauma, smelling a candle that reminds them of a safe place, and eating a cultural food that brings them pleasure. Another example of a culturally adapted grounding practice recommended by Dr. Newton would be modifying the more literal grounding activity of feeling one's feet and legs firmly planted to the ground (Punkanen & Buckley, 2021) to include asking clients to envision their ancestors (e.g., grandparents, aunts, uncles, etc.) securing their feet and then strengthening their legs, arms, and torso. In this way, clients are encouraged to access supportive presences of the past and feel rooted and lifted-up by these ancestors (Gutiérrez, 2022).

Breathing and Relaxation Exercises

Dysregulated breathing patterns can cause or worsen hyper-aroused states (Carter et al., 2013; Punkanen & Buckley, 2021). Breathing and relaxation exercises are effective because they help lower arousal triggered by the body's stress response. One of the more popular breathing exercises is called *diaphragmatic breathing* or *belly breaths* (Gutiérrez, 2022). Use of the diaphragm, which is a large muscle located at the base of the lungs, assists breathing by providing more power to the lungs and encouraging a pattern of deep inhalation and exhalation (Hopper et al., 2019). This has the effect of decreasing respiratory rate, improving blood flow, and lowering blood pressure, thereby reducing the body's stress response, and creating a greater sense of calm. While studies on the individual use of breathing exercises in the treatment of racial trauma are limited, existing research does support the use of various breathing techniques as part of broader culturally adapted CBT and mindfulness approaches (e.g., Hinton et al., 2013; Green et al., 2021). To lead clients in diaphragmatic breathing, instruct them to begin by placing one hand on their chest and the other hand on their stomach, just below the ribcage. Then, with their hands in place, instruct them breathe in, making the hand on their stomach push out as they do. The client should repeat this pattern until they begin to experience a sense of safety and calm back in their body (Gutiérrez, 2022). Relaxation exercises can also be used to regulate the body's stress response in similar ways as they too have the effect of reducing muscle tension, decreasing heartrate and blood pressure, and slowing breathing (Scotland-Coogan & Davis, 2016). Examples of various relaxation exercises include progressive muscle relaxation, pelvic floor relaxation, stretching, and yoga (Scotland-Coogan & Davis, 2016).

Culturally Adapted Cognitive Restructuring

Once clients have developed the ability to regulate symptoms that might interfere with higher-order processing, cognitive restructuring strategies may be implemented to reduce unhelpful thinking patterns that also contribute to their symptoms and ability to cope (van der Kolk, 2014). Core components of culturally adapted CBT such as enhanced psychoeducation and adapted cognitive restructuring are especially beneficial in achieving these aims, while being additionally supportive of broader empowerment goals connected to the treatment of racial trauma, including increasing critical consciousness (Banks et al., 2021; Bryant-Davis et al., 2021; Graham et al., 2013). For a review of these strategies, the reader is referred to Chapter 7.

As mentioned earlier in this chapter, Ehlers and D. M. Clark (2000) recommend several additional cognitive restructuring techniques specific to their treatment approach to PTSD. Techniques particularly relevant to liberation and African-centered cultural practices include reclaiming/rebuilding your life, which when applied in a culturally responsive manner is consistent with the problem solving, action-oriented nature of liberation psychology (Martín-Baró, 1994), written narratives, which are consistent with culturally derived storytelling practices (Chioneso et al., 2020), and imagery, which can be consistent with Black spiritual expression (C. B. Williams et al., 1999). *Reclaiming/rebuilding your life* refers to efforts designed to help the client resume activities they previously enjoyed and valued, along with activities consistent with their therapy goals (Kerr et al., 2023). In their first use, *written narratives* refer to complete written accounts of what happened during the original trauma from the time they realized they were in danger until the event was over, using past tense language. This is to encourage the client to recognize that the event is in fact over and just a memory (Resick et al., 2017). Reading the account out loud to the therapist and then every day is a way to encourage the client to experience their emotions and work toward extinguishing avoidance behavior. In a second iteration of the assignment, clients are directed to start writing from the point they recognized danger, continuing until the event was over, this time giving more detail about the worst parts of the trauma. These accounts are also read on a daily basis. Finally, *imagery* refers to the use of various imagery techniques to challenge negative appraisals and develop alternative perspectives (Kerr et al., 2023).

Case Illustration: Alaiyah

Alaiyah is a 27-year-old African American woman who sought therapy due to birth trauma. At 30 weeks of pregnancy, Alaiyah was hospitalized and placed on bedrest after developing high blood pressure and gestational diabetes. While in the hospital, Alaiyah encountered several instances of racial discrimination from hospital staff, including racially biased assumptions regarding single parentage and Medicaid participation, poor communication about medical decisions and treatment plans, delayed orders for an emergency C-section, and bias in pain management. Alaiyah explained that during labor, she experienced severe pain and blood loss, which lasted for nearly ten hours despite her complaints. It was only after the fetal tracing monitor indicated the baby's heartrate was in decline that an emergency C-section was ordered, and subsequent efforts were made to address Alaiyah's hemorrhaging. After delivery, Alaiyah continued to experience severe pain, which was largely dismissed by hospital staff. One doctor even expressed concern that Alaiyah might have been inappropriately seeking opioids.

By the time Alaiyah initiated therapy two months later, scores on the PCL-5 indicated that she suffered from PTSD. Symptoms included dissociation, frequent unwanted recollections of the sound of the fetal monitor as her baby's heartrate declined, flashbacks to the look on her husband's face as she was rushed into an emergency C-section, nightmares about her or her baby dying, avoidance of reminders of the event such as refusing to use toys or other gifts that were brought to the hospital after the baby was born, guilt, anxiety, and problems sleeping. Alaiyah additionally expressed anger and frustration about the racially biased treatment she received at the hospital, stating, "Their ignorance almost caused my baby to die." Scores on the Racial Trauma Checklist (RCL; M. T. Williams et al., 2022b) indicated that she had elevated scores on all three of the measure's subscales (i.e., Lack of Safety, Negative Cognitions, and Difficulty Coping), although her score on the Negative Cognitions subscale was the most elevated.

Alaiyah discussed her thoughts about the racially biased treatment of African Americans at length during her sessions. Alaiyah grew up in an upper-class two-parent household with two younger siblings. She described her childhood as difficult due to poor treatment from school staff, coaches, and peers. Although her neighborhood and school were racially diverse, Alaiyah noted disparate treatment of African American students when compared to White students. For example, Alaiyah and her sisters joined activities such as moot court during high school but were often challenged or dismissed by their peers when presenting propositions of the law or making arguments. When describing one specific instance, Alaiyah recalled feeling "furious" and thinking, "It's so unfair for them to treat me this way when I'm the smartest person here." Alaiyah reported having similar thoughts and feelings now in her career as an attorney, describing one particular incident with an attorney from opposing counsel who assumed she was an administrative assistant. According to Alaiyah, the encounter was "exhausting" and "just another example of Black people having to prove they belong." In response to her birthing experience at the hospital, Alaiyah stated that the event demonstrated, "Nowhere is safe for Black people" and she was now convinced that "You have to watch your back wherever you go, even when you're with people who are supposed to protect you."

Case Formulation

Following Ehlers and D. M. Clark's (2000) cognitive model of PTSD, the therapist in the case of Alaiyah conceptualized her client's psychological distress according to the three primary factors of the model: (1) negative appraisals, (2) trauma memories, and (3) maintaining cognitive and behavioral strategies. A diagram depicting this conceptualization is presented in Figure 11.2. Ultimately, Alaiyah blamed herself for the medical emergency during labor, stating, "I should've insisted that something be done before it was an emergency," "I should've known better," and "I know the statistics on Black women and maternal health." Alaiyah felt guilty, angry, ashamed, and overwhelmed by these thoughts, which resulted in new negative appraisals about her reactions such as, "I'm weak" and "It's my fault." Beyond the internal threats reflected in the previously identified thoughts, Alaiyah also had ongoing appraisals about external threats to her and her child's safety, for example, "Doctors can't be trusted," "The system won't protect you," and "I can't even say anything because if I do, I'll be labeled an angry Black woman."

Alaiyah's negative cognitions were extremely distressing and often accompanied by intense intrusions and arousal. Specifically, Alaiyah reported frequent dreams in which she and her baby did not survive the C-section. She additionally experienced intrusive and distressing memories of the birth that were commonly triggered by sensory cues that overlapped with sights and sounds from the event. One image was of the numbers on the fetal tracing monitor, which was triggered whenever Alaiyah heard beeping sounds, for example, from the microwave, from the morning alarm clock, or when passing construction sites. For Alaiyah, this memory of the prolonged warnings from the monitor signaling her baby's distress was a reminder of her failure to insist that action be taken during the event despite having the thought, "My baby is going to die." Another image was the look of terror on her husband's face by the time a decision had been

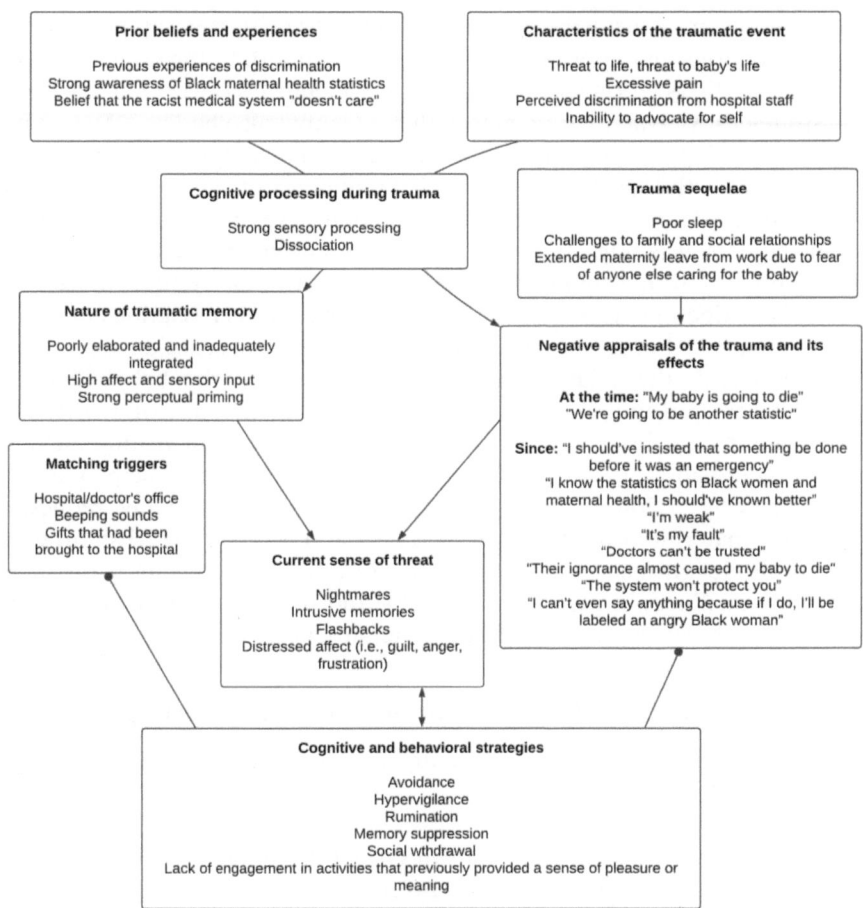

Figure 11.2 Alaiyah's Cognitive Model of PTSD. Round arrow heads denote "prevents change in." Adapted from Kerr, A., Warnock-Parkes, E., Murray, H., Wild, J., Grey, N., Green, C., Clark, D. M., & Ehlers, A. (2023). Cognitive therapy for PTSD following birth trauma and baby loss: Clinical considerations. *The Cognitive Behaviour Therapist, 16*, E23. https://doi.org/10.1017/S1754470X23000156

made to call for an emergency C-section. Unfortunately, Alaiyah thought of this moment every time she saw her husband. She described it as a cruel reminder of how much she and her husband were at the mercy of a racist medical system that "doesn't care." These intrusions were accompanied by difficulty with sleep, poor concentration, and an irritable mood.

While Alaiyah had vivid memories of certain parts of the baby's delivery, she also had difficulty recalling other parts of the event. For example, Alaiyah could not remember the exact moment she learned her baby would be okay or her husband's joy when holding the baby for the first time immediately after the delivery. This prevented Alaiyah from updating negative predictions and appraisals developed in response to the event and contributed to dissociation when discussing her memories (Kerr et al., 2023).

Strategies Alaiyah used to cope with her trauma also had an effect on her symptomatology. These strategies included avoidance, hypervigilance, rumination, and withdrawal. Alaiyah avoided reminders of the birth trauma, for example, refusing to use toys or other gifts that were brought to the hospital after the baby was born and attempting to receive all postnatal care for her and the baby from a midwife rather than a doctor. Her desire to keep the baby from doctor's appointments caused tension in her relationships with her husband and other family members, which led to a sense of social withdrawal. Eventually, Alaiyah was convinced to keep the baby's doctor's appointments, although not without a significant amount of worry. She often ruminated about mistreatment that could come from visiting the doctor with her baby, for example, being judged, ignored, refused help, or generally receiving a lower quality of care. Alaiyah additionally requested extended maternity leave from her employer and was concerned about what she would do when she had to return to work. She was constantly on guard for signs of illness in herself or the baby and did not trust anyone else to provide the baby with adequate care in her absence.

Activity 11.1: Case Formulation in the Case of Alaiyah

Review the negative appraisals presented in Figure 11.2, then respond to the following questions:

- What themes are evident in Alaiyah's negative appraisals?
- In what ways do these themes overlap with racial discrimination or disadvantage?

Treatment Plan

As mentioned previously, treatment in CT-PTSD focuses on modifying negative appraisals, elaboration of the trauma memory to include prior and subsequent experience and enhanced trigger discrimination in order to reduce reexperiencing of the trauma, and reduction in the use of dysfunctional behavioral and cognitive strategies (Ehlers & D. M. Clark, 2000). Recently, Kerr et al. (2023) applied this model to PTSD following birth trauma and baby loss and noted clinical considerations specific to this population, including cognitive themes surrounding the birth-related trauma and the need for early identification and treatment of PTSD. Accordingly, these considerations are taken into account in Alaiyah's treatment plan, which is presented in Table 11.1 and discussed in the sections that follow. Efforts to

Table 11.1 Alaiyah's Treatment Plan

Problem List
1. Intrusion, including flashbacks, nightmares, and dissociation
2. Avoidance of places, people, and objects reminiscent of the trauma
3. Poorly elaborated memory
4. Negative beliefs about self, others, and the world
5. Social, psychological, and occupational impairment
6. Hypervigilance and sleep disturbance
7. Racial discrimination

Treatment Goals:
1. Reduce intrusion and arousal
2. Decrease avoidance of places, people, and objects reminiscent of the trauma
3. Update trauma memories
4. Develop healthy thinking patterns and beliefs about self, others, and the world
5. Increase use of healthy, culturally derived coping strategies
6. Reduce impact to social, psychological, and occupational functioning
7. Increase use of advocacy and engagement with social support networks

Interventions
1. Psychoeducation
2. Reclaiming/rebuilding your life activities
3. Trigger discrimination
4. Written narratives
5. Site visits
6. Cognitive restructuring to challenge negative beliefs about self, others, and the world
7. Minority coping strategies such as expanding social networks and building community support, critical consciousness, self-care, activism, and embodied healing

address the unique experience of racial discrimination through empowerment and culturally derived healing practices are also included in the treatment plan.

Problem List

Statistics indicate that African American women experience low-quality and differential maternal healthcare when compared to women of other races (Centers for Disease Control and Prevention, 2023). One outcome of these experiences is worsened mental health. Markin and Coleman (2021), for instance, reported that gendered racial discrimination during childbirth may lead to posttraumatic stress reactions when proper support is absent, which is evidenced in the case of Alaiyah. Given the situational context of racial discrimination in Alaiyah's concerns, difficulties due to both PTSD symptoms and racial discrimination are identified on her problem list. This acknowledges and validates her lived experience as an African American woman, while also allowing for greater intentionality in addressing the racial aspects of her trauma in the goals and interventions included in Alaiyah's treatment plan.

Treatment Goals

Treatment goals in the case of Alaiyah focus on addressing the debilitating impact of PTSD in her life (Kerr et al., 2023). In consideration of the general goals of CT-PTSD (Ehlers & D. M. Clark, 2000), this includes an emphasis on (a) reducing intrusion, arousal, and avoidance symptoms, (b) restructuring personal meanings developed in response to the event, (c) elaborating trauma memories, and (d) increasing use of healthy coping strategies. To enhance cultural sensitivity in treatment, use of culturally derived coping strategies is also included, as well as increased use of advocacy and engagement with social support networks.

Activity 11.2: Treatment Goals in the Case of Alaiyah

Alaiyah's therapist chose to address racial discrimination in her treatment goals by focusing on advocacy and social support. What other specific strengths or coping strategies could Alaiyah draw from to counter the effects of racial discrimination (see Chapter 3)?

Interventions

Consistent with CT-PTSD, interventions in Alaiyah's treatment plan focus on the emotional, cognitive, and behavioral aspects of her trauma. However, interventions that directly address her unique experience as an African American woman are also emphasized on the treatment plan. In particular, Markin and Coleman (2021) suggest that therapy with African American women who have experienced childbirth trauma should highlight framing symptoms as understandable reactions to gendered race-based traumatic stress, as well as collaboration with relevant stakeholders to advocate for systemic change. About this, these authors suggest that strategies such as expanding social networks and activism can "strengthen the social fabric of the community," thereby providing affirmation, protection, and a source of empowerment (Markin & Coleman, 2021, p. 2). Strategies such as racial self-care may additionally promote qualities such as self-determination, self-preservation, and self-restoration in the midst of ongoing oppression. Culturally adapted embodied healing interventions such as the grounding, breathing, relaxation, and meditation techniques described earlier in this chapter also assist coping with the physiological aspects of racial trauma. Accordingly, these along with traditional CT-PTSD interventions are integrated into treatment planning in the case of Alaiyah.

Course of Treatment

Earlier, the significance of building a strong therapeutic relationship was discussed as it relates to the assessment of race-based traumatic stress. Consistent with traditional CBT principles, the therapeutic relationship is also emphasized throughout the beginning, middle, and end phases of treatment when working with African American women who have experienced birth trauma. Specifically, because the traumatic event for these women occurred within the context of interactions with healthcare professionals, special care and attention is needed in terms of reestablishing safety, trust, and a sense of collaboration in relationships with professional helpers. This includes addressing feelings of powerlessness that clients develop in response to having their concerns silenced or dismissed during childbirth, providing the support needed to process intense emotions, acknowledging cultural ruptures that occur in the relationship, and working to repair these ruptures (Markin & Coleman, 2021). The reader is referred to Chapter 5 for more information on cultural ruptures.

In terms of treatment delivery, CT-PTSD typically begins with one or two sessions that cover (a) psychoeducation focused on normalization of symptoms, (b) reclaiming your life activities, and (c) case formulation and orientating clients to the elaboration of trauma memory (Grey et al., 2009). Next, clients are guided in memory-focused techniques to access problematic memories that maintain a sense of current threat. This includes identification of hotspots and their most threatening personal meanings, usually in one session. The remaining sessions are spent addressing cognitive and behavioral strategies that maintain negative appraisals and working directly with trauma memories (Kerr et al., 2023).

On average, CT-PTSD lasts for 12 sessions, although there are shorter, more intensive formats (Grey et al., 2009; Wild et al., 2020). The sections below describe a course of culturally adapted CT-PTSD in the case of Alaiyah. Notice the acknowledgment of racial disparities in the delivery of healthcare among African Americans and their impact on Alaiyah's trauma, as well as the inclusion of environmental interventions such as advocacy and social support (see Chapter 8) in the therapist's approach. As you read, make note of any other cultural factors, interventions, or case formulation hypotheses that seem relevant to you for treatment with this client.

Beginning Phase of Treatment: Sessions 2 and 3

Alaiyah was a 27-year-old African American woman who presented to therapy with PTSD due to birth trauma, evidenced by scores on the PCL-5 (Blevins et al., 2015). Symptoms identified by Alaiyah during her initial intake session included dissociation, distressing recollections, flashbacks, nightmares, avoidance, guilt, anxiety, and problems sleeping. Alaiyah additionally expressed anger and frustration about the racially biased treatment she received at the hospital, with scores on the RCL (M. T. Williams et al., 2022b) indicating that she was elevated on all three of the measure's subscales (i.e., Lack of Safety, Negative Cognitions, and Difficulty Coping).

Based on Alaiyah's clinical presentation, Sessions 2 and 3 focused on key elements of initial sessions in CT-PTSD, including attention to the therapeutic relationship, identifying treatment goals, normalizing the client's symptoms, obtaining a history of the trauma, exploring the client's negative appraisals, identifying intrusions and how the client deals with them, conducting a thought suppression experiment, providing psychoeducation on factors that maintain PTSD, offering a rationale for trauma memory work, and introducing the client to reclaiming your life assignments (https://oxcadatresources. com/the-first-therapy-session/). To assist in this process, the therapist and Alaiyah reviewed an informational sheet discussing PTSD and the nature of trauma memories. An excerpt from this review is provided below.

Therapist: Alaiyah, I want to thank you for finding the courage to speak with me today given everything you experienced with your doctors.

Alaiyah: Yeah, it wasn't an easy decision.

Therapist: It makes sense that you would feel some reluctance in light of the racism you've encountered.

Alaiyah: I didn't know what else to do. I'm worried that I'm losing my mind.

Therapist: I understand your worry. I think it's important for you to know that women with birth trauma often experience the symptoms you describe. It's actually quite normal and common.

Alaiyah: Really? It feels like I'm the only one. Everyone in my family tells me I should just pray about it, which I've done, but I'm still struggling.

Therapist: I'm sorry to hear that. I know that sometimes our friends and family may say that prayer should be enough or that seeking professional help means you lack faith in God. Many of the clients I've worked with, however, have found going to therapy and learning additional coping strategies doesn't mean you have to eliminate prayer from your life. In fact, they can work together.

Alaiyah: That's good to hear.

Therapist: Mm hmm. You're not alone in this, I'm here to support you as you also rely on your faith and other support systems. Could we start by reviewing this information sheet to help you get a better understanding of PTSD?

Alaiyah: Sure.

Therapist: Great. One of the first points I'd like to emphasize is that PTSD is a normal reaction to emotionally painful events that are sudden, negative, and out of one's control. When these events happen within the context of racism, there can be an additional element of pain that occurs. Are you with me so far?

Alaiyah: Yes.

Therapist: Okay, good. Now, while each person's response to traumatic events is unique to that individual, there are some common reactions people tend to experience. These reactions include reexperiencing your trauma emotionally or through flashbacks, dreams, or bodily reactions; physical arousal; feeling like you're having an out of body experience; negative thoughts about yourself, other people, or life; and strong emotions like fear, anxiety, guilt, shame, anger, and sadness. [Each reaction was explained in depth].

Alaiyah: That describes a lot of what I've been experiencing.

Therapist: Right! And the reason people have these types of reactions has to do with the way the brain processes information during a traumatic event. Specifically, when people encounter situations that the brain perceives as dangerous, parts of the brain responsible for basic survival override the part of the brain where humans think and reason, initiating what's known as the fight-flight-freeze response. This involves a complex interaction of neuropsychological processes that have an effect on memory such that memories become fragmented, and the brain has difficulty organizing memories within their proper time, place, and context. This explains why certain reminders can cause you to reexperience the emotions and physical sensations of your trauma as if they are happening now, and why people with PTSD live in a constant state of threat that feels serious and current.

Alaiyah: I think "constant" is the right word to describe my feelings. It's like I can't trust anybody and I'm always on the lookout, especially when it's time for the baby's checkups. I really don't feel safe with the doctors. What if something goes wrong? How do I know I won't be brushed off like so many other African American women?

Therapist:	I hear the worry in your questions, Alaiyah. They really illustrate the additional pain added to the situation because of race.
Alaiyah:	Yeah.
Therapist:	Could you tell me more about what happened during the delivery so that I can get a better sense of your experience, particularly in terms of your experience as an African American woman?

As illustrated in the previous excerpt, traditional elements of therapy are enhanced through intentional cultural sensitivity in the counseling process. To build the therapeutic relationship, the therapist used skills such as validation and broaching, evidenced through statements such as, "It makes sense that you would feel some reluctance in light of the racism you've encountered" and "Could you tell me more about what happened during the delivery so that I can get a better sense of your experience, particularly in terms of your experience as an African American woman?" During the exchange, the therapist was also mindful of African-centered cultural values such as spirituality and social support, shown in the statement, "I'm here to support you as you also rely on your faith and other support systems." These skills contributed to the sense of safety felt in the session by signaling to the client that the therapist was comfortable discussing race and racism within the context of therapy. Use of these skills also increased the therapist's ability to obtain information necessary to conceptualize racially salient cognitions contributing to her current difficulties.

At the conclusion of the excerpt presented above, the therapist began an initial exploration of key details from Alaiyah's birth experience, including identification of symptoms, the worst moments in the event, and the meanings Alaiyah assigned to these moments, using questions such as, "What was the worst thing about your delivery?" "What were the worst moments?" and "What were the worst thoughts that went through your mind during those moments?" According to Alaiyah, the worst moments of her baby's delivery were listening to the baby's heartrate decline and when she was rushed into an emergency C-section. The thoughts that went through her mind at these moments were, "My baby is going to die" and "We're going to be another statistic." At the time, Alaiyah was frightened and overwhelmed. When thinking about the situation now, Alaiyah additionally reported feeling angry that "Their ignorance almost caused [her] baby to die." She also felt guilty and ashamed, stating, "I should've insisted that something be done before it was an emergency" and "I should've known better."

When exploring intrusions associated with the event, Alaiyah reported that her most frequent memories were of the numbers on the fetal tracing monitor and the look of terror on her husband's face when she was rushed into an emergency C-section. Her primary response to these memories was to try to push them away, which had not been successful. According to Ehlers and Wild (2015), attempts to avoid memories by pushing them away often has the opposite effect, causing more intrusions and blocking the processing of trauma. Therefore, the therapist carried out a thought suppression experiment to illustrate the paradoxical effect this strategy has on intrusive memories, developed a maintenance cycle diagram to visually depict the effect of this behavior (see Figure 11.3), and encouraged Alaiyah to instead work on letting the memories come and go. The therapist then reviewed other factors that contribute to the maintenance of PTSD beyond thought suppression and unprocessed memories, including negative appraisals and behavioral strategies such as rumination, hypervigilance, and avoidance. While discussing these factors, the therapist acknowledged that while typically viewed as maladaptive, some strategies such as hypervigilance may in fact be an adaptive coping strategy necessary to navigate the racially biased healthcare system and increase safety for Alaiyah and her baby (Roberson & Carter, 2022).

Alaiyah's initial introduction to therapy concluded with an explanation for trauma memory work and identification of reclaiming your life assignments. The reclaiming your life assignments involved naming activities Alaiyah enjoyed, as well as activities that would allow her to develop more satisfying relationships, given the current sense of isolation she experiences among friends and family (Ehlers & Wild, 2015). Alaiyah reported that prior to giving birth, she was an active dancer and regularly attended a Trap Cardio class that she had not returned to due to a desire to stay home with the baby. While Alaiyah did not currently feel comfortable enough to leave the baby to resume the class, she did acknowledge that she could engage the exercise using YouTube videos. To find support for her new experience as a

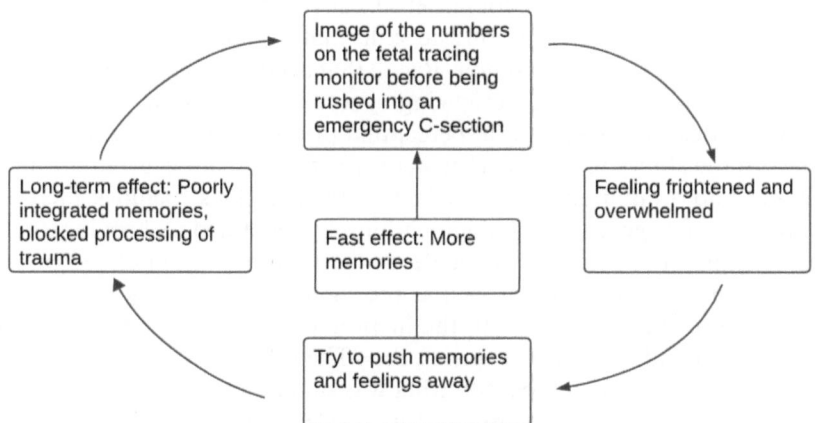

Figure 11.3 Alaiyah's Cycle of Thought Suppression. Adapted from Wild, J., Warnock-Parkes, E., Murray, H., Kerr, A., Thew, G., Grey, N., Clark, D. M., & Ehlers, A. (2020). Treating posttraumatic stress disorder remotely with cognitive therapy for PTSD. *European Journal of Psychotraumatology, 11*(1), 1–15. https://doi.org/10.1080/20008198.2020.1785818

mother, the therapist also provided Alaiyah with information for several baby groups in their community (Kerr et al., 2023). Finally, to help Alaiyah find social support for her unique experience as an African American woman, the therapist encouraged research and reflection on ways to increase her sense of belongingness and mattering, such as participation in culturally based community groups and institutions or attendance at formal or informal spaces that would offer counternarratives to negative self-appraisals developed in response to racism (Steele & Newton, 2023). Alaiyah stated that she would resume her bi-weekly trips to the hair salon and become more active in an organization for Black attorneys she belongs to.

Middle Phase of Treatment: Sessions 4 through 7

In Session 4, the therapist used information about hotspots in Alaiyah's trauma memory to provide further psychoeducation on the relationship between poorly elaborated trauma memories and PTSD and to introduce Alaiyah to trauma memory work. This included facilitating stimulus discrimination and preparing Alaiyah for work with her trauma memories by teaching her various mindfulness-based techniques to help regulate her stress responses, given her reported difficulties with dissociation.

First, the therapist normalized Alaiyah's dissociative symptoms by sharing research which shows that distortions in perception, gaps in memory and awareness, and flashbacks and nightmares are common reactions to trauma, and that this relationship remains in the presence of racial discrimination even when there is an absence of other trauma events over the course of a person's lifetime (Polanco-Roman et al., 2016). Next, the therapist taught Alaiyah stimulus discrimination and skills that would be useful for returning her attention to the here and now. Recall that according to Ehlers and D. M. Clark's (2000) model, reexperiencing symptoms develop as a function of strong associative memory and perceptual priming. *Stimulus discrimination* refers to the ability to differentiate between stimuli that occurred during the trauma and stimuli encountered in the present. This includes increasing awareness of triggers, which Alaiyah initially identified as beeping sounds, for example, from the microwave, from the morning alarm clock, or when passing construction sites, as well as the sight of her husband's face. Other triggers Alaiyah identified with the help of the therapist included visits to the hospital and certain toys. Using the "Then versus Now" technique, the therapist helped Alaiyah identify what was similar and what was different in her triggers during the trauma and now (Kerr et al., 2023). For example, Alaiyah noted the similarity between the sound of the baby monitor and her microwave and then identified differences, including the tone of the beeping, the purpose of the beeping, and the sound coming from an appliance in her kitchen rather than a monitor at the hospital.

Other emotional regulation skills useful for returning Alaiyah's attention to the here and now were also discussed in Session 4. Alaiyah described her dissociation as depersonalization experiences, noting feeling cut off from both her emotions and body at times. To help Alaiyah reconnect to the present moment while also drawing from African-centered principles such as interdependence and kinship ties during these experiences, the therapist guided her in the use of culturally adapted grounding exercises. Alaiyah had a particularly positive response to the grounding activity of feeling one's feet and legs firmly planted to the ground (Punkanen & Buckley, 2021). During this exercise, she liked to imagine herself as a tree, with her ancestors and other Black women who have also had traumatic birthing experiences serving as the roots and strengthening her physically and emotionally (Gutiérrez, 2022).

In Session 5, the therapist began narrative writing exercises. *Narrative writing* is an alternative to imaginal reliving that is often used during PTSD treatment when clients experience dissociative symptoms (Ehlers & Wild, 2020). It consists of three steps: (1) identifying hotspots and threatening personal meanings, (2) identifying updating information that does not fit with the personal meaning, and (3) incorporation of updating information into the hotspots (Kerr et al., 2023). Although Alaiyah's dissociative symptoms were somewhat mild, this technique was selected due to its ability to address gaps in Alaiyah's trauma memory, as well its consistency with storytelling traditions in the African American community. Chioneso et al. (2020) noted that over time, storytelling is an intervention that can be used to process events and reframe negative cognitions through the development of stories that challenge hegemonic cultural narratives. During the session, the therapist assisted Alaiyah in the initial retelling of her trauma story, focusing on key events, feelings, and cognitions, paying attention to hotspots. In Session 2's brief retelling of the trauma, Alaiyah identified listening to the baby's heartrate decline and being rushed into the emergency C-section as hotspots. As part of the narrative writing exercise, Alaiyah identified additional hotspots, which included doctors dismissing her concerns and losing consciousness at one point during the delivery. The meanings Alaiyah associated with these hotspots were, "I'm going to be another statistic" and "We're going to die." In clarifying these meanings, Alaiyah noted that her thoughts were focused on dying and becoming a statistic due to racism. Like other women with birth trauma, her emotions were fear (Distress = 100 percent; Nowness = 50 percent), shame (Distress = 80 percent; Nowness = 90 percent), and defeat (Distress = 100 percent; Nowness = 70 percent) (Evans, 2022; Kerr et al., 2023).

In Sessions 6 and 7, Alaiyah and the therapist worked on updating her trauma memory. This began with exploration of each hotspot and its personal meaning. During this process, the therapist was careful to validate

Alaiyah's experiences with racism, choosing to focus on challenging the negative self-appraisals. For example, Alaiyah had negative appraisals about her responsibility for the difficulties during the delivery (Ehlers & D. M. Clark, 2000), which included "I should've insisted that something be done before it was an emergency" and "I should've known better." These appraisals led to feelings of guilt and shame. During sessions, the therapist worked with Alaiyah to restructure these beliefs using techniques such as psychoeducation, pie charts, and Socratic questioning (Kerr et al., 2023). First, Alaiyah and the therapist reviewed research and other anecdotal stories on the maternal experiences of African American women. For example, the therapist shared findings from qualitative research which suggest that African American women experience a variety of inequities in maternal healthcare including dismissed pain concerns due to stereotypes, adverse birth outcomes, and negative mental health outcomes such as feeling alone, feeling misunderstood, doubting oneself/feeling incapable, loss of hope, and feeling angry (Adebayo et al., 2022; Alhusen et al., 2016; Evans, 2022). The therapist and Alaiyah also discussed tennis star Serena Williams's well-known traumatic birth experience, noting that even a woman with fame and resources was not immune to racially biased treatment in maternal healthcare. With this information, Alaiyah then completed a pie chart identifying other factors that contributed to the birth trauma including the fact that Alaiyah did speak out about her concerns and multiple trained professionals were there to identify an appropriate course of action. From a liberation perspective, the psychoeducation and pie charts were consistent with development of the critical consciousness needed for psychological empowerment and social change.

After reviewing the research and completing the pie charts, the therapist used Socratic dialogue the help Alaiyah develop an alternative view herself, emphasizing examining the evidence, devising alternative explanations, and gaining distance (J. S. Beck, 2020). Specifically, the therapist used questions such as, "Based on the research we reviewed and the factors described in your pie chart, what is the evidence for and against these thoughts?" "What's another explanation?" and "How would you respond to a friend if they were in this situation?" Through this dialogue, Alaiyah realized that essentially, she was "blaming the victim" and should respond to herself with compassion instead. Her alternative perspective became, "I did tell the doctors that something was wrong...my concerns were dismissed, and the doctors did not listen to me" and "Maternal health inequities are complex and not easily overcome...I did the best I could in the situation." To create an emotional connection to these updates, Alaiyah visualized holding her baby for the first time and hearing his cries in the delivery room. Table 11.2 presents a summary of Alaiyah's other hotspots and updating information.

Table 11.2 Alaiyah's Hotspots and Updating Information

Hotspot	Appraisal	Feeling	Updating Information
Doctors dismissing her concerns	"I'm going to be another statistic"	Fear, Defeat, Shame	"The biases that led doctors to dismiss my concerns are emblematic of racism among healthcare providers and should be addressed, but they are not my fault and thankfully neither my baby nor I died"
Listening to the baby's heartrate decline	"My baby is going to die"	Fear, Overwhelm	"My baby did not die"
Losing consciousness at one point during the delivery	"We're going to die"	Fear	"We survived"
Being rushed into the emergency C-section	"We're going to be another statistic"	Fear	"My baby and I made it through the surgery"
—	"Their ignorance almost caused my baby to die"	Anger	"I have a right to be angry about the racist treatment we received but my baby did not die"
—	"I should've insisted that something be done before it was an emergency"	Guilt	"I did tell the doctors that something was wrong...my concerns were dismissed, and the doctors did not listen to me"
—	"I should've known better"	Shame	"Maternal health inequities are complex and not easily overcome...I did the best I could in the situation"

Final Phase of Treatment: Sessions 8 through 12

In Session 8, Alaiyah began to incorporate the updating information obtained in the prior sessions into her revised trauma narrative. This included inserting the updating information into her written narrative for each hotspot, highlighting the new meanings in a different color, and reading the new narrative out loud (https://oxcadatresources.com/narrative-writing-2/). Alaiyah and the therapist also discussed ways she could support the new meanings through use of the senses, for example, mimicking the motion of holding the baby for the first time, looking at pictures of the baby shortly after his birth, and fast forwarding past the trauma to visualizations of the baby being happy and thriving now (Ehlers & Wild, 2020). During the session, Alaiyah reported significant declines in the distress and nowness associated with her hotspots. At the conclusion of the session, Alaiyah and the therapist also discussed ways she could remind herself of the updating information throughout the week, which Alaiyah identified as continuing to use the imagery discussed during the session and reading her updated trauma narrative.

In Session 9, Alaiyah reported that she was having fewer reexperiencing symptoms due to the trauma memory updating procedure discussed in prior sessions; however, she continued to be angry about the racism she experienced and was anxious about future visits to the doctor's office for the baby's check-ups. Accordingly, in Session 9, Alaiyah and the therapist agreed to explore her anger in greater depth. A primary intervention for anger when individuals experience as sense of unfairness, injustice, or being wronged is empathy (https://oxcadatresources.com/working-with-anger/). Broadly, empathy is a skill that has been recognized as essential to the therapeutic alliance when working with clients of color. Perceptions of therapist empathy and the strength of the therapeutic alliance, however, are both influenced by the therapist's ability to broach race during therapy with clients from diverse racial/ethnic backgrounds (Day-Vines et al., 2018; Fuertes et al., 2006). Therefore, the therapist utilized common microcounseling techniques to communicate empathy in the relationship with Alaiyah, such as reflection of feeling (e.g., "Alaiyah, I hear the pain in your voice") and reflection of meaning (e.g., "I understand that you felt powerless to protect your baby during the delivery, and you're worried about your ability to protect him in the future"). However, in addition to microcounseling skills, the therapist was also intentional in broaching the inter-racial, ethnic, and cultural aspects of Alaiyah's presenting problems (e.g., "I acknowledge that your birthing experience was negatively affected by racism in the healthcare system"). From the perspective of liberation psychology, these acts of empathy may be conceptualized as *acompaña-miento* (accompaniment), which refers to standing alongside clients and practicing radical empathy for the ultimate purpose of helping clients develop critical consciousness (Comas-Díaz & Torres Rivera, 2020).

According to the tenets of CT-PTSD, anger in PTSD is the result of reexperiencing symptoms that trigger irritability and low mood, as well as distorted appraisals about the trauma or the consequences of the trauma (https://oxcadatresources.com/working-with-anger/). Yet, for people who experience racism, subsequently developed beliefs about the trauma and its consequences are often accurate. For example, African American women who experience birth trauma may feel angry due to perceived racially biased medical treatment (Evans, 2022), and these perceptions are supported by extant research (Alhusen et al., 2016). Moreover, CT-PTSD suggests that with accidental trauma (which may be one way to conceptualize some traumatic birthing experiences), appraisals concerning malicious intent contribute to symptoms; therefore, Socratic questioning is recommended to guide clients in exploring alternative interpretations for the person's behavior. This recommendation may not be appropriate during therapy with individuals who encounter racism, as impact rather than intent should be prioritized in these cases in order to avoid minimizing or invalidating the individual's experience.

Another common approach to updating distorted appraisals in CT-PTSD is finding out information about context (https://oxcadatresources. com/working-with-anger/). While this may be appropriate when appraisals truly are distorted in nature, therapists should be careful in their application of this technique within the context of racism. For example, Alaiyah reported that after giving birth to her baby, she experienced intense physical pain but was initially denied adequate pain medication. In discussing this issue with hospital staff, one doctor expressed concern that Alaiyah might have been inappropriately seeking opioids. In response, Alaiyah had the thought, "These doctors are treating me like I'm not human." Traditionally, a therapist might help Alaiyah explore reasons for the doctor's assertion, such as the widespread opioid crisis or routine hospital procedures. Yet, given stereotypes about drug abuse within the African American community and research which shows that due to race-based physiological myths, many doctors are likely to underestimate pain in African Americans (Hoffman et al., 2016; Mende-Siedlecki et al., 2021), Alaiyah's thoughts and feelings of dehumanization seem valid.

While Alaiyah's perceptions leading to anger as a result of her birth trauma were accurate, rumination about the event led to a preoccupation with the injustice she suffered and maintenance of her trauma response. Accordingly, the therapist gently brought the pattern of rumination and its consequences to Alaiyah's attention and worked with Alaiyah to complete an advantage/disadvantage analysis (J. S. Beck, 2020), examining the advantages and disadvantages of continuing her preoccupation with the unjust and inhumane treatment she received versus finding alternative ways of coping. This included engaging Alaiyah in dialogue known as *deideologizing*, which encouraged Alaiyah to explore who benefited from her anger and who suffered the consequences (Comas-Díaz & Torres Rivera, 2020). During this process, the therapist also provided Alaiyah with information on research which has found that anger as a coping strategy in response to racism is associated with poorer wellbeing and greater psychological distress among African Americans (Pittman, 2011). Through this exercise, Alaiyah realized that ruminating about the injustice she experienced would not dismantle racism in the healthcare system, but instead would only prolong and worsen the effects of racism through its continued negative impact to her life (https://oxcadatresources.com/working-with-anger/).

Once Alaiyah decided to focus on alternative coping strategies, she and the therapist explored activities that would allow Alaiyah to express and process her anger. Aware of Alaiyah's interest in dance, the therapist suggested artivism as a way to cope. According to Mosley et al. (2021), *artivism* is defined as "using creative arts in the interest of facilitating Black liberation" (p. 31). More specifically, artivism is a form of activism that facilitates the resistance of racism through the creation of knowledge production that ideally leads to social change. Capitalizing on this idea, Alaiyah choreographed a solo dance performance, which she then shared on YouTube and TikTok, along with her story.

To address her anxiety about going to the doctor's office for checkups, Alaiyah and the therapist planned a site visit to the hospital where she gave birth in Session 10. According to Murray et al. (2015), returning to the scene of the trauma can achieve several therapeutic tasks within Ehlers and D. M. Clark's (2000) model, including stimulus discrimination, finding new updating information, reconstruction of trauma memories, and testing beliefs through behavior experiments. First, the therapist provided Alaiyah with a rationale for the site visit, explaining that returning to the site could help Alaiyah test her fears that being in medical spaces would produce flashbacks or dissociation systems she would not be able to manage (Kerr et al., 2023). The therapist also noted the opportunity to practice stimulus discrimination; that is, the ability to differentiate between stimuli that occurred during the delivery and stimuli encountered in the present during the visit to the hospital or future visits for checkups. To assist in these efforts, the therapist and Alaiyah reviewed the grounding and breathing techniques she was taught earlier in the course of treatment. Alaiyah and the therapist then met at the hospital together to conduct the site visit, with the therapist there to provide support, encouragement, and feedback throughout the experience (Murray et al., 2015).

In Sessions 11 and 12, the therapist and Alaiyah began summarizing what she learned in therapy and discussing how she could continue to make progress after termination, which in CT-PTSD is called creating a *blueprint* (Ehlers & Wild, 2020). This included use of specific questions such as "How did my problems develop?" "What kept my problems going?" "What did I learn during treatment that helped?" "What were my most unhelpful thoughts?" "What are the helpful alternatives/updated thoughts?" and "How will I deal with any setbacks in the future?" (Wild et al., 2020). To assist in this process, the therapist began by asking Alaiyah to summarize how her PTSD developed, which included identifying her trauma, threats she perceived during and immediately after the trauma and their personal meanings, feelings experienced during the trauma, initial gaps in memory of the trauma, and avoidance behavior after the trauma. Alaiyah and the therapist then discussed cognitive and behavioral strategies that maintained her PTSD, which Alaiyah identified as avoidance, hypervigilance, rumination, and withdrawal. The therapist also reminded Alaiyah of the role a lack of engagement in activities that previously provided a sense of pleasure or meaning also played in maintaining her PTSD.

After discussing how her PTSD developed and was maintained, Alaiyah and the therapist reviewed her most unhelpful cognitions, as well as the updating information and alternative thoughts that had been developed through the narrative writing exercise and use of psychoeducation, pie charts, Socratic questioning, advantage/disadvantage analysis, and deideologizing. During this process, the therapist and Alaiyah both emphasized the importance of critical consciousness and the danger of self-blame in response to racism, as well as the cathartic and empowerment benefits of (a) maintaining social connections with others, especially individuals who share similar social identities and can empathize with the lived experiences of African American women, and (b) engaging in social action through activities such as artivism or other forms of advocacy. As therapy ended, Alaiyah made a commitment to build on what she learned throughout the course of treatment, and developed plans for any setbacks that might occur in the future (https://oxcadatresources.com/wp-content/uploads/2020/10/Therapy-Blueprint-updated.doc).

References

Abdullah, T., Graham-LoPresti, J. R., Tahirkheli, N. N., Hughley, S. M., & Watson, L. T. J. (2021). Microaggressions and posttraumatic stress disorder symptom scores among Black Americans: Exploring the link. *Traumatology, 27*(3), 244–253. https://doi.org/10.1037/trm0000259

Adebayo, C. T., Parcell, E. S., Mkandawire-Valhmu, L., & Olukotun, O. (2022). African American women's maternal healthcare experiences: A critical race theory perspective. *Health Communication, 37*(9), 1135–1146. https://doi.org/10.1080/104 10236.2021.1888453

Alhusen, J. L., Bower, K. M., Epstein, E., & Sharps, P. (2016). Racial discrimination and adverse birth outcomes: An integrative review. *Journal of Midwifery & Women's Health, 61*(6), 707–720. https://doi.org/10.1111/jmwh.12490

American Psychiatric Association. (2013). *Diagnostic and statistical manual of mental disorders* (5th ed.). American Psychiatric Association. https://doi.org/10.1176/ appi.books.9780890425596

Banks, K. H., Goswami, S., Goodwin, D., Petty, J., Bell, V., & Musa, I. (2021). Interrupting internalized racial oppression: A community based ACT intervention. *Journal of Contextual Behavioral Science, 20*, 89–93. https://doi.org/10.1016/j. jcbs.2021.02.006

Beck, J. S. (2020). *Cognitive behavior therapy: Basics and beyond* (3rd ed.). Guilford Press.

Blevins, C. A., Weathers, F. W., Davis, M. T., Witte, T. K., & Domino, J. L. (2015). The posttraumatic stress disorder checklist for *DSM-5* (PCL-5): Development and initial psychometric evaluation. *Journal of Traumatic Stress, 28*(6), 489–498. https://doi.org/10.1002/jts.22059

Bor, J., Venkataramani, A. S., Williams, D. R., & Tsai, A. C. (2018). Police killings and their spillover effects on the mental health of black Americans: A population-based, quasi-experimental study. *The Lancet, 392*(10144), 302–310. https://doi.org/10.1016/S0140-6736(18)31130-9

Boswell, J. F., & Constantino, M. J. (2022). *Deliberate practice in cognitive behavioral therapy*. American Psychological Association.

Bremner, J. D. (2006). Traumatic stress: Effects on the brain. *Dialogues in Clinical Neuroscience, 8*(4), 445–461. https://doi.org/10.31887/DCNS.2006.8.4/jbremner

Bryant-Davis, T., Fasalojo, B., Arounian, A., Jackson, K. L., & Leithman, E. (2021). Resist and rise: A trauma-informed womanist model for group therapy. *Women & Therapy*. Advance online publication. https://doi.org/10.1080/02703149.2021.1943114

Bryant-Davis, T., & Ocampo, C. (2006). A therapeutic approach to the treatment of racist-incident-based trauma. *Journal of Emotional Abuse, 6*(4), 1–22. https://doi.org/10.1300/J135v06n04_01

Carter, R. T. (2007). Racism and psychological and emotional injury: Recognizing and assessing race-based traumatic stress. *The Counseling Psychologist, 35*(1), 13–105. https://doi.org/10.1177/0011000006292033

Carter, R. T., & Forsyth, J. (2010). Reactions to racial discrimination: Emotional stress and help-seeking behaviors. *Psychological Trauma: Theory, Research, Practice, and Policy, 2*(3), 183–191. https://doi.org/10.1037/a0020102

Carter, R. T., Johnson, V. E., Roberson, K., Mazzula, S. L., Kirkinis, K., & Sant-Barket, S. (2017). Race-based traumatic stress, racial identity statuses, and psychological functioning: An exploratory investigation. *Professional Psychology: Research and Practice, 48*(1), 30–37. https://doi.org/10.1037/pro0000116

Carter, R. T., Kirkinis, K., & Johnson, V. E. (2020). Relationships between trauma symptoms and race-based traumatic stress. *Traumatology, 26*(1), 11–18. https://doi.org/10.1037/trm0000217

Carter, R. T., Mazzula, S., Victoria, R., Vazquez, R., Hall, S., Smith, S., Sant-Barket, S., Forsyth, J., Bazelais, K., & Williams, B. (2013). Initial development of the Race-Based Traumatic Stress Symptom Scale: Assessing the emotional impact of racism. *Psychological Trauma: Theory, Research, Practice, and Policy, 5*(1), 1–9. https://doi.org/10.1037/a0025911

Carter, R. T., & Pieterse, A. L. (2020). *Measuring the effects of racism: Guidelines for the assessment and treatment of race-based traumatic stress injury*. Columbia University Press. https://doi.org/10.7312/cart19306

Centers for Disease Control and Prevention. (2023). Working together to reduce Black maternal mortality. https://www.cdc.gov/healthequity/features/maternal-mortality/index.html

Chavez-Dueñas, N. Y., Adames, H. Y., Perez-Chavez, J. G., & Salas, S. P. (2019). Healing ethno-racial trauma in Latinx immigrant communities: Cultivating hope, resistance, and action. *American Psychologist, 74*(1), 49–62. https://doi.org/10.1037/amp0000289

Chioneso, N. A., Hunter, C. D., Gobin, R. L., McNeil Smith, S., Mendenhall, R., & Neville, H. A. (2020). Community healing and resistance through storytelling: A framework to address racial trauma in Africana communities. *Journal of Black Psychology*, *46*(2–3), 95–121. https://doi.org/10.1177/0095798420929468

Clark, U. S., Miller, E. R., & Hegde, R. R. (2018). Experiences of discrimination are associated with greater resting amygdala activity and functional connectivity. *Biological Psychiatry. Cognitive Neuroscience and Neuroimaging*, *3*(4), 367–378. https://doi.org/10.1016/j.bpsc.2017.11.011

Comas-Díaz, L., & Torres Rivera, E. (Eds.). (2020). *Liberation psychology: Theory, method, practice, and social justice*. American Psychological Association. https://doi.org/10.1037/0000198-000

Cross, D., Vance, L. A., Kim, Y. J., Ruchard, A. L., Fox, N., Jovanovic, T., & Bradley, B. (2018). Trauma exposure, PTSD, and parenting in a community sample of low-income, predominantly African American mothers and children. *Psychological Trauma: Theory, Research, Practice and Policy*, *10*(3), 327–335. https://doi.org/10.1037/tra0000264

Davis, D. E., DeBlaere, C., Owen, J., Hook, J. N., Rivera, D. P., Choe, E., Van Tongeren, D. R., Worthington, E. L., Jr., & Placeres, V. (2018). The multicultural orientation framework: A narrative review. *Psychotherapy*, *55*(1), 89–100. https://doi.org/10.1037/pst0000160

Day-Vines, N. L., Ammah, B. B., Steen, S., & Arnold, K. M. (2018). Getting comfortable with discomfort: Preparing counselor trainees to broach racial, ethnic, and cultural factors with clients during counseling. *International Journal for the Advancement of Counselling*, *40*(2), 89–104. https://doi.org/10.1002/jcad.12304

Day-Vines, N. L., Cluxton-Keller, F., Agorsor, C., & Gubara, S. (2021). Strategies for broaching the subjects of race, ethnicity, and culture. *Journal of Counseling & Development*, *99*(3), 348–357. https://doi.org/10.1002/jcad.12380

Day-Vines, N. L., Cluxton-Keller, F., Agorsor, C., Gubara, S., & Otabil, N. A. A. (2020). The multidimensional model or broaching behavior. *Journal of Counseling & Development*, *98*(1), 107–118. https://doi.org/10.1002/jcad.12304

Ehlers, A., & Clark, D. M. (2000). A cognitive model of posttraumatic stress disorder. *Behaviour Research and Therapy*, *38*(4), 319–345. https://doi.org/10.1016/s0005-7967(99)00123-0

Ehlers, A., Clark, D. M., Hackmann, A., McManus, F., & Fennell, M. (2005). Cognitive therapy for post-traumatic stress disorder: Development and evaluation. *Behaviour Research and Therapy*, *43*(4), 413–431. https://doi.org/10.1016/j.brat.2004.03.006

Ehlers, A., & Wild, J. (2015). Cognitive therapy for PTSD: Updating memories and meanings of trauma. In U. Schnyder & M. Cloitre (Eds.), *Evidence based treatments for trauma-related psychological disorders: A practical guide for clinicians* (pp. 161–187). Springer International Publishing/Springer Nature. https://doi.org/10.1007/978-3-319-07109-1_9

Ehlers, A., & Wild, J. (2020). Cognitive therapy for PTSD. In L. F. Bufka, C. V. Wright, & R. W. Halfond (Eds.), *Casebook to the APA clinical practice guideline for the treatment of PTSD* (pp. 91–121). American Psychological Association. https://doi.org/10.1037/0000196-005

Evans, C. (2022). African American womens' experience of birth trauma. *Journal of Reproductive and Infant Psychology*, 1–10. Advance online publication. https://doi.org/10.1080/02646838.2022.2156988

Fani, N., Carter, S. E., Harnett, N. G., Ressler, K. J., & Bradley, B. (2021). Association of racial discrimination with neural response to threat in Black women in the US exposed to trauma. *JAMA Psychiatry*, *78*(9), 1005–1012. https://doi.org/10.1001/jamapsychiatry.2021.1480

Fischer, I. C., Bennett, M. E., Pietrzak, R. H., Kok, B. C., & Roche, D. J. O. (2022). Examining the associations between PTSD symptom clusters and alcohol-related problems in a sample of low-SES treatment-seeking Black/African American adults. *Journal of Psychiatric Research*, *154*, 261–267. https://doi.org/10.1016/j.jpsychires.2022.07.060

Foa, E. B., Ehlers, A., Clark, D. M., Tolin, D. F., & Orsillo, S. M. (1999). The Post-traumatic Cognitions Inventory (PTCI): Development and validation. *Psychological Assessment*, *11*(3), 303–314. https://doi.org/10.1037/1040-3590.11.3.303

Fuertes, J. N., Stracuzzi, T. I., Bennett, J., Scheinholtz, J., Mislowack, A., Hersh, M., & Cheng, D. (2006). Therapist multicultural competency: A study of therapy dyads. *Psychotherapy: Theory, Research, Practice, Training*, *43*(4), 480–490. https://doi.org/10.1037/0033-3204.43.4.480

Giordano, A. L., Gorritz, F. B., Kilpatrick, E. P., Scoffone, C. M., & Lundeen, L. A. (2021). Examining secondary trauma as a result of clients' reports of discrimination. *International Journal for the Advancement of Counselling*, *43*(1), 19–30. https://doi.org/10.1007/s10447-020-09411-z

Goldmann, E., Aiello, A., Uddin, M., Delva, J., Koenen, K., Gant, L. M., & Galea, S. (2011). Pervasive exposure to violence and posttraumatic stress disorder in a predominantly African American urban community: The Detroit Neighborhood Health Study. *Journal of Traumatic Stress*, *24*(6), 747–751. https://doi.org/10.1002/jts.20705

Graham, J. R., Sorenson, S., & Hayes-Skelton, S. A. (2013). Enhancing the cultural sensitivity of cognitive behavioral interventions for anxiety in diverse populations. *The Behavior Therapist*, *36*(5), 101–108.

Gray, M. J., Litz, B. T., Hsu, J. L., & Lombardo, T. W. (2004). Psychometric properties of the Life Events Checklist. *Assessment*, *11*(4), 330–341. https://doi.org/10.1177/1073191104269954

Green, C. E., DeBlaere, C., & Said, I. A. (2021). Mindfulness in Black church settings: A culturally-adapted group intervention for stress. *Journal of Psychology and Christianity*, *40*(2), 110–119.

Grey, N., McManus, F., Hackmann, A., Clark, D. M., & Ehlers, A. (2009). Intensive cognitive therapy for post-traumatic stress disorder: Case studies. In N. Grey (Ed.), *A casebook of cognitive therapy for traumatic stress reactions* (pp. 111–130). Routledge/Taylor & Francis Group.

Gutiérrez, N. Y. (2022). *The pain we carry: Healing from complex PTSD for people of color*. New Harbinger Publications, Inc.

Harnett, N. G. (2020). Neurobiological consequences of racial disparities and environmental risks: A critical gap in understanding psychiatric disorders. *Neuropsychopharmacology*, *45*(8), 1247–1250. https://doi.org/10.1038/s41386-020-0681-4

Harrell, S. P. (1997). The Racism and Life Experiences Scale (RaLES). Unpublished manuscript.

Hemmings, C., & Evans, A. M. (2018). Identifying and treating race-based trauma in counseling. *Journal of Multicultural Counseling and Development*, *46*(1), 20–39. https://doi.org/10.1002/jmcd.12090

Hinton, D. E., Hofmann, S. G., Rivera, E., Otto, M. W., & Pollack, M. H. (2011). Culturally adapted CBT (CA-CBT) for Latino women with treatment-resistant PTSD: A pilot study comparing CA-CBT to applied muscle relaxation. *Behaviour Research and Therapy*, *49*(4), 275–280. https://doi.org/10.1016/j.brat.2011.01.005

Hinton, D. E., Ojserkis, R. A., Jalal, B., Peou, S., & Hofmann, S. G. (2013). Loving-kindness in the treatment of traumatized refugees and minority groups: A typology of mindfulness and the nodal network model of affect and affect regulation. *Journal of Clinical Psychology*, *69*(8), 817–828. https://doi.org/10.1002/jclp.22017

Hoffman, K. M., Trawalter, S., Axt, J. R., & Oliver, M. N. (2016). Racial bias in pain assessment and treatment recommendations, and false beliefs about biological differences between Blacks and Whites. *PNAS Proceedings of the National Academy of Sciences of the United States of America*, *113*(16), 4296–4301. https://doi.org/10.1073/pnas.1516047113

Holliday, R. P., Holder, N. D., Williamson, M. L. C., & Surís, A. (2017). Therapeutic response to cognitive processing therapy in White and Black female veterans with military sexual trauma-related PTSD. *Cognitive Behaviour Therapy*, *46*(5), 432–446. https://doi.org/10.1080/16506073.2017.1312511

Hook, J. N., Davis, D. E., Owen, J., Worthington, E. L., Jr., & Utsey, S. O. (2013). Cultural humility: Measuring openness to culturally diverse clients. *Journal of Counseling Psychology*, *60*(3), 353–366. https://doi.org/10.1037/a0032595

Hopper, S. I., Murray, S. L., Ferrara, L. R., & Singleton, J. K. (2019). Effectiveness of diaphragmatic breathing for reducing physiological and psychological stress in adults: A quantitative systematic review. *JBI Database of Systematic Reviews and Implementation Reports*, *17*(9), 1855–1876. https://doi.org/10.11124/JBISRIR-2017-003848

Isen, R. (2022). The contribution of social media toward racial trauma and post-traumatic stress disorder in Black Americans: A forensic perspective. *The Journal of Forensic Psychiatry & Psychology*, *33*(5), 692–707. https://doi.org/10.1080/14789949.2022.2105250

Kabat-Zinn, J. (2013). *Full catastrophe living: How to cope with stress, pain and illness with mindfulness meditation*. Piatkus Books.

Kerr, A., Warnock-Parkes, E., Murray, H., Wild, J., Grey, N., Green, C., Clark, D. M., & Ehlers, A. (2023). Cognitive therapy for PTSD following birth trauma and baby loss: Clinical considerations. *The Cognitive Behaviour Therapist*, *16*, E23. https://doi.org/10.1017/S1754470X23000156

King, K. M. (2021). "I want to, but how?" Defining counselor broaching in core tenets and debated components. *Journal of Multicultural Counseling and Development*, *49*(2), 87–100. https://doi.org/10.1002/jmcd.12208

Kirkinis, K., Pieterse, A. L., Martin, C. Agiliga, A., & Brownell, A. (2021). Racism, racial discrimination, and trauma: A systematic review of the social science literature. *Ethnicity & Health*, *26*(3), 392–412. https://doi.org/10.1080/13557858.2018.1514453

Krieger, N., Smith, K., Naishadham, D., Hartman, C., & Barbeau, E. M. (2005). Experiences of discrimination: Validity and reliability of a self-report measure for population health research on racism and health. *Social Science & Medicine (1982)*, *61*(7), 1576–1596. https://doi.org/10.1016/j.socscimed.2005.03.006

Leahy, R., Holland, S. J. F., & McGinn, L. K. (2012). *Treatment plans and interventions for depression and anxiety disorders*. Guilford Press.

MacLean, P. D. (1990). *The triune brain in evolution: Role in paleocerebral functions*. Springer.

Malcoun, E., Williams, M. T., & Nouri, L. B. (2015). Assessment of posttraumatic stress disorder with African Americans. In L. T. Benuto & B. D. Leany (Eds.), *Guide to psychological assessment with African Americans* (pp. 163–182). Springer Science + Business Media. https://doi.org/10.1007/978-1-4939-1004-5_11

Malott, K. M., & Schaefle, S. (2015). Addressing clients' experiences of racism: A model for clinical practice. *Journal of Counseling & Development*, *93*(3), 361–369. https://doi.org/10.1002/jcad.12034

Markin, R. D., & Coleman, M. N. (2021). Intersections of gendered racial trauma and childbirth trauma: Clinical interventions for Black women. *Psychotherapy*. Advance online publication. https://doi.org/10.1037/pst0000403

Martín-Baró, I. (1994). *Writings for a liberation psychology*. Harvard University Press.

Mekawi, Y., Carter, S., Brown, B., Martinez de Andino, A., Fani, N., Michopoulos, V., & Powers, A. (2021). Interpersonal trauma and posttraumatic stress disorder among Black women: Does racial discrimination matter? *Journal of Trauma & Dissociation*, *22*(2), 154–169. https://doi.org/10.1080/15299732.2020.1869098

Menakem, R. (2017). *My grandmother's hands: Racialized trauma and the pathway to mending our hearts and bodies*. Central Recovery Press.

Menakem, R. (2022). *The quaking of America: An embodied guide to navigating our nation's upheaval and racial reckoning*. Central Recovery Press.

Mende-Siedlecki, P., Lin, J., Ferron, S., Gibbons, C., Drain, A., & Goharzad, A. (2021). Seeing no pain: Assessing the generalizability of racial bias in pain perception. *Emotion*, *21*(5), 932–950. https://doi.org/10.1037/emo0000953

Mosley, D. V., Hargons, C. N., Meiller, C., Angyal, B., Wheeler, P., Davis, C., & Stevens-Watkins, D. (2021). Critical consciousness of anti-Black racism: A practical model to prevent and resist racial trauma. *Journal of Counseling Psychology*, *68*(1), 1–16. https://doi.org/10.1037/cou0000430

Murray, H., Merritt, C., & Grey, N. (2015). Returning to the scene of the trauma in PTSD treatment–why, how and when? *The Cognitive Behaviour Therapist*, *8*, E28. https://doi.org/10.1017/S1754470X15000677

Pahl, K., Williams, S. Z., Lee, J. Y., Joseph, A., & Blau, C. (2020). Trajectories of violent victimization predicting PTSD and comorbidities among urban ethnic/racial minorities. *Journal of Consulting and Clinical Psychology*, *88*(1), 39–47. https://doi.org/10.1037/ccp0000449

Pan, X., Kaminga, A. C., Wen, S. W., & Liu, A. (2018). Catecholamines in posttraumatic stress disorder: A systematic review and meta-analysis. *Frontiers in Molecular Neuroscience*, *11*, 450. https://doi.org/10.3389/fnmol.2018.00450

Pittman, C. T. (2011). Getting mad but ending up sad: The mental health consequences for African Americans using anger to cope with racism. *Journal of Black
Studies*, *42*(7), 1106–1124. https://doi.org/10.1177/0021934711401737

Polanco-Roman, L., Danies, A., & Anglin, D. M. (2016). Racial discrimination as
race-based trauma, coping strategies, and dissociative symptoms among emerging
adults. *Psychological Trauma: Theory, Research, Practice, and Policy*, *8*(5), 609–617.
https://doi.org/10.1037/tra0000125

Punkanen, M., & Buckley, T. (2021). Embodied safety and bodily stabilization in the
treatment of complex trauma. *European Journal of Trauma and Dissociation*, *5*(3),
1–6. https://doi.org/10.1016/j.ejtd.2020.100156

Resick, P. A., Monson, C. M., & Chard, K. M. (2017). *Cognitive processing therapy
for PTSD: A comprehensive manual*. Guilford Press.

Roberson, K., & Carter, R. T. (2022). The relationship between race-based traumatic
stress and the Trauma Symptom Checklist: Does racial trauma differ in symptom
presentation? *Traumatology*, *28*(1), 120–128. https://doi.org/10.1037/trm0000306

Scheeringa, M. S., Weems, C. F., Cohen, J. A., Amaya-Jackson, L., & Guthrie, D.
(2011). Trauma-focused cognitive-behavioral therapy for posttraumatic stress disorder in three-through six-year-old children: A randomized clinical trial. *Journal
of Child Psychology and Psychiatry, and Allied Disciplines*, *52*(8), 853–860. https://
doi.org/10.1111/j.1469-7610.2010.02354.x

Scotland-Coogan, D., & Davis, E. (2016). Relaxation techniques for trauma. *Journal
of Evidence-Informed Social Work*, *13*(5), 434–441. https://doi.org/10.1080/237614
07.2016.1166845

Smith, J. R., & Patton, D. U. (2016). Posttraumatic stress symptoms in context:
Examining trauma responses to violent exposures and homicide death among
Black males in urban neighborhoods. *American Journal of Orthopsychiatry*, *86*(2),
212–223. https://doi.org/10.1037/ort0000101

Steele, J. M., & Newton, C. S. (2022). Culturally adapted cognitive behavior therapy
as a model to address internalized racism among African American clients. *Journal
of Mental Health Counseling*, *44*(2), 98–116. https://doi.org/10.17744/mehc.44.2.01

Steele, J. M., & Newton, C. S. (2023). *Black lives are beautiful: 50 tools to heal from
trauma and promote positive racial identity*. Routledge.

Sun, S., Crooks, N., DiClemente, R. J., & Sales, J. M. (2020). Perceived neighborhood
violence and crime, emotion regulation, and PTSD symptoms among justice-
involved, urban African-American adolescent girls. *Psychological Trauma: Theory,
Research, Practice and Policy*, *12*(6), 593–598. https://doi.org/10.1037/tra0000562

Trahan, L. H., Carges, E., Stanley, M. A., & Evans-Hudnall, G. (2016). Decreasing
PTSD and depression symptom barriers to weight loss using an integrated CBT
approach. *Clinical Case Studies*, *15*(4), 280–294. https://doi.org/10.1177/153465
0116637918

Tynes, B. M., Willis, H. A., Stewart, A. M., & Hamilton, M. W. (2019). Race-related
traumatic events online and mental health among adolescents of color. *Journal of
Adolescent Health*, *65*(3), 371–377. https://doi.org/10.1016/j.jadohealth.2019.03.006

van der Kolk, B. A. (2002). Posttraumatic therapy in the age of neuroscience. *Psychoanalytic Dialogues*, *12*(3), 381–392. https://doi.org/10.1080/10481881209348674

van der Kolk, B. A. (2014). *The body keeps the score: Brain, mind, and body in the
healing of trauma*. Penguin Random House.

Watson-Singleton, N. N., Black, A. R., & Spivey, B. N. (2019). Recommendations for a culturally-responsive mindfulness-based intervention for African Americans. *Complementary Therapies in Clinical Practice, 34*, 132–138. https://doi.org/10.1016/j.ctcp.2018.11.013

Weathers, F. W., Blake, D. D., Schnurr, P. P., Kaloupek, D. G., Marx, B. P., & Keane, T. M. (2013). Clinician-Administered PTSD Scale for DSM-5 (CAPS-5). National Center for PTSD.

Weathers, F. W., Bovin, M. J., Lee, D. J., Sloan, D. M., Schnurr, P. P., Kaloupek, D. G., Keane, T. M., & Marx, B. P. (2018). The Clinician-Administered PTSD Scale for DSM-5 (CAPS-5): Development and initial psychometric evaluation in military veterans. *Psychological Assessment, 30*(3), 383–395. https://doi.org/10.1037/pas0000486

Wild, J., & Ehlers, A. (2010). Self-study assisted cognitive therapy for PTSD: A case study. *European Journal of Psychotraumatology, 1*. https://doi.org/10.3402/ejpt.v1i0.5599

Wild, J., Warnock-Parkes, E., Murray, H., Kerr, A., Thew, G., Grey, N., Clark, D. M., & Ehlers, A. (2020). Treating posttraumatic stress disorder remotely with cognitive therapy for PTSD. *European Journal of Psychotraumatology, 11*(1), 1–15. https://doi.org/10.1080/20008198.2020.1785818

Williams, C. B., Frame, M. W., & Green, E. (1999). Counseling groups for African American women: A focus on spirituality. *Journal for Specialists in Group Work, 24*(3), 260–273. https://doi.org/10.1080/01933929908411435

Williams, M. T., Holmes, S., Zare, M., Haeny, A., & Faber, S. (2022a). An evidence-based approach for treating stress and trauma due to racism. *Cognitive and Behavioral Practice*. Advance online publication. https://doi.org/10.1016/j.cbpra.2022.07.001

Williams, M. T., Osman, M., Gallo, J., Pereira, D. P., Gran-Ruaz, S., Strauss, D., Lester, L., George, J. R., Edelman, J., & Litman, L. (2022b). A clinical scale for the assessment of racial trauma. *Practice Innovations, 7*(3), 223–240. https://doi.org/10.1037/pri0000178

Williams, M. T., Printz, D., Ching, T., & Wetterneck, C. T. (2018). Assessing PTSD in ethnic and racial minorities: Trauma and racial trauma. *Directions in Psychiatry, 38*(3), 179–196. https://www.monnicawilliams.com/articles/Williams_RacialTraumaPTSD_2018.pdf

Wolkin, J. (2016, June 15). *The science of trauma, mindfulness, and PTSD.* https://braincurves.com/2016/06/17/repost-the-science-of-trauma-mindfulness-and-ptsd/

Woods-Giscombé, C. L., & Black, A. R. (2010). Mind-body interventions to reduce risk for health disparities related to stress and strength among African American women: The potential of mindfulness-based stress reduction, lovingkindness, and the NTU therapeutic framework. *Complementary Health Practice Review, 15*(3), 115–131. https://doi.org/10.1177/1533210110386776

Index